HOLLY SCHUT

Midlife Momentum
LIVING WITH PURPOSE ON PURPOSE IN MIDLIFE AND BEYOND

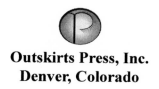

Outskirts Press, Inc.
Denver, Colorado

Midlife Momentum
Living with purpose on purpose in midlife and beyond
All Rights Reserved.
Copyright © 2011 Holly Schut
V4.0

Outskirts Press, Inc.
http://www.outskirtspress.com

ISBN: 978-1-4327-6954-3

Dedication

I dedicate this book to the ordinary but incredible people
God has placed in each chapter of my story.
You have raised me, taught me, encouraged me and loved me.
You have blessed me beyond words.

I give thanks for and to my mom, who in midlife went back
to school to fulfill her dream of becoming a nurse, to my
children and grandchildren, who are an inspiration and joy to
me every day, and to my husband Al who has loved and encouraged me unconditionally through this project and always.
To God be the glory!

Table of Contents

Acknowledgments

Brief quote from p. 119 from WISHFUL THINKING: A
SEEKER'S ABC by FREDERICK BUECHNER
Revised and Expanded. Copyright (c) 1973, 1993 by
Frederick Buechner.
Reprinted by permission of HarperCollins Publishers

Brief quote from p. 153 from CELEBRATION OF
DISCIPLINE: THE PATH TO SPIRITUAL GROWTH by
RICHARD J. FOSTER
Copyright (c) 1978 by Richard J. Foster
Reprinted by permission of HarperCollins Publishers

Exercise on Page 152 adapted from THE PATH:
CREATING YOUR MISSION STATEMENT FOR WORK
AND FOR LIFE by LAURIE BETH JONES
Copyright (c) 1996 Laurie Beth Jones
Used by permission of Hyperion. All rights reserved.

Introduction

What are your signs that midlife has arrived?

Signs: Is it the fact that the nest is empty…your parents are requiring more of your time…those extra pounds you put on over the holidays just won't come off…you women have gotten rid of every turtleneck and pullover sweater you ever owned in favor of something easier to take off when the hot flashes come, or are you simply bored with what you have been doing the last 25 years? Is there a holy restlessness stirring in your soul, calling you to search for more, to live a deeper, more significant life?

Whether you are an experienced business person, a teacher with 25 years in the classroom, a mom wrestling with an empty nest, or a person in your 40's, 50's or 60's ready for something fresh and wondering what is next, midlife is a time of transitions. Transitions mean change, and change is never easy. But for many of us this time has become an opportunity rather than a crisis. There is no script for when this restlessness begins to tug at us, or what it looks like. It often sneaks up on us without announcing its arrival.

Forty years ago you could expect to hit a midlife crisis at

about 40 years of age. The crisis was that life was passing you by. (Hey, who is over the hill at 40 anymore?) You only had XXX number of years left to accomplish what you had set out to accomplish. It was a time you began wrestling with your own mortality. But there have been significant cultural shifts that often move midlife back a decade: Expanding life expectancy, more years of education, marriage at a later age, first-born children come later in life: all these have delayed the onset of midlife for many.

The midlife crisis of yesterday is today an opportunity likely to happen in connection with the life circumstances mentioned above, and all of this is more likely to happen around the age of fifty. According to Gail Sheehy, an expert and author on the subject of life passages, 50 is the beginning of your "second adulthood." Your first adulthood, 25-50 is about establishing a career, building a family, becoming part of a community. This "second adulthood" will look very different from your first. When we realize that at 50 we could very likely live another 30/40+ years we need to explore what we want to be doing with those years, and why God might want so many elderly people around that long.

There is a movement afoot where people in midlife are stopping to reflect and search for what it is that they want this "second adulthood" to look like. There are some who tell us, "This is time for you! You have been taking care of others all your life (often true), now it's your turn." There is a healthy aspect to this, because self-care is a gift we not only give to ourselves, but to our families as well. But it is also easy to slip into a destructive, selfish approach to life. Others say that community service is what will make your life fulfilling. Again, this is an important aspect of what can make our next season of life meaningful, but is there a bigger picture we need to consider?

"I know the plans I have for you. Plans to prosper you and not harm, plans to give you a hope and a future," declares the Lord in Jeremiah 29:11. We are a participant in God's plan to love, redeem, and reconcile the world to himself. What an incredible thought. We are a part of something designed to change the world...for the better!

Midlife Momentum: Living with Purpose on Purpose in Midlife and Beyond is designed to aid those in midlife transitions, empowering them to live into the next season of life with meaning and purpose. In this process you are given the opportunity to: stop living on automatic and live with intention, reflect back on your lives and see how God has been at work in and through all of life's experiences, reclaim who you truly are, and listen to your own lives and to your Creator. The process leads to developing a mission statement for the next season of life, giving renewed hope and purpose.

When experienced in a group I have discovered that midlifing humor and care permeate the discussions as participants in retreats and seminars share their stories, goals and dreams. There is a camaraderie that develops as we realize we have so much in common, despite our differences. It can be a first step in the self-care we need in order to discover, "Who am I?" "Where is God leading me?" "What's next?"

Each and every one of us is an awesome creation. We are "Fearfully and wonderfully made." (Ps. 139:14 NIV) There are pressures in our younger years and first adulthood that strip us of who we truly are. Midlife can be that time of coming home to who we are created to be, launching us into a life of confidence, joy and purpose. Denise, a participant in a Midlife Momentum retreat said, "This experience has increased my expectation that the second half of my life will be better than the first." That is hope!

Sometimes we need a companion on the journey such as a life coach. A life coach is someone who is trained to listen for your heart's desire, and ask questions that help you make decisions and take action to make your goals and dreams a reality. It's not all downhill from here! There are places to go, people to meet, challenges to be undertaken, gifts to be developed, interests to be explored, people to be empowered, and needs to be met. God has amazing things ahead! (I recognize that God is not limited by gender, however, for ease of reading I have chosen to use the male pronoun when necessary.)

At the end of Sections 1 and 2 you will find questions encouraging you to apply what you are reading to your own life. In Sections 3 and 4 there are exercises and questions in each chapter. In Sections 5 and 6 you will find additional exercises as well as a training manual on leading a Midlife Momentum or Renewing Momentum retreat. I pray that they will be a blessing to all who use them.

So I invite you to join me on a journey. It is a journey into a new season of life: a journey of greater abandonment to God, into a fuller, richer life. We are here for a purpose!

Bio: Dr. Holly Schut: Masters in Religious Education, Dr. of Ministry

Holly is founder of Midlife Momentum, a certified life coach, pastor, wife, mom, grandma, and most importantly a child of God. Join me in this adventure!

For more information on retreats, seminars and life-coaching opportunities check out: www.midlifemomentum.com

SECTION 1
The Call to a Journey

Aslan threw up his shaggy head, opened his mouth and uttered a long single note; not very loud, but full of power. Polly's heart jumped in her body when she heard it. She felt sure that it was a call, and that anyone who heard that call would want to obey it, and (what's more) would be able to obey it, however many worlds and ages lay between.
From: The Magician's Nephew by C.S. Lewis

1

Get Off The Road

Enlarge the place of your tent, stretch your
tent curtains wide, do not hold back; lengthen
your cords, strengthen your stakes. Isaiah 54:2

Trust in the Lord with all your heart and lean not on your
own understanding; in all your ways acknowledge him,
and he will make your path straight. Proverbs 3:4 & 5

In my 56th year, the 8th year of the presidency of G.W. Bush I had a dream. (No this isn't political, but it does seem in Scripture that major events are often introduced something like this.) And this dream was not an ordinary dream. I knew this was a God-dream: God trying to get my attention and move me in a new direction.

The Dream: I am driving down a four lane highway. It is a beautiful sunny, summer day. I am in the country and the traffic is flowing smoothly at posted speeds. I am in the left lane, following a large dump truck. Suddenly I am in total darkness. I have no idea why. I don't know if the whole world has gone dark, or if it is just me. I don't know if others are trying to stop or slow down. I don't know what is on the side of the road, or if the truck ahead of me is stopping. All I can do is, to the best of my ability, GET OFF THE ROAD! I slow down, and ease off the road, heart pounding. As soon as I am off the road everything is light again, and I can see fine. I wait for my heart to settle down, check for traffic and gradually drive across the road to the other side. Once across the road I drive by a large V-shaped hole where it looks like someone has either just taken out, or is planting a new tree. I wake up and it is morning and time to get up.

Let me tell you my story. I am definitely a midlifing woman. I have two married children and in the last few years have become grandma 3 times. WOOHOO! My youngest son started his second year at Hope College in the fall of 2008. During my midlife transition, but before the grandbabies and empty nest, I went back to school to get my Doctor of Ministry degree. I discovered there were a lot of us midlifers in the program. This was a wonderful experience for me. I loved the collegiality, the intellectual stimulation, the opportunities to go deeper in faith and ministry. But one class in particular initiated a process of exploration and reflection that would enrich and refocus my life.

It was a small class of 4 men and 2 women. As part of our assignments for the class we were required to write our spiritual autobiographies, which I had done in the past. But, there was a significant difference this time, not in the writing of the story, but because of the sharing of our story in a small group of men and women who were all experiencing the transitions of midlife. As we shared our stories and encouraged one another I recognized how the process was preparing all of us for the next season God had in store for our lives. We recognized how God's grace had been at work throughout our lives. We began to value in new ways the good things, and the hard things we had experienced. We were able to reframe experiences from our past, and we released in each other the ability to dream about the future.

This was so powerful I decided to pursue taking the process further, and developed my dissertation around the theme of using spiritual autobiographies to aid women in midlife transitions. It worked, and I will tell you more of that story later.

At the time of my dream I was serving as associate pastor in a small town in the Midwest. My husband was the Senior Pastor. I was on staff part time working in congregational care and children's ministry. For three years I had been struggling with how God was calling me to use what I had learned and developed through my dissertation. I tried to work at it, "on the side" as I continued the rest of my ministry, but I was feeling more and more restless. My New Year's resolution in January 2008 was that I really would cut back to working half time and spend 20 hours a week developing a new ministry called Midlife Momentum.

The first week of January I took my son back to Holland, Michigan for his second semester and to network with some colleagues at our denominational seminary. The second week I led a retreat for parish nurses in a nearby city. These two weeks I was forced to only work part-time at the church, but I was feeling fragmented, unable to do well at either "job."

Then I had "The Dream." After getting out of bed I needed to prepare for the congregational prayer time in our worship. I turned to the book of Isaiah and began reading at chapter 42. When I got to verse 18 my heart began to pound, much as it had in my dream. I read these words:

"Hear, you deaf; look, you blind and see!
Who is blind but my servant, and deaf like the messenger I send?
Who is blind like the one committed to Me,
Blind like the servant of the Lord?
You have seen many things, but have paid no attention:
Your ears are open, but you hear nothing."

I couldn't believe what I had just read. Later that day I told my family about the dream and the Scripture. I knew I needed to act on what God had revealed to me that morning, but still wasn't sure what that looked like. (Sometimes we can be really dense! Thank God for his patience!)

On Thursday evening our consistory (leadership board) was meeting, and I joined our prayer team to pray while they met. "Lord, send your Spirit to move among our leaders. May they sense you presence and your leading. Help them to be obedient…..." (God really does have a sense of humor). He allowed me to pray this way for a time and then firmly spoke to my heart. He was not just at work downstairs where the consistory met, but he was moving upstairs where I was praying the very things that needed to be happening in my life.

I stopped the prayer time and told the team I needed to go downstairs and resign. The Spirit had firmly told me to resign **that night**…resign effective the end of March! Having taken us all by surprise, one of them asked, "Holly, how do you know that was God?" After assuring them I knew it was from God, the team asked if they could pray for me before I went downstairs. I agreed and they began to pray, but I didn't hear a word they were saying. Immediately I began to think about options. Maybe I should resign the end of the summer. After all, once Easter was past the schedule at church would lighten up and

I could probably REALLY work part time, and still get paid through the summer. Yada, yada, yada! Caleb had just started private college. It would really be nice to have that pay check! Yada, yada, yada!

I told them they had to stop praying and I had to go downstairs immediately and resign! I called my husband out of the meeting and told him I was going to announce my resignation. Somewhat in shock, he nodded and said, "If that is what you need to do, you better do it." (Thank you, Lord, for speaking peace into Al's response.)

God was definitely calling me to live out what I was hoping to lead others to do:

> Surrender myself to the plans and purposes God has for my "Second Adulthood."
> Step out in faith, even if it is scary. (Where will the money come from? Who will want what I have to offer? What if I am a failure? What if I am wrong about this?)
> Live intentionally with joy!

So I invite you to join me on a journey. It is a journey into a new season of life: a journey of greater abandonment to God, a journey into a fuller, richer life. Together we will discover how aging is not a matter of becoming less, but rather, of how God is working, calling us to become more.

2

Beginning the Journey

Come, all you who are thirsty,
Come to the waters;
And you who have no money, come, buy and eat!
Come, buy wine and milk without money and without cost.
Why spend money on what is not bread,
And your labor on what does not satisfy?
Listen, listen to me, eat what is good,
And your soul will delight in the richest of fare.
Isaiah 55:1-2

It was a cold, dark, November evening when 13 midlifing women made their way to a retreat center on the shores of Green Lake in Wisconsin. How significant was it that none of the women, other than myself, the facilitator, had been here before, or that we arrived after dark? Even the lights illuminating the name of the retreat center and its driveway were not functioning. Fortunately the road dead-ended right into the retreat center's gates. There was really no other way to go, but through those gates. No one really knew what they were getting into during the next 20 hours.

As we drove through those gates we were entering a new

place, a bit like the children in *The Lion the Witch and the Wardrobe*, by C.S. Lewis.

"I wonder if there's any point in going on," said Susan. "I mean. It doesn't seem particularly safe here and it looks as if it won't be much fun either. And it's getting colder every minute, and we've brought nothing to eat. What about just going home?"

"Oh, but we can't, we can't," said Lucy suddenly; "Don't you see?"

And how significant was it that the next afternoon we would leave during a crisp sunny fall afternoon? In those few hours we would be enriched by getting to know new friends, old friends better, ourselves deeper, and God's presence in our lives more fully.

These were very trusting women. They had been recruited to experience a retreat that would launch a process of life reflection, storytelling, and writing parts of their own spiritual autobiography. This would hopefully culminate in discerning God's purposes for the next season of their lives. They knew they were guinea pigs for my dissertation project.

Jackie deserved special credit! She didn't know any of the other women. In fact, she only knew me because we had run on treadmills side by side at the local fitness center. One day as we chatted she talked about some typical midlife issues and I invited her to join the group. When she was preparing to come to the retreat her husband asked her who she would be spending the next 24 hours with. She acknowledged that she didn't really know any of us. "What if they are a cult?" he asked. From that day on as she left for follow-up sessions following the retreat, she would report that she was on the way to her "cult group".

For the purpose of the project 6 of the women knew each other very well, over a long period of time, and were all from the same church. The other 6 knew none of the other women well. In this group, the participants were from 5 different churches, representing five different denominations. The purpose of the two different groups was to see if the process was more effective with women who knew each other well, or if there was more freedom to do the exploring and storytelling with people who didn't know your past and wouldn't have connections with the people in your stories.

On that crisp November night we lit the fireplace, put on the coffee and hot chocolate, and began an adventure. We filled that lodge with chatter, laughter, tears, prayer and hope. (Who was still young enough to crawl up to the top bunk??)

Twelve recruits, between the ages of 45-60 opened themselves up to:

- ➤ discussing the issues that midlife raises for most of us
- ➤ exploring who God had created them to be
- ➤ discerning how GRACE had been at work throughout their lives
- ➤ preparing to live out the next season of their lives with God-given purpose and JOY.

In fact, the Scripture that guided our process came from the Apostle Paul in 1 Corinthians 15:10. Paul is defending himself to the church, against arguments that he wasn't really an apostle. He declares, "By the grace of God I am who I am and God's grace to me has not been in vain." (NKJV) Paul realized that there had been much good and much bad in his past. But more importantly he knew that grace had been at work in and through all of it, redeeming the bad, weaving it into the good, producing the person God created Paul to be.

By the time we left the next afternoon, the level of trust and confidentiality built was so strong it really didn't matter if the participants had known each other before or not. Following the retreat the two groups met independently for four two-hour sessions, after which the total group came back together for a celebration ceremony. While the two groups functioned differently in those follow-up sessions, both were very open and effective. Both "worked" in helping the participants listen to their lives and the Spirit of God, and to each other, as they sought God's purposes for the next season of their lives.

At the first session of the retreat "not being needed as much" surfaced as one of the greatest difficulties in midlife. As they enjoyed the camaraderie of the process they were able to look forward to the future with less fear, more confidence and greater trust in the God who had been with them throughout their lives to that point. Prior to the project they all knew in their heads that these issues were common to many women, but until they heard each other's stories it was not a reality. Naming the fears they were experiencing or anticipating helped them get a handle on those fears and empowered the women to move beyond them.

At the conclusion of our two months together several of the participants had made significant decisions. A kindergarten teacher for 30 years, Gert decided to take early retirement to pursue other things in which she was interested, and to spend more time with her family. Two of the participants went back to school to train for new careers. Nancy gained the freedom to retire and spend additional time caring for her aging mother. Denise, a recent widow, realized that her difficult life experiences with a husband suffering from schizophrenia had prepared her to be a support for other families wrestling with mental illness. Two women were wrestling with a deep call to a more defined ministry.

These women realized that their jobs did not define who they were, and their pasts, while informing their futures, did not dictate or determine the futures God had in store for them. All twelve of the participants said the process had positively impacted how they would deal with the opportunities and difficulties of midlife.

Although the initial project focused on women 45-60 in rural Wisconsin I have discovered that the process crosses a number of boundaries. In the past three years retreats and workshops have included couples, discipleship groups, ministry worker retreats, and participants 39-80 years of age, though I recommend setting about a 20 year age range for each particular event in order to keep the life issues similar. I have also had the privilege of leading events which included people from Ireland, Egypt, Korea, Australia, Malaysia, China, and Canada as well as from the east coast to west coast of the US.

I hope that as we share a journey through this book you will be encouraged to stop…listen to your life and your Creator… find a few friends (new or well-worn) to walk with you…. trace the work of grace in your life… and share the joy of knowing that the One who formed you in your mother's womb (Psalms 139) has amazing plans and purposes for the next season of your life. All that has come before can be woven together to prepare you for the adventure in Kingdom living that God has before you.

I give a hug of thanksgiving to each of the initial women who opened themselves up to me, and the process, that has become so much a part of Midlife Momentum, and Renewing Momentum for the post-midlife participants.

1. What made you consider reading this book?
2. If you had the momentum what would you love to do?
3. Where do you sense you need to "Get off the road"?
4. What encouragement do you think God wants to give you today?

SECTION 2

How Do We Know We Are In Midlife Or Beyond?

There is a time for everything,
and a season for every activity under heaven:

a time to be born and a time to die,
a time to plant and a time to uproot,
a time to kill and a time to heal,
a time to tear down and a time to build,
a time to weep and a time to laugh,
a time to mourn and a time to dance,
a time to scatter stones and a time to gather them,
a time to embrace and a time to refrain,
a time to search and a time to give up,
a time to keep and a time to throw away,
a time to tear and a time to mend,
a time to be silent and a time to speak,
a time for love and a time to hate,
a time for war and a time for peace.
Ecclesiastes 3:1-8

3

The Need To Get Directions!

*When the pleasures and/or security of remaining in the comfort
zone always outweigh the joy of growth, life starts ending.*
Laurie Beth Jones

Denial is more than a river in Egypt!

*There is a time for everything, and a season for
every activity under heaven. Ecclesiastes 3:1*

I wonder how many times I have heard retired friends say,
"I'm busier now than when I was working." For most of us the
questions will not be, can we stay busy but rather, what will we
stay busy with? What will commandeer our time and energy?
Will we be intentional, or will our retirement years slip away
like sand through an hour glass? And who will determine how
we spend these years? We are created with a longing and need
to have meaning and purpose. It is the psychological need of
midlife and beyond, to make meaning of our lives and to pass
on blessings to the next generations. Eric Erickson calls this the
"generative stage".

It is good news that many of us do get this chance to live

generatively, while a generation ago as people approached midlife there was a much greater sense that time was running out. People felt that if they had not made a significant contribution, if they had not reached success by their mid forties, they had better hurry. Life was slipping away. With our expanded life span Gail Sheehy invites people into their "second adulthood". She notes that during the years from 25-50 people are busy establishing families, finishing education, and building careers, but when they reach 50 there is a major shift in responsibilities and focus. Now the realization in this transitional time is that they may have decades of time following midlife in which they have the opportunity to deepen the meaning of their existence, enrich relationships and invest in causes greater than their own survival or success. They have the opportunity to discover anew who they are created to be and how they can invest the years ahead. Having this sense of mission and purpose is critical in living well, finishing the race, and pressing on toward the goal of our calling. (Phil. 3:12-14)

There is a striking story about an aqueduct which carried water from the mountains down to Segovia Spain. The aqueduct was built around 100AD and had faithfully and efficiently carried the water down the mountain for 1,900 years. Mid-twentieth century there was a decision made to stop using the aqueduct to preserve it for its historical value. They stopped the flow of water, built a new system and within a few years the ancient aqueduct began to crumble. When it was no longer fulfilling its purpose even this inanimate object began to die. The aqueduct now undergoes constant surveillance and preservation, and once again carries water.

What happens if we refuse to take the time to ask questions concerning our life's purpose? There are many statistics that tells us midlife can be either a crisis or an opportunity, depending on our ability to stop, reflect, pray, and listen to our lives and the Spirit of God at work in our lives.

Let's look at some of the statistics that let us know how important this intentional reflection is.

1. Divorce rates for those in midlife are on the rise. For women, the message from the world is, "Now that you are in midlife it is time to take care of you. You have been a caregiver for the past 25 years. It is your turn." There is value in this message, because we know that you can only give if you are also replenished; and truthfully women, we have not done this very well in the past. However, the general tenor of this message can lead to an unhealthy selfishness. We need to enter into this quest with Spirit guidance.

It was amazing to me, as I read the secular books written by women in the 1980's, and 90's, how many of these women ended up leaving their spouses, and some their families as well, as they sought to find themselves. It can be so foreign for women to think about what they want and need, that many women may decide prematurely that their mate does not have a place in their new life. Sue Monk Kidd, in her novel *The Mermaid's Chair,* tells one woman's story of living through this process. It is a helpful read for women whose hunger for more in their second adulthood has kicked in.

This is not the same issue as women who in midlife finally gain the strength and power to leave an abusive marriage, or deal with a marriage that has been dead or destructive for many years. There are circumstances where it is right and healthy for women to say, "Enough!" They no longer will subject themselves to this kind of destructive behavior and dehumanizing treatment. Midlife can provide the window and impetus to leave and begin a new season of life.

It is encouraging that in the books I have read, written by women and published after the turn of the century, there seems to be a greater focus on making meaning and finding a purpose or cause to which they want to commit in midlife and beyond, rather than the more self-centered approach of simply asking, "What do I want for me?" This is a challenging and tricky balancing act as we seek health and wholeness. It is critically important for you to find the true you, the authentic self, in order to be able to live into your God-given purpose. God desires that you be fully you. Just be careful and prayerful of what you think you want or need to discard in the process.

Women are not alone in opting out of a long term marriages in midlife. For men as well, leaving the marriage may look easier or more interesting than doing the hard work of reconnecting with one's spouse on a whole new level once the kids have left the nest. Often the marriage has been taken for granted for so long that the concept of reviving and working on it looks like just plain hard work. What is the allure in that? In marriage counseling sessions we often here comments such as, "It is just such hard work." "If we loved each other it wouldn't be this hard." Unfortunately that perception is all too prevalent! Love equals romance in our society, and romance should just come naturally. Attraction = romance = love. How immature we can become in these middle years! This is where commitment not just to your wife, but family, friends, society in general and your faith community impacts how you will respond to major transitions in your married life. Our faithfulness and integrity, commitment and willingness to do the hard work matter on so many levels. We need to fight the individualistic opinion that what I do in my life isn't anybody else's business.

How many years has it taken to get into the ruts in which we find ourselves? How long will we work at getting out of those ruts and discovering a whole new dimension to our marriage? Statistics reveal that while divorce rates on a whole have declined significantly from a peak in 1981 divorce rates among boomers continue to lead the way. In fact 1 out of 4 divorces are among couples who have been married more than 20 years.

We are not the same people who said, "I DO" 20+ years ago. Both spouses have changed, grown, and evolved while the children have grown up and we have been busy with careers. Not only is self-discovery an important task in midlife, but spouse discovery is also crucial. Midlife offers the opportunity to re-engage on a deeper level.

2. Depression rates begin to rise in the late 40's and 50's. The precipitating issue for women is often identity, especially as they are dealing with the empty nest and struggles with midlife marriage; while men are most susceptible when facing job loss or being passed up for younger colleagues, losing prestige or dealing with retirement.

For years the perception was that women suffered from depression more than men. However, today that assumption is very much in question. While women tend to seek professional help and use more prescribed medication, the reality is that men more often choose to self-medicate through alcohol and street drugs, sports, adrenaline producing activities, and withdrawing from family and friends. Dr. Archibald Hart, author of *Unmasking Male Depression,* helps us in understanding what is happening with the men who are dealing with changes and loss. Hart claims that 100% of us deal with "run of the mill" depression at some time or other. Most of us recognize, if we are honest, that we all feel a little crazy at times, or experience lingering sadness, or are overly irritable. But acknowledging it is depression is particularly difficult for men.

While women struggling with depression often experience the sadness, men are more likely to get irritable. And once caught in depression it becomes difficult for us to recognize what is happening, especially for men, who are used to masking or filtering out the emotions with which they need to deal.

Jed Diamond has actually written a book called, *The Irritable Male Syndrome,* where he identifies four triggers for male depression:

1. Fluctuating testosterone levels
2. Biochemical imbalances
3. Loss of masculine identity
4. Stress

Hart would add to this list:

5. Addictions
6. Messing with our internal clocks
7. Adrenaline. In an adrenaline driven society we experience tremendous shifts in our adrenaline levels. After an adrenaline high one becomes more prone to depression.
8. Turmoil in shifting family roles and situations.

All of these factors show up in midlife for most men. Diamond makes the point that in our culture we specialize in specialists when it comes to health care. No one deals with the whole person. Irritable male syndrome is a complex issue because it deals with physical, spiritual, emotional, mental, and relational dimensions of our lives. He also stresses that Irritable Male Syndrome is not a disease but a signal that something is out of balance in our lives.

Diamond provides us with some warning signs to look for in our relationships which may point to depression, or irritable male syndrome. They are:

1. Rise in criticism
2. Expressions of contempt
3. Defensiveness
4. Stonewalling or withdrawal, and refusal to communicate.

Believe it or not, Hart tells us that depression is a healing emotion if we co-operate with it, listen to it, learn from it and deal with it.

For both men and women we need to overcome the perception, particularly in smaller communities that getting help with depression means weakness. We need to bury the stigma associated with getting the help we need to be healthy emotionally and relationally. We need courage to be all God wants us to be, and sometimes that means co-operating with depression and searching for the imbalance causing it.

3. Suicide rates: Between 1999 and 2004 the suicide rates for women between the ages of 49 and 54 increased 31%, while for men it was 20 percent.(US Department of Health and Human services) The suicide rate for men in retirement is second only to teenagers.

These statistics and more indicate that there is a great need for addressing the changes and accompanying fears that are inevitable in these years. Our very health and well-being are dependent upon it. If we are going to stop the crumbling of our lives (remember the aqueduct?) we will need to figure out what our purposes are in our second adulthood, and begin to determine how we are going to carry the water from the mountain to the city in midlife and beyond. Research shows that people who have a calling greater that their own happiness live longer, are healthier, enjoy better relationships, and are in fact happier than those who focus on achieving that happiness. One day as I was perusing some books at Barnes and Nobles I was taken aback by books that seemed to claim that the purpose of life is happiness. This goal is too small! I firmly believe we are called and equipped for more.

In contrast I was encouraged to think bigger and deeper by someone who suggested that when we create our mission or purpose statement we would do well to realize that we serve a purpose which is always part of a bigger picture. For example, rather than saying *my purpose in life is to* motivate and mobilize the boomer generation for greater impact on their spheres of influence, I would do well to realize, *I serve the purpose of* motivating and mobilizing the boomer generation. This helps me realize it isn't just my purpose. God is calling us to be a part of something much bigger than ourselves. We have companions on this journey, people to learn from, and to learn with, who are also serving a purpose connected to ours. Our purpose doesn't originate with "me," but rather with the God of all callings and purposes.

4

Reading the Road Signs

Yesterday my little girl was walking through the snow
with her friend as she headed to kindergarten. Today she
bundles her son up and sends him off to his kindergarten.
And the seasons continue to change.

My husband has an extreme case of doubting the road signs as we travel, and despite getting teased unmercifully for it, he continues to second guess the compass in the car, the maps, the garmin and yes, the signs along the way. Before the days of the GPS we were on a trip to Salem, Massachusetts where we were going to visit a museum about the Salem witch hunts. We had never been in the state or the city before. We got to a "T" in the road, which had a sign with an arrow telling us to go left. Al, all too true to form was still going to turn right. "What are you doing?" I queried, "I don't know," he respond, "It just feels like we should go right." "Al," I said, "The people who actually live here say we should go left." Whether we like them or not we should pay attention to signs along the way, especially when we are navigating in unfamiliar territory.

What is happening in our lives, families and culture that creates the turbulence we experience in our forties, fifties and sixties? What does midlife feel like? Change....change....and change, which equals unfamiliar!

Time is a slippery concept. We just came back from a 10 day vacation time with our family. On one hand it seemed like we had been gone for months...on the other hand we couldn't believe it was over already. Aging is like that. On one hand people are experiencing that life is like the grass that withers and the flower that fades. Life is fleeting (Psalm 90:5-6, 103:15). On the other hand we are faced with the potential of 30-50 years of life after the nest empties, and 20+ years if we retire at 65. At this point in history, life expectancy has risen to 78.3 years in the United States. (United Nations List, 2009) In 2006, if you were 68 years old and living in relatively good health, you could expect to live another 17 years. (National Vital Statistics Report) Information presented by Charles Arn at the Catholic Charities' 15th Annual Life Long Wellness Conference in 2003, revealed that 700,000 women are widowed each year, and will be widowed an average of 14 years. Forty-five percent of women over 65 are widowed. While many women are aware that statistically they will probably outlive their husbands, these figures urge women to prepare for a life of meaning outside the role of wife. The life expectancy for men is rising and the span of years between the deaths of spouses is diminishing, however, it is wise to remember that one spouse or the other will almost always need to learn how to live well alone. This is a formidable task, and one we can do a better job of preparing for without getting morbid.

As our life span increases and cultural shifts occur we discover ourselves in a recently evolved season of life, much like adolescence in the last half of the 20th century. Prior to World War II the passage from childhood to adulthood was much shorter. As this passage expanded in time we found ourselves with a never before defined stage of life, adolescence. In the latter half of the 20th century and early 21st century we began dealing with another new stage. Demographers talk about this stage including those who are between the ages of 50-75, and describe them as neither old, nor young. Check out the shelves at your favorite bookstore and you will realize that currently we have many options for what we might call this stage of life, but whatever the name, this stage is filled with unique changes, challenges and transitions.

Because it is something new in the culture no one is quite certain what navigating this season of life should look like. We are the first generation that has seen our parents on average live well into their 70's, 80's and many into their 90's and 100's. Listen to Willard Scott, of the Today Show, as he celebrates those having birthdays over one hundred. It is quite a phenomenon. On top of being in so many of our personal transitions we are a transitional generation. I often feel I want to rewrite the words that Tevye sings in *Fiddler on the Roof*. Instead of crying out "Traditions" I believe our song cries out "Transitions". And like Tevye we are learning to live into a new world.

Allen Sullender, in his book, *Losses in Later Life*, sheds much light on why there is such turbulence and the potential for life crisis as we age. There is no denying that we continually face change, and all change involves loss. However, as we continue to age beyond fifty these changes and losses roll up onto our shores like waves intensifying in a storm. We need skills and perspective to navigate these swells of loss in healthy, depth-enriching ways. Yes, God can work good out of these loss experiences for all who love God and are called for his purposes. (Rom.8:28)

Unfortunately in western society many of the "bones" of our culture are shifting and changing rapidly. Religion, family, and work no longer command the loyalty and respect they once did. Our value systems are in constant flux. For many there is no foundational framework, no anchors to hang on to as they face this sea of changes. In their book, *The Search for Meaning,* Thomas and Magdalena Naylor and William Willimon speak of the "incredible consequences of meaninglessness" in western society. They attribute America's health problems, crime, addictions, suicide and waste of leisure to this void of meaning. As Christians we have an anchor to hang on to; a rock to stand upon in the midst of the storm. The world needs to know a relationship with God brings strength for the journey, wisdom for the decisions, and hope for tomorrow.

If loss is inevitable, a primary task in this season is to prepare for it. What are the losses which begin to accumulate? How do we know we are in our second adulthood? What should we be doing?

5

Road Sign:
Shifting Family Role

*I remember my son's big wheel speeding down the driveway;
now he's buckling car seats into the back seat.*

*If I could do life over again, what would I change?
I have today, and unknown tomorrows to live life well.*

Grandparents are the family historians. They are the
keepers of the collective memories, the repositories of
stories, and the connecting link between generations.
Richard Morgan in Remembering Your Story

Male and female, we all deal with shifting roles and priorities in our family relationships and systems. These are primary sources of our identity and therefore must be addressed
in healthy ways.

Most parents deal with losses of an empty nest. There is
no longer the rhythm of our teenager's comings and goings,
the busyness of attending our teen's events; even the stress of
wondering where they are and what they are up to comes as

a loss. They are no longer as dependent upon us: eating our foods, spending our money, needing our support in relationships and school issues, calling for help with the car, and on and on. Women especially, often feel that a huge part of their identity has been stripped away as their children leave for college, become adults and discover their independence.

If you talk with college counselors, faculty or administrators one of the new challenges for colleges and universities is the phenomenon of "helicopter parents." As their teenagers head off to college parents today have a plethora of ways to stay in touch with their sons and daughters. Between cell phones, emails, facebook and whatever the next new thing is, parents are often communicating with them on a daily or more often basis. Colleges are dealing with parents who "hover," overprotecting, inserting themselves into their kid's problems, not allowing them to grow up and be responsible. A generation ago we had to stick it out, work through roommate issues, deal with professors we didn't like. We had to grow up. And our parents had to let go.

An additional challenge in today's world is that we may end up having "boomerang kids," sons and daughters returning home after the nest had once been empty. Economics, delaying marriage into the late twenties, 30's and beyond, continuing education beyond college all create situations where young adults find themselves living "at home" again. A recent phenomenon for American families is the concept of parents living with their adult children. While more traditional and expected in other cultures, this is a relatively new response in American culture to the current economic situation.

How can we prepare for these transitions? Is there a way of alleviating fears and accepting the shifts in family relationships? It is important to realize we are grieving the loss of a time in our life. Even if they return to the nest for a time, neither they, nor we, will be the same. This is one of the tasks of midlife. One of the most helpful, simple steps may be to listen to peers who are a step or two ahead of us. Look for parents who seem to have gone through the transition well and seek their counsel. Seek healthy community. Recognize that there is a time and energy void you have the opportunity to fill with things you may have put off for many years. Decide to invest this reserve in significant ways in your community or congregation, your friendships and extended families. We do survive it, and often find joy on the other side of this transitional bridge.

One of the most consistent responses to the question, "What do you enjoy most about being in midlife (or beyond)?" is, "I enjoy the adult relationships I have with my children!" Over and over again there is a discussion about the blessing of having our relationships with our offspring mature into one of mutual respect and friendship. If we let go well, they can come back with freedom as adults.

I was talking recently with our 21 year old son who is away at college. We talk about once every week or two, and email occasionally in between. I told him of a friend who talks with her 23 year old son about 5 times a day, and waited for his reaction, which was, "Yea, I like our relationship." I like it too. Do I miss him at times? Of course! But I also know he doesn't need me 5 times a day, or every day. And that is good! Our goal as parents is to train up our children to become God-loving, independent, strong, adults able to live into all God is calling them to be. That means our roles must shift as they grow. It will be a huge blessing to our children if we learn to do that well.

And while our roles with our children are shifting so are roles with our parents. We are the sandwich generation: dealing with our children and grandchildren, and helping our parents as they are aging and require more of our time and attention. We need to help with decisions about moves out of the family home, into apartments, care facilities, or our own homes. We wrestle with schedules as we accompany them to appointments. There is a complex dance we do as we balance assisting, and allowing independence; and a few toes get stepped on along the way.

Whether we do this gladly as a response to all they have done for us or reluctantly because they have not been able to parent us well, it takes time, energy and patience. At some point in the process we lose the parent who has been taking care of us, and now that role belongs to us. There are no perfect parents…or children. Be gracious. The longer we can find ways to allow our parents to invest in us by praying for us, encouraging us, giving us hugs, the sweeter will be this transition. I wonder if one reason for the fifth commandment, "Honor your Father and Mother," is because it is critical in the emotional health of our parents, but also in our own emotional health as we continue to advance in age.

Sometimes sooner, sometimes later we lose our parents and recognize we have become the elder generation. This too is a shock to our identity system. We become the torch bearers in the family. How well will we do that? Will we carry the role of elder with dignity and purpose; passing on blessings to the next generation, being an encourager, a support, providing wisdom and modeling courage to the next generations? Will we mentor and model what it means to live a life worthy of our King?

A major shift and celebration for many in midlife is becoming grandparents. For some this takes on different forms such as: grandparents, step-grandparents, surrogate grandparents (Many children grow up a considerable distance from their biological grandparents and need you.) great aunts and uncles etc. Grandparenting provides opportunities to model and mentor and love. What messages will we communicate?

I have a friend named Jane who lived an hour and a quarter from her parents as her children were growing up. She was incredibly thankful to her parents for the model of servanthood and purpose they were demonstrating to their grandchildren as they went on mission trips and were involved in community support groups and agencies. As her children got older they accompanied their grandparents on some of these trips and activities, introducing them to people in other countries, enabling them to see the kingdom of God in a variety of places. Jane's sibling however, who lived closer to her parents were not so appreciative. They felt their children were being cheated because grandpa and grandma were not always able to be at their soccer games or school events. They were not on call to babysit whenever a need arose. In truth, they were not the typical grandparents of their community. They were living very intentional lives, which Jane realized would significantly impact the grandchildren's future for good. Is it bad to go to your grandchildren's events? Of course not! Is it healthy grandparenting to make your grandchildren the center of your universe and the dictator of your calendar? No, not really. This is a challenging message to send. How can one speak against spending time with your grandchildren?

During a recent parenting class one of the issues raised was dealing with grandparents who over-indulged their grandchildren and basically over-grandparented, much like helicopter parenting. If as Joyce Rupp asserts, one of the tasks of midlife is grieving the loss of parenting children, one wonders if over-grandparenting is, in part, a denial of the end of the parenting stage.

Many boomers come from large families. Fifty years ago it

was not uncommon for families to have 5, 10 or more children. Often there was a twenty-year span between the first and last child. When the first child left home, married and had the first grandchild there were still several siblings at home that needed to be parented. This continued through several siblings. No grandchild could commandeer all of grandpa and grandma's attention. With the arrival of smaller families where two or three children are born within a few years there are many more grandparents who have launched their last child before the first grandchild is born. Now grandparents have more time, energy and resources to "spend" on their grandchildren, which can mask the grief over the empty nest.

Healthy grandparents are an incredible gift in the lives of young people. Intentional living requires that we look honestly at how we are doing, and what we want to communicate to these much loved people in our lives.

6

Road Sign:
Our Work World is Shifting

The Third Age (51-75) can become a time of choice with regard to returning talents and gifts to society and the world. It is a time to launch out in new directions, unimpeded by the stress of the workaday world. Richard Morgan

During a retreat one of the first activities assigned is to answer the question, "How do you know you are in your second adulthood?" Inevitably we end up talking about how different our work life is, with some of the responses being: I look around and realize all of the people I work with are younger than I am, I am no longer the expert because there have been so many changes, I can share wisdom with my younger co-workers, I can't keep up with the younger ones, my options are limited, etc.

Also raised are discussions about what we want our "retirement" years to look like. According to Chuck Underwood the very word "retirement" is a taboo word for the boomer generation. Very few boomers feel they are worn out when they reach retirement age, so they are looking for ways to stay active, engaged and/or meaningfully employed either in their current career, or in a totally new venture. The title of Lloyd Reebs book, *From Success to Significance* really sums up the journey in our work life. For many in midlife there is a soul-shift occurring, and climbing the ladder, financial success, and name recognition are no longer sufficient. The bigger questions become, "Do I have an impact on my sphere of influence? How does God want to use me in the kingdom?"

Milt Kuyers, chairman and C.E.O. of GMK Companies wrote an article entitled *"Don't Retire Me, Lord,"* in which he talks about the biblical imperative to use the gifts God has given us throughout our lives. He has been blessed with the gift to make money, and the companion gift of generosity to give it away. Mr. Kuyers wrote, "If I'm financially able to retire without needing a supplementary paycheck, I could then work for pay and contribute my paycheck in its entirety to one or many of God's causes within the church." He continued to say, even if it meant working at McDonald's or as a greeter at Wal-Mart he would consider it a blessing to be able to contribute that much more to the kingdom. We all have different gifts and passions, so determining how God is calling us to impact the kingdom in our second adulthood will look different as well. For some, the opportunity to retire may mean time, energy, relationships and resources to engage in totally new ventures.

In the New York Times in 2004 there was an article called, *Your Second Midlife Crisis* which addressed the issue that in their 60's and 70's people were still wrestling with what they wanted to accomplish in the remaining years of life. This phenomenon has led to vacation options during which people can try on new careers, such as ranching or being a chef, as well as the birth of volunteer organizations such as SCORE, a senior corp of retired entrepreneurs who mentor young entrepreneurs. The possibilities are limitless when we open our eyes to the needs around us.

For men in particular, these shifts in the workplace produce great stress on our sense of identity. Many women jokingly speak about what it will be like, and how they will handle it if their husbands are not off to work each day. However, in actuality, it isn't a joking matter. There is much fear around filling our days with meaning and purpose, rather than feeling useless and in the way.

Chuck Underwood, in *The Generational Imperatives* reports that in a survey taken in 2005 by Merrill Lynch, 83% of the 3000 boomers surveyed planned to work beyond normal retirement, and 56% of them anticipated working in a new profession. Boomers do not plan to ride silently into the sunset.

In a conversation with a colleague who had retired 3 years earlier he asked about the work I was doing. When I told him I was helping people in midlife navigate transitions and live with meaning and purpose his response was, "Holly, I need that now." The lure of retirement, he claimed, was freedom. But after a couple of years of this freedom, and resisting invitations to get involved because of fear that it would take away that freedom, he came to realize that freedom without commitment couldn't offer the meaning and purpose he so much desired. He was ready to reengage and desired help in finding significant ways to channel his energy and passions.

One of the greatest blessings of our second adulthood is the ability to intentionally determine where your heart, soul and strength need to be invested, and then doing something about it, with passion!

7

Road Sign:
We look in the mirror

*The gray head is a crown of glory, if it is found in
the way of righteousness. Proverbs 16:3*

*Wrinkles should merely indicate where smiles have been.
Mark Twain*

*Aging is mandatory, but growing old is optional.
I've known 90 year olds who don't think old.*

The mirror tells us we are no longer young. We may not be
old, but we can't deny that we no longer look 30. What is happening to our bodies?

1. Menopause arrives with its accompanying flashes and
    flushes. The symptoms vary greatly from one woman
    to another, but all deal with the fact we are no longer
    childbearing age. (And if men are not going through
    male menopause why is Al sleeping so poorly because
    he just can't get the right temperature?)
2. We don't have the endurance we once had. The first

time we probably acknowledge this is when our kids can outplay us at whatever sport it is we taught them. Remember the days when we held back to let them win? Then came the stage where we could play full out, and finally we arrive at the age where they leave us in the dust. And the next thing we know our 5 year old grandchildren can outrun us in a shot. Humility is a great virtue, and God seems to delight in developing it in us.

3. Our skin, joints, muscles and our bones all become challenged as the years pass. I remember reading in bed one night when I accidentally glanced to the side and saw my white, flabby, age spotted arm lying there. Of course the lighting and particular angle must have contributed to how shocking it looked to me, right? Diet and exercise become increasingly important if we want to stay fit, enjoy life and mobility and take on new challenges. It is inspiring to see the accomplishments of our peers in triathlons, marathons and Senior Olympics, but it doesn't come without discipline. For those of us not so athletically inclined it is still crucial that we increase our exercise.

4. With the onset of menopause women's risk of heart disease takes a huge jump. High blood pressure and cholesterol levels often increase dramatically within one or two years. This is of special concern since women are less likely to survive after a heart attack or surgery.

5. Visits to the doctor for yearly checkups elicit new questions and concerns about osteoporosis, diabetes, prostate levels, all reminding us we are aging, and the doctors keep getting younger!

6. The old saying, "What goes up must come down"

certainly doesn't seem to apply to the numbers on our scales. Weight comes on so easily and off so hard! Remember, doctors tell us that as post menopausal women we need to eat 500 less calories per day just to maintain our current weight.

It is very important that we be as intentional about our health as we are about our time if we want to live full and enriching lives in our second adulthood. We have a responsibility to our families and to our God, for we are the vessels God chooses to inhabit, that he might work through us to impact the world with his love. In I Corinthians 6:19 Paul instructs us, "Do you not know that your body is a temple of the Holy Spirit, who is in you, whom you received from God? You are not your own; you were bought at a price. Therefore honor God with your body."

8

Road Sign:
Someone Has Hi-jacked
My Mind and Emotions!

I still have a full deck, I just shuffle slower. Author Unknown

Nobody grows old merely by living a number of years. We grow old by deserting our ideals. Years may wrinkle the skin, but to give up enthusiasm wrinkles the soul. Samuel Ullman

Again this road sign varies from one person to the next, but I chuckle at how many of us in our 50's fear we have early onset Alzheimer's. The fear was mine, and I discovered I wasn't alone. Our brains may become sluggish from sleep deprivation, and there is a menopausal fog that can descend. Our mental files fill up with names, dates and data, which then become more difficult to recall, but research assures us that while there may be some mental functions which decline with aging, it is illness rather than aging which is the major contributor to the significant mental losses some experience. Most of us can look forward to being bright, alert, mentally competent and continually learning as we continue to age. I love to check out the comics in the daily paper to see how they help us to laugh at ourselves as we deal with many of these aging indicators.

Just looking in that mirror is an emotional experience some mornings! All change creates stress, whether it is positive or negative change that is occurring, and this stress impacts our emotional abilities to cope. Debate also continues on how menopause hormonally impacts our emotional systems, or whether it is the symptoms of menopause, such as sleeplessness which throw our emotions into orbit.

The challenge of figuring out "WHO AM I?" as we let go of old roles and identities and try on new ones is an emotionally charged experience. Joyce Rupp, in *Dear Heart, Come Home: The Path of Midlife Spirituality* and Sue Monk Kidd, in *When the Heart Waits: Spiritual Direction for Life's Sacred Questions* both share their midlife journeys with incredible openness and intimacy. I felt like they were dear friends mentoring me on my own journey. They helped me to understand what I was living through, and make progress on my own journey. I recommend them to you.

And remember those losses that are piling up? We need to give ourselves a break, grieve in healthy ways, do some serious self-care and learn to enjoy life again. Self-care at this stage is a gift not only to ourselves, but to our family and friends as well. Breathe deeply, seek professional help when needed and trust God to bring you through these turbulent waters of midlife. Please believe me when I say there is no shame in needing help in navigating these midlife waters. For some of us a counselor can help us examine what we are going through and what factors contribute to the struggle. For others, a life coach, someone who walks alongside to ask important questions, help us clarify our identity, and sort through our dreams and goals can be a great help.

Do you want some GOOD NEWS!? In a study conducted at the University of Chicago by Bernice Neugarten it was reported that 75% of postmenopausal women interviewed said they felt better after menopause than they had for years! I can attest to it myself. I feel like I have gotten myself back. Women entering and experiencing midlife need to hear this good news, since most of us can anticipate living at least one third of our lives after menopause.

Psalm 139:14 says, *"I praise you because I am fearfully and wonderfully made; your works are wonderful, I know that full well."* This verse acknowledges that God is our creator and has done an amazing job of creating us. The wonders of God's creation continue to bring me to a place of awe. There are doctors who describe a literal rewiring that takes place in our brains beginning in our 40's to prepare us for the changes we will experience in our second adulthood. Our brains know that the old systems and ways of living will not work for us as we face a whole new world of relationships, shifting roles, and realities. God is getting us ready for the next season of life, for he has incredible things planned for us if we are willing to step out in faith and live into the challenges and purpose which will bring us joy and meaning.

9

Road Sign:
Wisdom, Experience
and Confidence!

Give instruction to someone wise, and they will be wiser still.
Teach the righteous and they will increase their learning.
Proverbs 9:9 (Author's version)

And we, who with unveiled faces all reflect the Lord's glory, are
being transformed into his likeness with ever increasing glory,
which comes from the Lord, who is the Spirit.
II Corinthians 3:18

Another question participants in a seminar consider is,
"What are the best things about your current age?" Almost
without fail the answer is, "I don't worry so much about what
other people think. I have more freedom to be me." Another
response is, "I have wisdom to share. My kids and co-workers
come to me for advice. I have lots of experiences that have
given me wisdom." Rare are the people who would like to go
back to living through their 20's and 30's.

Arriving at our second adulthood gives us perspective on

what we have already lived through; which in turns gives us the wisdom to live into the future with greater confidence and peace. This afternoon I spoke with my sister. This is 2010 when the economic situation in the States is anxiety-producing for many people. In her place of employment they have announced another level of layoffs coming. Last year she had tried for a promotion, which she was denied. At the time she was very disappointed and frustrated with the system. Her words to me today were very different as she commented, "Once again God knew what he was doing. At the time I was angry that I didn't get the job, but if I had I would be one of those getting laid off. Right now my current job is pretty secure. I am really thankful." She continued reflecting on how often that pattern is repeated in life. It is in looking back on life that we see how in the hard times of life God continues to be at work, shaping, forming and leading us. In looking back we reframe our experiences, celebrate our perseverance and growth, and see the wisdom we have banked through life experience.

Self-knowledge is also an important factor in our maturing into wisdom carriers. On the one hand we recognize that we cannot be all things to all people, having limited abilities and our own certain personalities. We have learned there are some things to be accepted and with which we must live. On the other hand, we also realize that we are not the same people we were fifteen years ago. Hopefully we have changed and grown, developed new interests and abilities, and often mellowed in relationships.

But these are choices we make. Will we choose to be flexible, expanding, wisdom carriers, or will we become ornery, aging curmudgeons? Will we bring life and light to relationships and events, or will we bring stress and fear? Will we bring encouragement and hope as we focus on others, or will we be judgmental and negative, holding others back from being all

God wants them to be in order to keep the world the way we want it? We have all known both types of these people. Who will we choose to be?

God desires that we continue to flourish! Listen to these words from the Apostle Paul, "Now the Lord is the Spirit, and where the Spirit of the Lord is, there is freedom. And we, who with unveiled faces all reflect the Lord's glory, are being transformed into his likeness with ever-increasing glory, which comes from the Lord, who is the Spirit." (II Corinthians 3:18) Ever increasing glory! I like that. This is God's plan and purpose for our lives; that we should become more and more like Christ. Now that is a goal worth striving for!

We will not live in denial. There will be thoughts about growing older, the need to deal with lessons learned, with bodies aging, with roles shifting, and relationships changing. We desire to do that well. The issues of mortality will be faced, but one can absorb these truths in light of God's plan and go on. In fact, midlife, with the freedoms it brings and the wisdom we have gained can launch us into exploring things for which we discover we carry a spirit-given passion. We have the time, energy, relationships and resources to impact our world in significant kingdom expanding ways, and we become more Christlike in the process.

1. How do you know you are in midlife? (Or the season you are in)
2. What are the best things about your present season of life?
3. What are the most difficult things about this season?
4. What are the unique opportunities?
5. What challenges do you most need support in meeting?

SECTION 3
In Search of Self at Midlife

O Lord, You have searched me and you know me.
For you created my inmost being: you knit
me together in my mother's womb.
I praise you because I am fearfully and wonderfully made; your
works are wonderful, I know that full well.
My frame was not hidden from you when
I was made in the secret place.
Psalm 139

By the Grace of God I am what I am, and his
Grace to me was not without affect.
I Corinthians 15:10

10

God is Good, But is He Safe?

"Then he isn't safe?" said Lucy.
"Safe?" said Mr. Beaver; "don't you hear what Mrs. Beaver
tells you? Who said anything about safe? 'Course he isn't
safe. But he's good. He's the king, I tell you."
C.S. Lewis: The Lion the Witch and the Wardrobe

I have come that they might have life, and have it abundantly.
John 10:10

There are foundational building blocks we need to consider if we are going to journey into the next season of our lives in such a way that we will experience the "abundant life" Jesus came to bring us. For starters we must realize this is a spiritual journey. The hunger for meaning and purpose is birthed in us by a higher power. In order for us to live into abundant life, filled with meaning, connecting us to eternity, we need to know the Holy Uncreated One. No matter how long we have been a spiritual seeker there is always more to know, experience and love about God.

The basic starting place in launching this journey is to realize, **Our vision of God is too small!** This is true no matter who we are. Graham Cooke tells us, "Our vision of God *always* requires an upgrade to enable us to see who we are going to become in the next season." (Italics mine.) God does not call us to small lives, so we will need to believe in the greatness of God, and believe God has intimately committed himself to empowering us to live into our call.

In the story, *Prince Caspian*, by C. S. Lewis there is a beautiful picture of the child Lucy finding the lion Aslan, the Christ figure, after a long time had passed since they had last been together.

> "Aslan, Aslan, Dear Aslan," sobbed Lucy. "At last."
>
> The great beast rolled over on his side, so that Lucy fell, half sitting, half lying between his front paws. He bent forward and just touched her nose with his tongue. His warm breath came all around her. She gazed up into the large wide face.
>
> "Welcome child," He said.
>
> "Aslan," said Lucy, "You're bigger."
>
> "That is because you are older, little one," answered he.
>
> "Not because you are?"
>
> "I am not. But every year you grow, you will find me bigger."
>
> For a time she was so happy she did not want to speak.

I invite you to imagine lying between the paws, or being held in the arms of God, looking into that loving, but somewhat terrifying face and realizing there is so much more to our God than we can fathom. Yet God holds us, and breathes his Breath upon us, calling us close to Him, sending us into the next adventure. In the book, Lucy was given the task of following Aslan, even if none of her siblings would believe her, or follow her. What adventure is God calling you to embrace, and are you ready to lie between the paws and let God infuse you with his Breath, his Spirit?

What is there that we cannot do IF God calls us to do it? Will he not supply all we need to be all God wants? In Ephesians 3:20-21 the Apostle Paul blesses us with this benediction, "Now to him, who by the power at work within us, is able to accomplish abundantly more than all we can ask or imagine, to him be glory in the church and in Christ Jesus to all generations, forever and ever." (NIV) Do you see a spiral happening here? The more we grow, the bigger our understanding of God, which means we trust him for greater things to be done *through the power at work within us!* When we see God at work in these amazing ways our perspective of God grows, enabling us to step into greater adventures with God.....You get the point.

If we want to soar to new heights we need to experience more of God's love, power, intimacy and knowledge. One more story...when our youngest son, Caleb was about 3 years old we were lying on the bed doing our bedtime prayers and we began a silly game of, I love you more than...the stars in the sky, more than a hundred hugs, etc. Then Caleb said, "I love you more than a pickle," and he began to giggle and giggle. About two weeks later I was at a retreat which was culminating in communion. As I approached the table I sensed God saying to me, "I love you more than a pickle!" It made me smile. It made me cry. God loves me more than I love my son. God's love for me is intimate, fun-loving, real, and greater than I can imagine!

But never fall into the trap of believing God is predictable or particularly safe...God is good, God is King!

MIDLIFE MOMENTUM

1. What have you discovered about God in this last year?
2. In what way do you need your belief to grow?
3. If you were going to experience something new with God what do you think it would be?

11

Catching the Wind

Let's go fly a kite, up to the highest heights, and send it soaring.
Up through the atmosphere, up where the air is clear.
Let's go fly a kite!
Mary Poppins

Those who wait on the Lord shall renew their strength,
they shall mount up with wings as eagles, they shall run
and not be weary, they shall walk and not faint.
Isaiah 40: 41

How many of you are kite fliers? My mom used to love to fly kites with us in the spring. I flew kites with my kids, and now with my grandkids. It is a magical thing to run into the wind, and let the string out, feel the tug as the kite catches the wind, and then watch as it soars overhead. A couple of times Caleb and I have gotten our kites all the way up, as far as the string would go; so high the kite was a tiny speck in the sky. I encourage you to go fly a kite!

This January I had a kite flying on my balcony, though I

had to bring it in when the wind got too strong. As I looked out my office window on those freezing, snowy, North Dakota days I could see my kite flapping on the porch of our apartment. It was my reminder. It reminded me that my life cannot soar without the wind of the Spirit taking it to the HIGHEST HEIGHTS. The kite flies out there because it is amazing how often I need to be reminded that I am totally dependent on God for: strength, energy, creativity, persistence to keep on keeping on, dependent on God for people to walk with me, and the list goes on and on. When I lose that focus I rapidly spiral into frustration, weariness, and anxiety. (The kite also reminds me that spring will come!)

So today, I invite you to "Go Fly a Kite!"

The kite invites us to: run into the Wind, look up to our Source, and launch something new for the kingdom of God and for the joy of living! It invites us to fly! There is no kite flying if there is no wind. You may have a kite, string, and a tail, but without the wind you are out of luck. I like the image of having to run into the wind, leaning into it with expectation.

In the second chapter of Acts we see the followers of Jesus gathered together in a room in Jerusalem praying. Jesus had been crucified, buried, risen and had appeared to them after his resurrection with instructions for the next part of their journey. Now they are waiting for the promised gift of the Holy Spirit. Jesus told them to stay put...stay in Jerusalem until the Spirit came upon them. When that happened they received power to witness as to who Jesus is and how much God loves the world. They had a mission, but they weren't ready to fulfill it until they received the Spirit. In much the same way we are not ready to live our purpose unless we realize that we are dependent on the Spirit catching our kite, providing the power and guidance we need.

Every one of us is a creation of God, called to living for the King; called to give up living small lives. We are free! We are empowered by the very breath of God! We are loved and claimed by our heavenly Father! What does God want me to do with this freedom, this fresh beginning in midlife?

God wants to take our kites places beyond our imagination. In Ephesians 3:20 we read, "Now to Him who is able to do immeasurably more than you can think or imagine, by His power at work within us...." (NIV) If that is where God wants to take us it is going to require leaning on God, drawing near to him. In our weakness we will tap into God's strength. Wait on the Lord, and think on these questions.

1. What heights would you like to explore?
2. What roadblocks stand in the way of going after those heights?
3. How do we gain the courage to let out more string and fly higher?"

12

New Creation

Fear not, for I have redeemed you; I have summoned you by name; you are mine. When you pass through the waters, I will be with you; and when you pass through the rivers, they will not sweep over you. When you walk through the fire, you will not be burned; the flames will not set you ablaze. For I am the Lord, your God, the Holy One of Israel, your Savior. Isaiah 43:1-3

Therefore, if anyone is in Christ, he is a new creation; the old has gone, the new has come. II Corinthians 5:17

Once we take our view of God to a new level we need to take a new look at the **new creation**. This is what God declares concerning us in II Cor. 5:17-18, "Therefore, if anyone is in Christ, he is a new creation; the old has gone, the new has come! All this is from God, who reconciled us to himself through Christ and gave us the ministry of reconciliation." By nature we are sinful, deserving of judgment and in need of a Savior. But Hallelujah! God provided the answer in His Son Jesus Christ, who took our judgment and became our Savior. Then God went above and beyond all we could ever hope and imagine and made us a new creation, filling us with the very

Spirit of Christ!

In I Corinthians 15:10 Paul describes himself with this statement, "But, by the grace of God I am what I am, and God's grace to me was not without effect. No, I worked harder that all of them, yet not I but the grace of God that was with me." This is part of Paul's response to the church in Corinth as he recounts his role among all those who saw the resurrected Christ, and defends his place among the disciples. Unfortunately, even in the early life of the church there was a plague of competition and jealousy. Some were saying that Paul had no authority to teach and exercise leadership in the church, in part because of his background.

But Paul had received grace. I have received grace. You have received grace and God does not waste his grace. He has lavished it on us, showers us with it, and it doesn't come back empty. For all who claim the name Christian this is the truth! Once we have known the love and power of God in our lives we are never the same. TRUTH

I would argue that there are two types of grace at work in our lives. There is saving grace, and there is also the grace of "Christ in me." It is amazing how easy it is to take "Christ in me grace" for granted. We are glad God is around when we need him. I am thankful I know my eternity is secure. But, way too often my relationship with God focuses on "ME." On the other hand, "Christ in me grace" builds a church, develops ambassadors of the King, matures Christlike children of the heavenly Father, people trained and fit, growing into the fullness of Jesus, changing the world, loving God above all and their neighbors as themselves. Wow! That's not just about me. It sounds scary, challenging. It is going to take submission, commitment, and sacrifice! I have been saved for a relationship with God, but also for a purpose in the Kingdom.

If God is not wasting grace on me, how can I make sure I don't waste it as well? There certainly seem to be times when we make the journey toward Christlikeness longer and more difficult than it would have to be if we paid a bit more attention to how God is working in our lives.

When we were first married Al was a journeyman tool and die maker, a tradesman, and I was finishing a teaching degree. Just prior to the birth of our second child we experienced a call to ministry which involved moving out of state so Al could go to college. Throughout college Al was able to work semi-full-time in his trade while going to school. Despite growing up in a denomination that was only beginning to open up to women in professional ministry, by the time we headed to California for seminary we believed both of us needed to attend. However, our house in Michigan didn't sell, finances were non-existent, and we fell into the typical pattern of me, the wife, trying to work full-time so Al could go to seminary. I was miserable in a job I hated, and couldn't do well. I had lost a piece of my identity because I wasn't using my gifts in ministry, my kids were in school and daycare for the first time, and we were adjusting to a new part of the country. Then our home was broken into and I lost symbols of who I was. My class ring, wedding rings and gifts of jewelry were stolen. To put it mildly, I was stressed!

We firmly believed God had moved us out there, yet nothing seemed to be working. Suddenly there was an awakening, and we realized we were trying to live someone else's plan. God called us back to the unique plan for our lives.

Al and I both began working part time. He could make as much in 10 hours as I was making working 40. The next semester we were both taking classes and loving the experience; and we were both involved in ministry at a church in which we were interning and worshiping. Two years later we found ourselves back in Michigan, living in the house we were never supposed to sell.

It is abundantly more exciting and fun to live when I am looking for those signs of God's presence, provision and power! These signs look different in each of our lives. Sometimes we don't recognize them until we stop to reflect, intentionally looking for, and seeking to interpret signs that God is at work moving us into the plans he has for us.

If you were writing a story about a time in your life when you seemed to take the long way around to get to where God was taking you, I wonder what that story would be.

When Saul/Paul looked back on his life he could give thanks for the family in which he was brought up; and being from Tarsus was a good thing, making him Jew and Greek. He recognized the excellent education he had gotten, knowing the law and the prophets. In many ways he had been favored by God, but he also had to deal with the fact that he had become an angry, violent persecutor of the followers of Jesus. When you put that whole package together you have a man, chief among sinners, by his own account, whom God had chosen to be an apostle to the gentiles, and a writer of Scripture. God took the good and the bad, redeemed it all through Jesus, and gave Paul an incredible assignment for the kingdom.

Few of our assignments will seem as significant, in comparison to Paul's, but that doesn't really matter. The key is, "Are we living into our assignment?" In Ephesians 2:10 Paul declares, "We are God's workmanship, created in Christ Jesus to do good works, which God prepared in advance that we should walk in them." (KJ) Psalm 139 is a declaration that God formed us in our mother's womb. He knows our days, and we can never flee from God's presence. Scary??? Sometimes, but how incredible!

You may think that too many bad things have happened in

your life. The wounds are so deep, the memories too painful, the mistakes too severe, the sins too many. That is where the stories of Scripture are so amazingly encouraging. Very few of God's greatest heroes look good by the world's standards. Some were murderers, others liars, some were unfaithful followers, some tried to run away from God's calling, many struggled with depression. God doesn't seem to mind lavishly spreading His grace to the least likely candidates, making them chosen vessels of the great Good News and the love of God. I like the way God chooses to work!

1. Where have you been growing most in the past year?
2. Name three ways your past has shaped and formed you.
3. What do you celebrate the most about the new creation God is working in you?

13

Let's Journey Together

Paul says that the gifts of the Spirit were given by the Spirit to the body in such a way that interdependence was insured. No one person possessed everything. Even the most mature needed the help of others. The most insignificant had something to contribute. No one could hear the whole counsel of God in isolation.
Richard Foster in Celebration of Discipline

Be in Community! Many of us boomers, especially men, have grown up with a strong work ethic, and a very strong belief that independence and rugged individualism are great virtues; to which I think we need to say, WRONG! We are created for relationships. We are created for community. If we truly want to become all God has created us to be we will need others to help us along the way. Why would we think that if Jesus needed 12+ disciples and an entourage of women to support his ministry that we should have to do and be what God has created us for on our own?

I encourage you to read Romans 16 to get a glimpse of the many people who enabled Paul to accomplish the ministry to which he was called. It is a beautiful picture of how the Body of Christ, "joined and held together by every supporting ligament, grows and builds itself up, in love, as each part does its work." Ephesians 4:16.

Does that mean it was easy to learn how to be this Body? Of course not! If we follow the story of the life of the church in the book of Acts we hear of arguments and rifts as they figure out how to minister in the world with very real people. Life happens, but so does GRACE. And the Spirit continues to lead and teach.

Not only is there a lot we need to learn about how to be this Body of Christ, there is also a lot we need to unlearn.

We need to learn how to receive help, as we unlearn rugged individualism. If we are a disciple of Jesus Christ, God has a mission for us that is more than we can do on our own. Again, God does not call us to small things. There may be a thousand small steps, but the mission is beyond our own abilities. That is the kind of God we serve. Remember, we are ambassadors for the King, we are reconcilers to the world, we are light in the darkness. I don't know about you, but I want help with that! And throughout Scripture God has demonstrated that the call is not limited to spiritual superheroes. We will need God's help, and often God provides that help through other people, even as he empowers us through his Holy Spirit.

We also get to be the answer to the prayers of others. I find that rather awesome! Our son, Caleb and a friend were beginning their freshman year at Hope College. They had decided to visit a variety of churches on Sunday mornings, seeking a church home where God might want them to serve and worship. On their second Sunday they found New Community Fourth Reformed. As they sat in the pew and checked out the bulletin they read this prayer request, "Pray that God will send us musicians." Approaching the pastor after the service they said, "We think we are the answer to your prayers." For the past three years they have been blessed to be a part of this church family, leading worship and working with youth, and the team from Hope is growing, as is the church.

We need to learn the value of accountability, as we unlearn insisting that "our business" is nobody else's. This can be very scary! It means I have to trust someone enough to share areas of my life where I know I might fail, and will probably stumble. Accountability partners are a source of encouragement, but they also have permission to call us on those things to which we are being less than faithful. I am currently in a mutual life-coaching relationship with someone I've never met, and who lives hundreds of miles away. But every Wednesday we talk, and every other week I am going to have to give account of whether I am working on goals, and taking action steps. Accountability relationships take on many forms, but a key to effectiveness is giving those partners permission to ask the hard questions.

As Christians we are a people of vows. We take baptismal vows, marriage vows, and vows when we join a church and profess our faith. If we are going to be disciples of Jesus Christ we need to live with integrity and fulfill those vows. I need help in that, and I'm guessing so do you. That is why God had this wonderful idea of putting us in community. God is with us, and God is with us through the people we live with, talk to, like and even those we don't like quite so much. Never in Scripture does God tell us, "Stand on your own two feet." "Pull yourself up by the boot straps." He does tell us to, "Love one another." Pray for one another." "Lean on one another." "Save enough so you can give to others."

Learning to live in community is not easy. Not only do I need to work on accepting it more, I also need to learn to offer it, and to model it. It will prepare us for eternity.

Here are four foundational questions for becoming who

God has created and intended us to be.

1. How will your understanding of God grow as you discover your purpose and passion?
2. Who are you becoming as the new creation? What areas of your life are being transformed?
3. Who will be a part of your journey, providing support and accountability?
4. What do you need to "unlearn?"

SECTION 4

Navigation tools for the Journey
Creating Space
Seeking Sweet Spots
Exploring Pathways
Life Reflection
Storytelling
Wondering
Discerning Core Values
Creating a Mission Statement
Visioning

14

Creating Space To Listen

The Soul is like a wild animal — tough, resilient, savvy, self sufficient, and yet exceedingly shy. If we want to see a wild animal, the last thing we should do is to go crashing through the woods, shouting for the creature to come out. Parker Palmer

We are a people in a hurry. We are a people who have been seduced into believing that there is a quick fix to every problem, an answer to every question, a someone responsible for every situation. We don't like having to wait, wrestle, or live in the unknown and with the mysteries of life and faith. In our culture it has become very difficult to listen to our life or the Spirit. We are better at crashing through the woods than walking quietly, sitting in silence, making the time and space to allow our souls to show up.

I recognize the audacity of inviting people to come to a retreat, or join a 6 week study group in order to discern their mission for the next season of life. Occasionally the process creates a great Ah Ha moment, which is incredibly fun to share in, but for many others it is more likely to create a "Hmmmm?" moment. It may be the beginning or continuation of a search and listening process that goes on for weeks, months, even years.

Have patience, midlifing child. If you create the time and the space, your life and the Spirit will speak; maybe in a whisper, perhaps in a shout of recognition, but speak it will.

Sue Monk Kidd, in her midlife journey discovered the imagery provided by a butterfly. Early one spring she found a cocoon, and found herself watching and waiting for the arrival of the butterfly. As she waited the lifecycle of the caterpillar came to represent her own stages in midlife of leaving the old life, entering a time of transformation and emerging into a new creation. She knew it was a process that couldn't be rushed, and just as with a butterfly breaking out of the cocoon, no one could do the work for her without causing damage to the new creation. Another interesting fact was that not all caterpillars work on the same schedule. It seems some caterpillars put off weaving their cocoon for quite some time before entering the transformation process. It appears that even caterpillars have trouble letting go of the past and the familiar to enter into a beautiful free new life.

Kidd also parallels the transformational journey with the exodus of the people of God out of slavery in Egypt and into the Promised Land. While in Egypt as slaves (caterpillars) they cried out to God for deliverance. God sends Moses to lead them out through the wilderness (cocoon), to a land promised to them generations before (butterfly). The wilderness was hard, and soon the people were lamenting the fact that God had rescued them from slavery, and they wanted Moses to take them back to their oppressors. What they didn't realize was that they needed wilderness time to be transformed into a nation, to build strength, identity and a relationship with their deliverer. The wilderness was the time and space they needed.

In a Midlife Momentum event there are certain elements used to create this kind of time and space, allowing transformation to take place. Obviously, the longer the retreat the easier it is to allow time and space for reflection, introspection, and listening. While the process can be adapted to many settings it is helpful to be able to "get away" from our normal surrounding and responsibilities in order to focus our attention. I find that even if I am home alone the distractions keep coming: the phone rings, the laundry calls, the mail arrives.

In a previous chapter I talked about catching the wind of the Spirit, using the analogy of a kite. In order to fly a kite one of the things needed is an open field: no trees, no wires, and no buildings blocking the wind. You need space. How do you create an open field for the catching of the Spirit in your life? This looks different in each of our lives. For many it means daily time with God and Scripture, best done in the early morning before the rest of your day begins. But I would encourage you to figure out when and how you best find the time and space for your open field. Our daughter Acacia and husband Ephraim are not morning people and have two small children who don't need much sleep. They discovered an open field when they began using the lunch hour to meet at their church for a time of prayer and seeking God's leading in their lives.

Birdwatching has become an open field for me. It is a quiet time, surrounded by the beauty of God's creation. In that time and place I enjoy being with God and listening for the voice of the Spirit, which I often sense through the design of creation. One of my first discoveries in watching birds was that you often look for birds close to the ground, not up in the trees. God seemed to be saying to me, "I'm on the ground, in the ordinary experiences and people you encounter…look for me there." I learned to "scan," watching for movement and color, listening for the calls. And I heard God speaking into my heart, "Be alert. Keep scanning to see where I am at work.

Look for movement, light. Listen for my call." I encourage you to explore new ways to be with God.

Routine and discipline are helpful in developing and fine tuning our listening abilities and expectations. However, we can also expect God to intervene in our days in surprising and fun ways. My grandson was about 3 years old as I was launching Midlife Momentum. We were playing a form of tag and he was running circles quite literally around me. As I stopped to take a rest Diedrick declared, "Grandma, you know you can't quit up on this!" And in the persistent voice of my grandson I heard the voice of the Spirit saying, "Holly, you know you can't quit up on this!" I still have that admonition posted on my refrigerator and read it often, especially when I doubt my calling and am wondering if I can do what I so strongly sense God calling me to do.

While the Midlife Momentum process can be experienced individually there is incredible power in sharing the journey and hearing one another's stories. In order to do that you need to create a safe community where there is a stated policy of confidentiality and acceptance. In my original work for my Doctor of Ministry degree I worked with two subsets of participants. In one group all of the participants had known each other for about 20 years, while in the other group none of the participants knew each other well. My goal was to see if it was easier to share your stories with those who knew you well, or with strangers. It was so interesting to see that although the groups functioned differently, both groups freely shared their stories and supported one another. They recognized they were on their own unique journey in a faithful, supportive company.

As participants continue to evaluate their experience a common theme is that they discover their own stories as they listen to one another. In the words of one participant, "The most meaningful aspect was receiving grace from each other. Isn't it amazing what we all have in common?" While it is not particularly designed to be therapeutic the Midlife Momentum experience has been healing and strengthening for many.

"Holly, you didn't really teach us a lot, but you provided a process to help us listen to what God is speaking into our lives." I consider this comment, given at the end of a retreat, one of the best compliments I have ever received. My goal is not to tell anyone else what God is saying to them, but to create a place, an environment, that invites people to listen to God and to what God wants to say to them through their very own life. When that place is created, and the process takes place in a safe community, powerful insights occur and participants are blessed with the encouragement and prayers of fellow journeyers. For me there are few things as exciting as seeing what can happen when this comes together.

Using strategies to create this safe environment is important. However, prayer, gentleness, honoring one another's story, and modeling by leadership should never be underestimated or forgotten. Obviously there are many factors that will affect the intimacy and community formed, some within our control, but many a gift we receive as together we live into it.

You will find some of the techniques used in the training manual in the back of the book.

1. What is one new way to create an open field for listening to God?
2. What brings you peace?
3. When do you feel most fully alive?

15

Finding our Sweet Spot

"Narnia, Narnia, Narnia, awake. Love. Think. Speak.
Be walking trees. Be talking beasts. Be divine waters."
C.S. Lewis in Magician's Nephew

"This is what I was created for!" Caleb at 19 years old
"Squares are just too hard! I was born to draw rectangles."
Diedrick at 5 years old

The place God calls you to is the place where your deep gladness
and the world's deep hunger meet. Frederick Buechner

Our son, Caleb spent the summer between his freshman and sophomore years of college as a counselor at Mount Hermon, a camp in northern California. It was an incredible summer for him. He was surrounded by the beauty of the mountains, ocean, and giant redwoods. He was living with other young disciples. He was able to use his gifts in music, and in drama. He was able to share the love of Jesus with children from strong Christian homes, and from broken families. One child had to leave mid-week for a custody hearing. Another one of his campers had a father in jail for murder. It stretched him and opened his eyes to the needs in our world. When he came home at the end of the season he summarized his experience in these words, "THIS is what I was created for." Caleb had found his "Sweet Spot", that place where his deep gladness met the world's great needs, which is how Fredrick Buechner defines vocation, or calling.

"Sweet Spot" is a sports term. It refers to that place and timing where the bat, the ball, and the power of the hitter come together in exactly the right way causing the ball to take off and fly farther. It also happens in golf with the ball, the club face, and the swing of the golfer. For me it has become an analogy in life where timing, people, places, events and the presence of God all come together to produce the perfect conditions for us to take off and fly. But more importantly, it is when we live intentionally, allowing our personalities, gifts, passions and calling to line up, giving us the experience of a life filled with meaning and purpose.

Will being a camp counselor always be that "sweet spot" for Caleb? Probably not. But, in the summer of his 19th year, he knew he was exactly where he should be, using his God-given gifts, living out his passion, allowing his personality to shine, growing in grace and knowledge, touching people with the love of God. WOW! Isn't that where we all want to be? I know I do!

Part of the challenge of growing in Christ is that finding our "Sweet Spot" isn't a once and done experience in life. We need to learn to constantly live into God's calling for our lives. Each season of life offers us new dreams and challenges, new opportunities to use the gifts, passions, life experiences and personalities God has created, and continues to create in our lives. And yet, once we do the searching and listening to discern our life-long calling we can more easily see how it can be reshaped and reframed for each season and circumstance in life. Building blocks for the future are being created in our present.

In the first few months of our marriage my husband Al and I decided on a name should we ever have a daughter. We would name her Acacia. We were reading through the biblical book of Exodus and encountered the chapters when the Israelites were instructed to build the Tabernacle in the wilderness. They were told to use acacia wood and overlay it with gold. Repeated over and over the name captured us as a beautiful name for the daughter who would be born two years later.

Acacia grew up with an increasing desire to spend time in Africa, firmly determined to do so by the time she was in junior high. While in college she spent a year studying in Nairobi, Kenya where she saw for the first time the acacia trees growing on the plains. Her name in the Maasai language is Olorei. She fell in love with Africa, and later with Ephraim, a young man from Ghana, West Africa. She and Ephraim are now preparing to launch an Non-Governmental Organization that will establish educational resource centers in Africa. When she first returned from Africa she declared, "My name was predestined." Acacia had found her sweet spot, and recognized it was a calling from God. She has been busy living through the building block times for the next season of their lives.

It is a constant temptation for many of us to get so busy with careers, family, school, in other words LIFE, that we move from day to day without evaluating whether we are living with purpose and ON PURPOSE. The current of life is flowing and we are simply trying to stay afloat, while avoiding bashing into boulders or dropping over waterfalls. Who has time to think about "Sweet Spots"?

While in generations past a familiar proverb claimed, "cleanliness is next to godliness," today's proverb might read, "busyness is next to godliness." Our reputations may be at stake if others do not perceive us as extremely busy, overwhelmed with life people. Is this truly the abundant life Jesus came to offer us, or are you hungry for more depth?

My goal is to encourage you to find that place where your deep gladness meets the world's deep needs.

1. If you had a week to do exactly what you wanted to do, what would it be? Where would you go? (Not sure you know? What would it be if you did know?)
2. What would it be if you did not spend the week with any family members?
3. What would you like to learn more about?
4. What keeps you from doing it? What steps can you take to begin experiencing it, perhaps on a smaller scale?

16

Doors, Windows and Ways

If one door closes God opens a window. Proverb

Whether you turn to the right or to the left, your ears will hear a voice behind you, saying, "This is the way, walk in it."
Isaiah 30:21

Many of us have used the proverb above when someone doesn't get that job they wanted, or they get fired from the one they have, or we don't get into the college of our choice, or...... It is a comment to encourage and give hope. "This isn't the end" we communicate, "There are other options." And in the midst of the struggle we pray that God is there providing and directing. But for those of us on whom a door has closed, a way has been shut off, we often assume that if we had just done things differently, or better; if there had been more justice done on someone else's part, the door might still be open. Especially for us Americans, if something goes "wrong" we feel a strong need to blame someone, or at least figure out a logical reason why. Plus, we are quite sure that we must fix the situation.

I have been intrigued by the work of Parker Palmer in his book, *Let Your Life Speak*. In this small but powerful book he talks about open and closed doors as WAY OPEN and WAY CLOSED. I like this imagery since a door often opens or closes to a room, a defined space, while a WAY is a path, a part of a journey. We don't start down a path and see the end in most cases. There is an element of trust needed to choose a path and discover where it will lead. Some ways, Parker tells us, close and we need to put them behind us, turn around and see which ways are open before us.

Palmer makes a profound statement that is foreign to our natural perspective as we navigate through life's surprises, disappointments, decisions and changes. He claims, "There is as much guidance in way that closes behind us as there is in way that opens ahead of us." We learn as much about ourselves from WAY CLOSED as we do from WAY OPEN. Way closed, that barrier or door that closes does not mean that God is not answering our prayers, but rather God may be leading us in a direction away from one thing before He can lead us to another.

Let me give an example. I am the only one in my immediate family who can't sing. Door Closed. My husband is a great tenor, my daughter a soprano, both of my sons sing and play guitar. Alas, I cannot sing well. For many years I was "not so secretly" jealous. I wanted to be able to bless God with songs of praise. Then I discovered liturgical signing. I had learned some basic signing and began working with junior and senior high girls putting sign language to songs of praise. (We also discovered a great website: aslpro.com) What a ministry of praise we discovered! This WAY OPEN also enabled me to build a mentoring relationship with the girls in our group. My life has become so wondrously rich from this ministry on so many different levels. Signing continues to be a favorite way for me to bring God praise in worship, and provides an entree into the lives of children and young people in a fresh new way. Would

I have discovered this WAY if I could sing well? Perhaps, but I no longer am frustrated with my singing ability, and recognize that my limitation in one area released a potential for greater blessing and impact by exploring a new "way."

Gerry, a man in his 50's, had a way dramatically closed in his 40's. Although I have only recently met him I am truly inspired by his story, his attitude, his perspective, and his faith. When in his late 40's, Gerry fell in a work accident. The fall left him a quadriplegic with very limited use of his hands. In the 10 years since his accident He has become an advocate for those with disabilities, as well as helping develop recreation and camping facilities on Vancouver Island, British Columbia. Ah, way open!

When I was in Australia earlier this year I met a 40 year old Irishman who has been in Australia for about 15 years. Again, his story is amazing; both in how God has opened the way for him in ministry, as well as in how ways have been closed. James grew up in war-torn Belfast, and became active in the IRA even as a child. Following a move to Australia he met Jesus and his life was transformed. As a Christian pastor James made plans to return to the area in which he grew up to be the love and presence of God where there is so much hatred. His wife's unexpected pregnancy delayed his plans as he sensed God saying, "The time is not right." James sees this WAY CLOSED as a timing issue rather than a permanently closed way. But he has peace as he continues to discern ways God is guiding him and his family. Way open!

Palmer says, "When I resist way closing rather than taking guidance from it, I may be ignoring the limitations inherent in my nature—which dishonors true self no less than ignoring the potentials I received as birthright gifts." I think this presents a deep challenge for us as we seek to love and understand ourselves as God's creation. Can we learn to honor ourselves by saying, 'These are my limitations.' 'These are the things I am not good at, and it is okay.' without abdicating responsibility for work poorly done, or blaming God when we fail to put forth our best effort? In order to do this well we need to put ourselves humbly before our God, listening with all the honesty, integrity and trust within us. It is rather frightening to face our limitations and be that honest with ourselves, but it also creates a fresh, glorious freedom to let go of unreal expectation and seek the doors through which God wants to develop the potential with which we have been gifted.

In the story of my Irish friend James, the way that closed was not a closure for all time, but guidance that said, "This is not the time. Wait on me." Lord, grant us wisdom and mercy that we might listen, and learn, and rejoice that you love us so much you invest your presence in us every day.

Palmer speaks of our tendency to keep pounding on those doors which close, rather than opening ourselves to the possibilities that are present as we turn from that path and seek a new way of being. Few of us are forced to make the radical changes that Gerry had to deal with when he became a quadriplegic. In his story we recognize the determination to be healthy and whole while in a wheelchair. Gerri has a meaningful life that contributes to the well-being of society in general, and has a purpose for which to live and deal with his disability. His limitations contribute to making him an inspiration, because his potential has been released as he works in so many ways to make life better for all of us with handicaps. Yes, one of the things he has already taught me is that nearly all of us will someday, in some way live with handicaps; whether that be hearing loss, vision, mobility, or cognitive loss. He has a head start on me and is working hard to make our lives better.

Can we learn to honor our true selves by accepting our limitations and celebrating our potential? I truly believe that is one of the gifts that living 50, 60, 70+ years gives us. We can stop fighting what we can't do and invest in what we can do. We can live intentionally!

1. What possibilities do I want to explore?
2. What are my limitations? What gifts do I not have?
3. Are there doors I need to stop banging on?
4. What other ways may be open before me?

17

Becoming

Praise is becoming for the upright. PS 33:1(NASB)

It is fitting for the upright to praise Him. PS 33:1(NIV)
What Becomes you?

Do you remember hearing people say, "Oh, your hairstyle is so becoming"? Or, "That color is very becoming on you." It is a phrase we do not hear much today, so if you do remember it, it may be another indicator we are in midlife. It's a compliment. That "something" brings out the best in you. The opposite also happens when we get the wrong hairstyle, or wear clothes that definitely are not appropriate for our bodies. They are "unbecoming" to us. Been there, done that? Take out some of those old photo albums and have a good laugh. There are times when the pressures of the culture make us do, or buy ridiculous things.

As we begin a Midlife Momentum retreat I often ask, "What color is your favorite color to wear?" And then a second question, "What style of clothes are you most comfortable wearing?" In the 70's and 80's color analysis became a big business. Did you ever host a color analysis party in your home?

Today on the web there are 846,000 results for a google search of "color analysis season." Initially I thought these questions might only work with women, but I have found it crosses gender lines. The men have some strong feelings about how they dress as well. Why bother to spend time on this?

First of all, a question or two is always needed to introduce participants to one another. Often this is true even if they think they know each other, or have been a part of the same church for decades. Secondly, this simple question often tells us much about those in the group, and sometimes about ourselves. There are some who like their sweats the best, and the more ragged the better. Others feel best in something crisp and sharp, black and whites. There is a lot more than clothes involved in these answers. There are no right or wrong answers, but the answers do give glimpses into personalities and preferences. Thirdly, it goes back to the issue of what "becomes" us. What brings out our best? What "fits" us well?

II Cor. 3:18, tells us we are being, "transformed into the likeness of Jesus." Eph. 4:13, encourages us by saying we are, "becoming mature, attaining to the whole measure of the fullness of Christ." And in I John 3:2-3, we read, "but when Christ appears, we shall be like him." These are just a few of the Scriptures that refer to us growing up into, or becoming like Jesus. That is the goal of the Holy Spirit at work in us, and it is a big job! We are all in the process of "becoming" something, whether we realize it or not. Every choice that we make, every conversation we have, every relationship we develop becomes a part of who we are. We have the choice of being intentional about becoming our best, or living day to day "by accident," or in our default mode. Our default mode represents all those choices we make without giving thought to our options. It is what we do automatically if left to our own habits and whims, including the habit of choosing based on what others will think.

Once we have done some work on discovering our true selves and realize who God is calling us to be, we can partner more effectively with the Spirit. What will it look like in my particular life to become more Christlike? We can get caught into thinking that we should all look alike; or we should all look like whoever we have decided is the most spiritual person we know. If only I could be like….. But no matter how wonderful that person is God doesn't want two of them. There is a design and plan, uniquely created for you by the Creator. Christ chooses to clothe himself with the unique personalities, gifts and passions of His followers. Look at how that is depicted in the life of God-followers throughout Scripture! There are no two alike in their gifts, or in their weaknesses, and they all have them. This should be an encouragement and a warning to each one of us. There is a well-known rabbinical story of a distraught rabbi named Zusya. Being a man of the Torah he often lamented that he wasn't more like Moses. Eventually he realized that when he got to heaven God would not ask him why he had not been more like Moses, but instead would ask, "Why were you not more like Zusya?" Those who model Christlikeness in their lives, who demonstrate the love and light we are all called to be are an inspiration to us, but let it be inspiration to become all God has uniquely called us to be.

As we look at the question of what "becomes" us it should help in decisions we make, all the way from the clothes we wear, to volunteer appeals, or to job opportunities before us. In Deuteronomy 30 Moses calls on the people to make a choice between life and death, blessing and curse. The choice for life meant loving and obeying God. That choice would have to be lived out in a thousand choices along the way. Choose you this day, growth or stagnation, life to the fullest or emptiness, purpose or the treadmill of life onto which so many of us can be lured by a thousand different voices.

We were on vacation in Massachusetts a few years ago and went to Salem, the center of the witch hunts of the 1690's. As we looked around the town we came upon a very old cemetery. On the gravestones they often listed the cause of the person's death. The one that jolted my attention was one that read, "He died on a treadmill." In those days treadmills were used to generate power or grind the grain, often using prisoners, slaves or animals to do the work. Today when we think of treadmills we are more likely to think about running and running, but going nowhere. I, for one do not want to die on a treadmill, literal or figurative! Evaluating ways we have chained our identities and lives to a treadmill are important experiences in learning to live intentionally.

Susan Scott, author of *Fierce Conversations* notes, "One of the most painful realizations upon reaching forty or fifty or sixty can be that you have no discernable identity, that somehow your identity has been compromised. It's not that your credit card or social security number was stolen, it's that an internal voice is whispering, insisting, 'This isn't you. This isn't enough of you. Parts of you are failing to show up.'"

So how do we stop this identity vacuum from continuing? How do we talk with ourselves, hold meaningful, or as Scott says, "fierce" conversations with ourselves and ask the deep questions which will help our true selves surface? It begins with resolve, for it takes courage to go down this path, knowing it will lead us somewhere that involves change, revelation, and also awakening and hope. You may truly discover you like who you find! Of course there will be aspects of you that need work, healing, polishing, becoming, but there is a wonderful, God-created you inside that needs to be discovered. Sometimes we have no idea what we are looking for, yet we know something more is waiting for us.

Susan Scott provides helpful exercises enabling us to access those parts of ourselves which have been well-hidden, or up to this point just too overwhelmed by life to come out. During those exercises she realizes we don't think we know the answers to many of her questions, so the question she keeps coming back to is, "If you did know, what would the answer be?"

I've been thinking about how often I respond to a question, or an inquiry about my preferences with a statement such as, "I don't care (much)," or "I don't know (because I'm not sure if you would like another option better)." Unfortunately, but as is often the case for women, I have been socialized to believe my desires aren't important, and everyone else needs to be kept happy. "Where would you like to stop for lunch?" What would the answer be if I was willing to set my desires on the table? How about that little Indian restaurant downtown? It has taken me until my 50's to acknowledge and live out my belief that in a healthy marriage both partner's desires are legitimate. I don't always have to get my way, but I can certainly verbalize, and when needed lobby for my desires and preferences.

After 40, 50, or 60 years of living we have many habits and patterns of thinking and behaving that keep our true selves securely tethered to what has become safe, predictable and often a treadmill.

What choices do you make every day that impact whether or not you are having a treadmill experience in life? When you open the refrigerator do you choose to eat things that make you healthier? When you open the closet door can you pull out clothes that you feel good in, or have you always bought what is "in," or what is the cheapest. When you turn on the radio or TV, what messages are you putting into your mind? When someone calls and asks you to fill a volunteer spot, what criteria do you use to determine if this will help you "become," or if it will drain you of energy that God would have you use in other ways?

When we hold before ourselves the realization that we are choosing to become all we can be in Christ it frees us to make better decisions. We can look at our birthright gifts: that personality, those gifts, passions, and the calling that God has created in us to see how each choice either does, or does not "become us". Does it help you to be who God wants you to be? Does it fit well with who you are becoming? If it does and the timing seems right give it a whole hearted yes. If it does not, then feel guiltless freedom to say no. Remember, this can affect choices from what you are going to eat or wear, to choices about whether you will help in the local food pantry, take a new position, or go into missions in Ecuador.

The Holy Spirit is in the business of making us a new creation and he longs for our surrender and cooperation. The Spirit wants to be our counselor, guide, and friend. He isn't out to trick us. Many times the answer to life's greatest questions about our future lay deep within us, in who God has created us to be. The good news is that when we choose well, it feels right. Does that mean we will never make mistakes? Of course not, but that is when we rejoice that grace is at work, redeeming our errors, shaping and forming us through the good times and bad, helping us to become more like the Master.

1. What color do you enjoy wearing the most? What color clothes seem to draw the most compliments? Or, what color clothes dominate your closet?
2. What style of clothes do you feel most comfortable in?

What style of clothes call your name?

3. What decisions are you making today that either will, or will not help you become more fully you?
4. What would you like to say to your Creator today?
5. What questions do you need to ask yourself?

18

Tracing Grace

From the beginning, our lives lay down clues to selfhood and vocation, though the clues may be hard to decode. But trying to interpret them is profoundly worthwhile. Parker Palmer

Listening to other's stories is a gift we offer them. But we also receive a gift as we realize that every story is in some way the story of us all. Richard Morgan

When Joseph, son of Jacob was in midlife he was able to look back at how God had been at work in his life preparing him for his life purpose in midlife and beyond. Here is a quick synopsis in case you are not familiar with the story. (Or, better yet find a good Bible story book or look up Genesis 37-50.) This story tells us how the people of God arrive in Egypt, from which Moses will deliver them after 400 years.

Joseph was the favored of the 12 sons of Jacob, demonstrated by the special coat he was given by dad. Joseph was also the one chosen by God to save his people from a famine throughout the region in about 1,900 BC. Joseph, as a child, was spoiled and definitely not beloved by his brothers. On top of that, in his teenage years he had two visions which indicated that one day his family would all bow down to him. When he proceeded to tell the family about these dreams the resentment grew to the point that the brothers ended up delivering Joseph into the hands of Egyptian slave traders, while telling their father he had been killed by a wild animal.

Though he was taken to Egypt as a slave, God worked in many amazing, but uncomfortable ways to bring Joseph into a position of leadership in the land. When God revealed through dreams that a famine was coming in seven years, Joseph was charged with preparing the country for it. The famine came, and so did Joseph's brothers, seeking food to keep their families alive. Not expecting to see Joseph in Egypt, they did not recognize him when they came before him to make their request for food. When they discovered it was Joseph and realized he was in a position to have them killed they were terrified. However, Joseph recognized he had been put in this specific position by God to save his people, and was willing to forgive his brothers.

As we look back on the life of Joseph we recognize God's presence with him, but still wonder, "Why did he have to go through so many difficult experiences?" Somehow God knew exactly what would build the character Joseph needed to fulfill God's plans for his life, and for the future of the people of God. Grace is woven through the good and the bad, the failures and successes. Here are scenes from Joseph's life:

1. Favored child
2. Thrown in a pit
3. Sold as a slave by his own brothers
4. Rose to a position of responsibility in his master's house
5. Stood firm against temptation and was lied about

6. Ended up in prison
7. Rose to a position of responsibility in the prison
8. Forgotten by others he had helped
9. Interpreted dreams for Pharaoh
10. Put in position of leadership in the land
11. Prepared the land for the famine
12. Provided the food for his family

On our Midlife/Renewing Momentum journey we take the time to reflect back on life. The goal is to trace the path of grace all through our lives, realizing that through the good times and hard, the ups and downs, the successes and failures, grace has been at work: shaping, molding, and developing our character for a purpose. As I persist on this journey leading groups through the process, God reveals to me glimpses of how he has prepared me for my future, and sowed seeds that would germinate years later.

One of my favorite exercises during a retreat or seminar is to use a guided imagery experience to explore our river of life.

River of Life: To begin this exercise, imagine that you are walking through a forest. You come to a stream and find Jesus waiting there, with a canoe. He invites you to get into the front of the canoe, while he takes his place behind you. He tells you that this is your river of life, and he wants to take a look at it with you. You push off from shore and Jesus guides you down the river.

As you go he calls your attention to different things in the river. Look for boulders....twists and turns..... rapids.....low hanging branches.....whirlpools....deep quiet places...places where the river flows swiftly.....dams....

sandbars....places you need to portage.....do other streams feed into your stream? Are there places where water is siphoned off your river to feed into other streams, to irrigate? What kind of countryside do you pass through: woods, meadows, canyons? Do you see any life in or around your river? What does Jesus say to you about your river?

You come to a sandbar. Up ahead the river disappears around a bend. Jesus brings the canoe up on the sandbar and gives you a hand out. He gives you a hug, and as he hugs you, you realize that he melts right into you.

Now take time to capture the river on paper using crayons, pencils, etc. Some of you may choose to write a poem or story instead.

As an example, let's imagine that you are drawing a river that reflects Joseph's river of life. How would you picture his childhood as a favored son? How about the tension that grows as he gets older? I'm thinking a stretch of whitewater might depict the time when he is thrown into the pit and then sold as a slave. I'm also thinking about a canyon as he spends years in a prison for a crime he didn't commit. And what does the river look like when he is elevated to a position of leadership in the country? Or when his brothers stand before him asking for food, not realizing this is the brother they sold into slavery?

Do you get the idea? Grace, woven through the fabric of life, often seeming to disappear for a time, but always at work shaping, forming, developing character, accomplishing God's purposes.

As we have done this exercise we process together recognizing many things about our river:

1. Everyone's river is unique.
2. But, there are so many similarities in our struggles.
3. We were never alone.
4. Getting around one boulder helped us navigate the next challenge.
5. For some a dam represented something blocking their way. For others a dam represented a source of power. For yet another the dam was a place where the river slowed and they could be rescued.
6. The waterfalls have been places of danger for some, while for others waterfalls have been beauty that fed their stream.

As the river flows, so flows the grace of God, always creating, redeeming, healing and loving us into the next season of life. Many become aware that it is often through struggles that life changes direction, personal growth happens, and character and strength are found and formed.

1. Where are the major turning points in your river?
2. What does Jesus want to say to you about your river?
3. What does your spirit rejoice in as you take this journey?

19

I Did It! I Love It!

*When we lose track of our true self, how can we pick up the trail?
One way is to seek clues in stories from our younger years, years
when we lived closer to our birthright gifts.*
Parker Palmer in Let Your Life Speak

*For you created my inmost being; you knit me together in my
mother's womb. I praise you because I am fearfully and wonderfully made; your works are wonderful, I know that full well.*
Psalm 139:13

In search of our true selves we journey back, to rediscover
the self that has often gotten left behind as we move from one
season to another.

During one of our Midlife Momentum exercises we reflect
back on memories of things we loved to do, our successes, accomplishments and awards, favorite people, places, and activities; looking for threads which run through our lives, giving
us clues to our passions, gifts, personalities and calling. We
are searching under rocks and in crevices for this fearfully and
wonderfully made creation we are. This is not easy work! We
aren't used to thinking deeply about who we are.

I DID IT! I LOVE IT!

As I began reflecting back I realized that my first clear memory was when I was 5 years old. I went to a three room country school, and when you were 5 you could visit once during the year, so you would know what first grade was going to be like. (So much for preschool and kindergarten.) I remember that visit so clearly. Janice was the girl assigned to let me sit beside her for the day. She was wearing a beautiful blue dress with a big square collar. I fell in love with school that day, and have loved academia ever since. This first memory begins a thread of education that flows throughout my life and the lives of our children. We often say we are education rich, though we may not have a lot of "toys."

When I was about 8 years old I attended a mission conference. At these conferences several churches came together to worship, eat, and hear what God was doing through our missionaries around the world. As children we had our very own mission speakers. One year we had a woman who had been a missionary to China until they were refused entry. She told us of the Chinese children she worked with, and taught us to sing Jesus Loves Me in Chinese. I was enthralled. I even wrote to her later and asked her to send me the words in Chinese, so I could teach it to my friends. It was my first call to ministry. Did I realize it at the time? No, I just knew I wanted to teach children to sing Jesus Loves Me in China. I have never been to China, however I have taught children in several states and in Haiti to sing and sign Jesus Loves Me. I also have a beautiful Chinese daughter-in-law, and my very own Chinese-American granddaughter. Reflections of God's grace and how He has been shaping me continue to be uncovered as I relish this process of seeing God's plans unfold.

As I introduce this exercise I ask participants what they loved to do when they were 11. This helps get the wheels turning, but it is also true that at about this age we begin to put different parts of ourselves up on a shelf. By the time we are 11 we discover that some of the things we love to do are not considered "cool" by peers, or we discover other interests we pursue. As we get into high school social life and extra-curricular activities may take up so much time we add more bits and pieces to the shelf. Once we exit our teens there is getting an education, finding work, volunteering, and any number of other opportunities, many of which develop new interests and abilities. Along comes marriage and the baby carriage…more things are up on the shelf.

None of this is bad. It just means that at midlife we have the opportunity to go back and take a look at the things we have put on the shelf, see how they are a part of our true selves and decide which things need to be dusted off, re-evaluated and integrated back into our lives. What has been left behind that we want to reclaim?

Palmer says it like this, "We arrive in this world with birthright gifts—then we spend the first half of our lives abandoning them or letting others disabuse us of them…If we are awake, aware and able to admit our loss—we spend the second half trying to recover and reclaim the gift we once possessed."

As I conduct seminar after seminar I am amazed at how challenging it is for people to focus on their achievements, joys and gifts. Somehow we have been conditioned into an unhealthy imbalance between pride and humility. Rare are the people who feel "comfortable in their own skin;" who recognize both their gifts and limitations, and can celebrate who they are created to be. As participants push further in it becomes a treasure hunt for true self.

I DID IT! I LOVE IT!

1. What did you love to do when you were 11?
2. What gifts, relationships, activities have you put on the shelf?
3. What would you like to add to the shelf?
4. What would you like to take down, dust off, and reclaim?

20

Mentors Who Have Come Before Us

*I wonder as I wander down many paths
and with many companions.*

The Word of God is Living and Active. Hebrews 4:12

*Our story merges with God's story whenever we perceive God
as the "silent companion" in life's journey. Richard Morgan*

I wonder. Do you? I have learned to wonder a lot more since I began working in the area of children's ministry and began leading Young Children and Worship, a program developed by Jerome Berryman and Sonja Stewart. It is a way of being in worship with children that can open our hearts to new ways of reading Scripture and encountering God. It is about allowing the stories of God to intersect with our stories. It shows us a way to be IN the stories. Wondering opens the windows to our souls, and allows the Spirit to awaken us to the living, active Word and work of God.

As I have learned to share the stories of Scripture this way I have come to know the people of the Bible in deeper, richer ways. They really are characters! They have so much to teach us about living a life of faith. It can be challenging for us to hear their messages given 2000 years of time, a totally different culture, and our silly assumptions that we are more advanced, deal with different problems, and have nothing in common with these ancient people.

During most retreats I hand out a sheet with a list of biblical characters and the Scriptures that tell us their stories. Our goal is to turn these men and women into our mentors. Participants choose a person from the sheet, work alone or with a partner to read the passages and then respond to wonderings, such as, "I wonder what dangers (Miriam) faced on her journey." "I wonder what challenges (Mordecai) would encourage us to embrace." After a time of pondering we introduce our mentor to our retreat companions and share our responses to these wonderings, with the goal of discerning what it is they would want to say to us today if they were sitting at the table with us. Often while the participants work on this I take time to be still, prepare for the next step, and evaluate how things are going.

In March 2008, while conducting a retreat, I decided to quickly choose one of the women on the list for myself. I picked someone with only a few verses. I didn't recall exactly who this person was as I began the study. All it said on my sheet was "Woman with a fever," and then it gave three Scripture passages: Matthew 8:14-15, Mark 1:30-31, Luke 4:38-39. Ah, synoptic Gospels, all three passages basically the same simple story of Peter's mother-in-law, who was sick with a fever. Jesus came into her house and healed her. She got up and served Jesus and his followers. What would she say to me today? How much insight can there be in 2 or 3 verses with such a simple, short story?

It just so happened (umm, right) that in the next month I would travel to Ohio to visit our daughter and her husband,

and to Sydney, Australia to visit our son and his wife. I am a mother-in-law. Not only that, but our son-in-law is from Ghana, West Africa, and our daughter-in-law is from London, but of Chinese ancestry, which means there are cultural differences in many things we do; such as how fast we go, what we eat, and of course, how we parent. The list goes on and on. But these beautiful young people have so enriched my life! What does Peter's mother-in-law have to teach me?

I began thinking about what it must have been like for her to have Peter as a son-in-law. He was after all bold, impetuous, one who often speaks without thinking, a leader. I wondered how she felt when Peter left his nets and boats to follow Jesus. "Hey, you are the bread-winner in the family!" "Excuse me, but who is going to provide for me and my daughter if you leave your livelihood?" "Who is this itinerant prophet running around Galilee disrupting our family?" Why would Peter risk leaving his family and work to travel all over creation following this "Messiah"? Remember, this was early in Jesus' ministry. There were still lots of questions about who he was, and if he was who they hoped him to be. As his mother-in-law I can imagine she was none too thrilled to have her daughter left home while Peter was on the road with Jesus.

Now imagine what happened to her understanding of Jesus when he came into her home and healed her of the fever! I believe peace came to that home. Maybe there is something to this Jesus. Maybe Peter should leave his nets and follow Jesus. Maybe he is the Messiah! Now she becomes part of the support team for her daughter and son-in-law, instead of feeling sorry for herself and her daughter. I believe that after this encounter she can engage positively in a household that knows they need to live in obedience to God, even if it means living a life of total faith in an itinerant preacher.

So I considered my visits to our married children and I knew that this woman with the fever would tell me much about trusting God with my children's lives. "Encourage your son-in-law and daughter-in-law, in their work, in their marriages, and as parents. And support your children and their spouses as they seek to follow the Messiah. Let them know you believe in them." I gave thanks that it is indeed true that they are whole heartedly seeking God. I also realized it wouldn't always look the way I might expect it to. Cory and Elisa were already ministering in Australia, while Acacia and Ephraim would be heading for Ghana in the future. It is okay! I need to be a part of their support teams as they follow God to the ends of the earth. But it also means being respectful of who they are, where they come from and how they live out daily life. I want to bring encouragement, hope, joy, and empowerment when I come into their homes. I want to be a blessing that helps them to be all God is shaping and forming them to be. I want to be a great mother-in-law! And this is what Peter's mother-in-law encouraged me to embrace.

I was once again reminded of how living and active the Word of God is in our lives. It was an SKT moment. SKT= Socks Knocking Time. Do you know the phrase, "Knock their socks off" as an encouragement to people who are about to perform? It is a fun little message we send to one another in our family before someone performs in drama, music or forensics. SKT. But there are also many moments when God "Knocks our socks off." God took these few short verses about Peter's mother-in-law and not only reminded me of how I need to love and encourage my son-in-law and daughter-in-law; He also let me know that he is intimately aware of exactly what is on my calendar, how I need to grow, and where I need insight. I recognized that some of those stories we read over so quickly are rich with meaning and power and are the means by which God desires to speak to us in very real ways. They have Spirit inspired power to impact our lives and holiness at just the right moment, if we slow down long enough to listen. God is so amazing!!

No matter which person we choose to look at through this exercise we discover an amazing story behind the story. Take a look at two of my favorite people in scripture: Elizabeth in Luke 1 and Mordecai from the Book of Esther. We know both of them because of their relationship to more well-known people. Elizabeth is the mother of John the Baptist, and the cousin of Mary, mother of Jesus. Mordecai is the cousin who raised and advised Esther, who would become the Queen of Persia. They are invaluable behind the scenes older people mentoring and investing in the lives of God's chosen young people. Teach us, they can! For I believe this is an area where each one of us, as experienced midlifers, can be used to impact the kingdom and the world. There are young people all around us who need someone who believes in, affirms and blesses them.

Wondering about these stories makes them come alive. When I speak with someone who is more concerned with answers than with questions and wondering I share with them the image of an open window. As long as we are seeking God, seeking truth, and willing to live in the mystery it is as if the windows of our soul are open to the Spirit. As soon as we believe we have the answers, know the solutions, or can explain God the window closes, communication is cut off and the air becomes stale. One of the hallmarks of being a child is the ability to wonder. Is there anything more beautiful than a child's face filled with awe and wonder? I'm guessing this is one of the attributes that Jesus loved so much when he told us it is essential for us to be childlike if we are going to belong to the kingdom.

1. What biblical or historical person would you like to have as a mentor?
2. What do you want to ask him/her?
3. What do you believe she/he would say to you today?
4. Who would you like to have lunch with?

21

Exploring Our Core Values

If your behavior contradicts your values, your body knows, and you pay a price at a cellular level. Susan Scott
Above all else, guard your heart, for it is the wellspring of life.
Proverbs 4:23

Have you seen the television commercials for NBC with the theme, "Characters welcome"?

When our son Cory was about eight years old we were eating in a restaurant. At a nearby table a boy about five years old was getting a lot of attention by acting out in ways that were not necessarily naughty, but too rambunctious for the restaurant setting. I commented to our family, "Boy, he is a character." To which Cory responded, "That's what I like to be, a character." He was absolutely right. He loved to be a character. Sometimes it got him in trouble. Sometimes he didn't have the maturity to rein it in when needed, but his heart was good, and he just loved to add life to the party. It was fascinating to see him identify this characteristic or value in himself. He valued fun, and he valued performing. This theme has played itself out in wonderful ways through music, drama, forensics, and youth ministry.

Core Values are the themes in your life that flow through

every area of life, determining who you are at the heart level. You can't really fake core values. They will show up. You can be working on improving them on a consistent basis, because you realize you fall short of living up to them, but if they are not important to you it won't last.

Core values are difficult to explain. We rarely think about how they shape our lives. We are more likely to work on them in reference to our work or organizations in which we participate. But if we realize it is important to recognize their power to shape our businesses and the success of organizations, think how important it is to evaluate how our values impact our personal and family lives. It is a key factor in living intentionally.

It takes some time and thought to discern and develop a list of our core values. The challenge is to think intentionally about values you feel are non-negotiable for you. Even though they will flow through all areas of your life it may be helpful to apply some of them to particular areas of your life. Take the time now to write down at least two core values you hold in each of the following areas. Don't over analyze at this point, name whatever comes to your mind. What things, attitudes, characteristics are most important to you in the following areas?

1. Family and relationships:
2. Professional/work:
3. Health and wellness:
4. Emotional:
5. Spiritual:
6. Financial:
7. Personal development:

After identifying your core values in each area see how they flow through the other areas of your life.

For example:

1. Under professional you may note INTERGRITY as a core value. It will mean that your co-workers, employers, employees know that they can trust you. Your word is good. You will do all you can to be honest and forthright. The good news is that if integrity is a core value in your professional life your family will also know this is the kind of person you are. Your church family will know they can depend on you. Your friends will know they can trust you. You won't have integrity in your business if it isn't heart and soul who you are.

2. Under spiritual life you may note LORDSHIP OF CHRIST as a core value. It will mean that you recognize Jesus as Lord, King, Sovereign in your life. Your life will be surrendered to the will of God for you. The good news is that if this is true your family will be raised to know that God is the ultimate authority in your family. In your business every decision that is made needs to go through the scrutiny of deciding if this move will bring glory to God. Will it live up to the King's standards? When it comes to health and wellness you will need to take good care of this physical body that belongs to the Lord.

Do you remember this little nursery rhyme? "There was a little girl, who had a little curl, right in the middle of her forehead. When she was good, she was very, very good, and when she was bad, she was horrid." Like me, are you surprised sometimes by the words that come out of your mouth, or the response you have toward someone? Are you ever embarrassed by your actions, or lack of action? My husband Al and I jokingly use this phrase when we are surprised by each other, "Who are you and what have you done with my husband/wife?"

It is important to remember that we have both actual and preferred values in our lives. Actual values are those that we have integrated well into our lives, and most of the time we live according to them, for good or for ill depending on the value. Preferred values are those we think we should have, or would like to have, but we are still striving to achieve them at a consistent level.

It will be helpful to go back to your list of values and rate them on a scale of 1 to 10. A one means this is a value I recognize as important, but I have never developed it in my own life. For example, I may realize having a small group, or deep friendships where I experience true community is important and biblical, but, "Hey, I'm a very private person, I don't let people get that close." Community would rate pretty far to the left under preferred values. If, on the other hand you believe community is important and have established a strong support group where you listen, care and hold one another accountable, you hold community as an actual value and it is about a nine or ten.

Preferred		Actual
1	5	10

As I was working on my dissertation for my Doctor of Ministry degree I knew that I was on to something significant. I also sensed that God was calling me to integrate this work on midlife/second adulthood transitions more fully into my life and ministry. I liked the idea. When I was leading the retreats or talking with others about what happens in midlife I got excited, felt the adrenaline pumping, and knew I needed to do more. However, we had a son preparing to go to college and it didn't seem financially reasonable for me to resign from a position that would be paying the tuition to embark on a journey that would need seed money and probably wouldn't be generating any income for a while, if at all.

Now I would never have told you that financial security, according to the world's standards, was one of my core values. In the realm of finances I believe that God is my source and obedience to God comes first...and yet, here I was dragging my feet and refusing to take the leap into Midlife Momentum based, at least in part, on money.

I would never have told you that worrying about what people think about me is a core value...and yet, I was fearful of what would happen and what people would think if I resigned from my church position to launch a ministry I believed God was calling me to start and it went nowhere. What if I failed? My preferred values in this realm would be confidence and courage to do what I believe I am called to do regardless of what others think.

Values I claimed were my core values were definitely doing battle with some actual values that still had power over me. Taking a good look at our values can be hard work and a little too revealing at times to leave us comfortable. But if I want to claim integrity as another core value (which I do) it means I need to wrestle, do battle, and allow the Spirit to show me where the lines of my inner life are not plumb.

Here is another fun exercise that has proved helpful in evaluating which values we are living by.

On a sheet of paper write as many "proverbs" as you can think of, such as:

A bird in the hand is worth two in the bush.

EXPLORING OUR CORE VALUES

Waste not, want not.
He who laughs last, laughs best.
The early bird catches the worm.

In preparations for some retreats participants do a bit of homework. One such assignment asks those planning to attend to make a proverb list ahead of time. One woman decided it would be fun to engage her mother, who was living in a nursing home, in the exercise. As they reminisced and began developing their list others overheard their conversation and got involved. Other residents and their families and caregivers all started to add to the list. The woman asking for the proverbs even had people calling her at home as they thought of more. By the time she came to the retreat she had a list of 157 proverbs. It is a fun exercise. After compiling the list we take a second look to determine: What are the values embedded in these proverbs, and are these values I choose to embrace, or are they values which need to be "ditched"?

For example, a value embedded in "A bird in the hand is worth two in the bush" is caution. We shouldn't take chances. Play it safe. Hang on to what you have, rather than going for more. I'm quite sure that overall this is not a godly value. I don't see God playing it safe when he chooses a people, sends a Savior, or entrusts us with Kingdom work. Jesus tells a parable of a master who entrusts his servants with his property by giving them his money, and then going on a journey. When he returns each servant must give account of what he has done with the money entrusted to him. The only servant who got in trouble was the servant who "played it safe" and hid the master's money in the ground, not risking the possibility of losing what had been entrusted to him/her.

There are many proverbs that we have heard all of our lives

so we assume they must be good or true, but a closer look may tell us they need to be rethought and eliminated from our core values. The next step in the exercise is to see which of the proverbs is something you agree with and live out (positive actual), which you think represent good values which you need to work on (preferred), and which represent values you need to "ditch."

As participants do this exercise one of the discoveries occurring is that these proverbs often represent values they have inherited from their families of origin. These become well ingrained values we never stop to evaluate, and they often hold us hostage without announcing their presence.

I've been putting more work on the values aspect of our identity recently as I grow in my awareness of how these values impact our actions and decisions. Why is it that important? According to Susan Scott in *Fierce Conversations* your health and well-being, as well as our relationships, success, and joy depend on integrity. This means I need to live my values. Scott claims, "If your behavior contradicts your values, *your body knows,* and you pay a price at a cellular level. Over time, depending on the severity of the integrity outage and how long it's been going on, your immune system will weaken, leaving you increasingly vulnerable to illness." (Italics mine) She goes on to explain that each individual, marriage, and organization has an immune system. It is critical that we seek to live in alignment with the values we claim, and often believe we hold.

As you work on defining your core values do not settle for those expected of you by others, instead look for those that hold you captive; that excite you in your inner being, when nobody is noticing.

These are exercises you may want to come back to as you think more deeply about who you are and where God is taking you in this next season.

1. What value do you most want to work on?
2. What value do you most need to "ditch"?
3. Which value sneaks up and surprises you at times?
4. What inherited values need to be evaluated? We all live with many values inherited from our families of origin, some healthy, some not so healthy.

22

Discerning Our Passions

Recollection becomes a matter of priority only when we have experienced one too many times the tastelessness of a passionless life.
Gordon MacDonald

I know I can give up my TV time for something so exciting and right for me. Carol

My comfort zone cannot compete with the joy I have as I live into my passion, scary as it may be!

When our son Cory was about 8 years old he saw a documentary on the Anastasis, one of the Mercy Ships of Youth With A Mission (YWAM). It told how these ships had been transformed from old cruise ships into hospitals which would dock in third world countries to provide medical help otherwise not available to many of the people so desperately in need of doctors, nurses, medicine and surgery. Doctors and nurses would fly in for two weeks or a month at a time to share their time, skills and hearts with the people they met in these ports. It showed the conditions of some of the people coming to the ship for help. The next day Cory and I were in the car together when he began to sob. I had no idea what was wrong and why he was sobbing so. When I asked him, he responded, "I just keep seeing those kids on that program last night."

At eight Cory's young heart was broken by the suffering he was seeing. When he was 19 he spent 6 months on the Anastasis as it traveled to Togo, Benin, and Ghana. Later he returned to YWAM as staff to work, not in the medical field, but with youth who were at a point in their lives when God was challenging them to become world changers in the name of Christ.

Those tears, shed by an 8 year old provided a glimpse into Cory's passions and God's purposes for him.

In order for us to live into God's calling for our lives we have to know that it is connected to the issues, people, and places, about which we are passionate. God has planted those passions in us. Your passion will not be exactly like mine. You can't live out my passion, and you must not expect everyone else to get excited about the same things that you do, no matter how important they are. This is an emotional challenge when you are passionate about something and others don't seem to understand the needs. How can you not care about children in India or Uganda who have no place to sleep? How can you not get involved in providing educational opportunities to help children in Ghana find a way out of poverty? How can you not see the importance of mobilizing the boomer generation to; feed the hungry, clothe the naked, bring hope to those in despair, and be the presence of God in a lost and broken world, so loved by God? We need to be actively passionate about what God is calling us to and allow the Spirit to awaken a passion in others. Perhaps God will use us, and their passion will dovetail into ours, making us partners in a greater purpose...perhaps not. We are uniquely created and impassioned.

Often we can be overwhelmed by the needs around us, and the challenge becomes finding our unique calling: that place of passion where God has created us to live, serve and love. Not every need is a calling. If we try to address every need out of guilt or compassion we will be ineffective, frustrated and worn out very quickly. The following questions may help you determine where your passion lies.

List at least 10 things for the first 3 questions, about 5 for the 4th, and only one for the 5th question.

1. What brings you JOY? (10)
2. What brings you to tears? (10) (Tears of joy or sadness)
3. What makes you angry? (10) Do you have righteous indignation about an injustice?
4. When is it you feel fully alive? (5)
5. If you knew you would not fail what would you attempt for the Kingdom of God? (1)

After you have allowed these questions to stir in your soul for at least a day or two come back to your responses and see if there are things you would add. Then answer this question:

What is the first step you need to take to address the passion that surfaced through question 5?

As people answer question 5 they often speak in very broad strokes, such as: feeding the hungry, bringing people to Christ, world peace, etc. While it seems totally impossible, the question of first steps helps people realize that if they have spoken from their passion there is a way to get involved in helping to make it a reality in some smaller way.

DISCERNING OUR PASSION

Carol recognized that her passion of helping young people at risk connected to her joy of horsemanship and she signed up to be part of an organization that uses horses in their work with at-risk teenagers.

Fran realized that her passion to provide housing for single moms trying to get their lives together meant her first step involved researching the work of others in this area and learning from them.

Prior to doing an exercise on passions Carol's group was talking about Steven Covey's quadrants for establishing priorities in our lives: important and urgent, important but not urgent, urgent and not important, and not urgent and not important. As we talked we listed all of the things which take up our time and which are not important, TV being a major time eater. As Carol recognized her passion to help kids while working with her horse she declared, "I can easily give up my TV time for something so right for me." It had clicked, and she knew she wouldn't be volunteering out of a sense of obligation or guilt, but out of a passion and joy in knowing she was doing what God was calling her to do.

Does it always become this clear the first time we wrestle with these questions? No, for some it takes time and patience to see what your life wants to say to you. Remember the deer we were seeking in chapter 14? You need to allow a time and place for your spirit to speak. It doesn't always come out on demand, but God will honor your search.

Return to the questions you pondered earlier in this chapter.

1. What brings you JOY?
2. What brings you to tears of sadness/tears of joy?

3. What makes you angry?
4. When is it you feel fully alive?
5. If you knew you would not fail what would you attempt for the Kingdom of God?

23

Crafting a Mission Statement

"I know the plans I have for your", declares the Lord,
"Plans to prosper you and not to harm you, plans to give
you hope and a future." Jeremiah 29:11

Balance!

But as long as you know you're nobody special,
you'll be a very decent sort of Horse, on the whole.
C.S. Lewis in The Horse and His Boy

Some of us have been a part of helping an organization or
church craft a mission statement, but few have tried to actually figure out, "What in the world am I here for?" In the first
adulthood we are kept so busy birthing families, careers, hob-
bies and interests that we don't give much thought to, "Why
am I getting up this morning?" We have schedules to keep, and
often not just our own schedules but children's as well. Then
the nest empties. The job may no longer seem as significant as
it once did. We wonder where the romance has gone from the
marriage. We are so busy, but not sure what we're busy with, or
if we want these things to eat up our time.

What impact is my life having? STOP the merry-go-round! I don't want to keep going around in circles, I want my life to count!

If you have gone through the Midlife Momentum process you have looked at who you are in this season of life. You have recognized how God has been shaping and molding you in the past, and have discovered what you are passionate about. By now you should realize that you have an awesome God who has created and known you from before your birth, gifting you with abilities and a personality uniquely your own. You are indeed fearfully and wonderfully made! (Psalm 139) Then God has added a special calling and has given His Spirit so that you can live out this calling with joy and meaning. You are blessed to be a blessing! (Genesis 12:1-3)

In this chapter we will try to pull all of this together and develop a mission statement that simply and clearly declares what you sense God is calling you to be and do in this next season of life, or in your second adulthood. A word of warning; this isn't a once and done process. It may take time: weeks, months, perhaps years before you feel like you have "nailed it." But take heart, there is joy in the journey, as well as in the wrestling. However, even when you have nailed it you need to continue to seek and listen, for each season offers fresh opportunities, as well as limits on what we are called to be. In other words this mission is not carved in stone, but must be malleable. We are clay in the potter's hands, and the clay never gets hard and brittle, for the Potter brings us to new challenges and experiences throughout our lives. We need not fear that once we can no longer accomplish one purpose God is finished with us. That was but one building block of the many which will shape the life God is calling us to live.

Developing a mission statement helps us to focus our time,

energy, and thoughts. It gives us a valuable tool for making decisions, and helps us escape the tyranny of the urgent. In many ways defining a mission can be a redeeming act. Doug Shapiro and Richard Leider in their book, *Repacking Your Bags,* discuss the fact that for many people the number one deadly fear is "Having lived a meaningless life." Laurie Beth Jones in, *The Path,* adds, "Finding one's mission , and then fulfilling it, is perhaps the most vital activity in which a person can engage."

Laurie Beth Jones (LBJ) has helped many individuals and corporations develop a mission statement. In her book, *The Path: Creating Your Mission Statement for Life and Work,* she not only explains the difference a life lived with purpose can provide, but gives exercises and examples of how to create our own mission statements.

According to Laurie Beth Jones there are three keys to an affective mission statement:

1. It needs to be short and concise; no more than one sentence long.
2. It should be easily understood.
3. You should be able to recite it by memory under stress.

While it may seem easy to come up with a single sentence, in reality it is very challenging to be able to do the introspection and word-smithing to focus one's mission into one simply understood sentence, but it is also extremely helpful. It becomes a guide to our decision making, helping us to "Become" who we are created to be. It enables us to prioritize our time and resources. It is a tool of self-knowledge, shaping our identity. LBJ says, "(it) acts as both a harness and a sword—harnessing you to what is true about your life, and cutting away all that is false." It provides freedom to be your best true self, and provides protection from being driven to be what you or others demand that you be.

As you develop your mission statement we will pull together things you have learned or remembered about yourself throughout previous exercises and meditation. The following process is adapted from *The Path: Creating Your Mission Statement for Work and for Life,* by Laurie Beth Jones. Answer the following questions.

1. What do I love to do? What are my gifts? Think of three action words you identify with. _____

   _____

   It may be helpful to brainstorm as many action words as you can to create your list. Your list may include anything such as: acting, baking, communicating, coordinating, listening, embracing, praying, providing, motivating, etc. Remember, this is a beginning place. You may want to come back to this exercise several times as you develop your mission statement. As I developed my mission statement it took several months to land on the action words I finally chose, and none of those words were on the original list I was working with. This exercises helped me specifically think about those things I wanted to focus on and am uniquely called to do.

2. What are the key core values and characteristics you determined back in chapter 21? _____

   _____

3. What cause or group of people are you most passionate

about working with/for, as discerned in the chapter 22?

_____

_____

Your challenge now is to take these elements and shape them into a one sentence statement. For example: My mission is to motivate and mobilize (action words) the boomer generation(with whom) for greater impact in the kingdom and their world. (passion that comes out of my core values: helping people live with God-given purpose)

As I crafted this statement I was truly surprised to discover how this fit into my whole life, and yet had been radically modified in my own midlife. A life-long mission in my life has been to help people live into their God given purpose, whether that is as a parent, youth group leader, pastor, friend, mentor, etc. In fact Al and I were affirmed in our parenting when one of our children said to us, "I realized that we grew up believing that we needed to help change the world. Most kids aren't parented that way."

Suddenly I discovered that in midlife I had a particular call and passion to enable those in midlife transitions, helping them to discover the power of living into God's purposes for their next season of life. Often people wrongly assume that if God is calling them to a mission it will mean they will have to do something totally different with their lives. My personal example reflects that sometimes it is primarily a more intentionally focused mission.

Perhaps you are afraid that God is going to call you to do something you have no desire to do. I really doubt the effectiveness of that kind of call, and firmly believe our God is much wiser than to use that tactic to accomplish his purposes. Instead, I love the story of Byron Easterling as he tells it in

Dream Big, Dream Often: A Journey Into Transformation. Byron discovered that God was calling him to the world of professional golf, which he had for many years assumed was too "worldly" a vocation in which to serve God, and so he has been a minister, motivator and worship leader in the church. Even Byron's mom had said, "Byron, you will do more for the Lord on the professional golf tour than you ever will in vocational ministry." Finally, as he was approaching midlife Byron realized he needed to allow God to release the dreams and desires of his heart, just as he had been traveling around the world seeking to release destinies and dreams in the lives of others.

Perhaps you fear that God will call you to do something you do not feel capable of doing. Well, you are definitely on to something here! Graham Cooke puts it this way, "You carry a profound and unfathomable call on your life, placed there by God Himself. It is fresh and new and completely beyond your natural ability to accomplish – God has called you to do something you cannot possibly do…It's a gift God has given each one of His children. In fact, your inability to accomplish it is exactly why He has selected you to carry that call." We are not called to live small lives. God has chosen to abide in each one of us to accomplish His purposes. Ephesians 3:20 says, "Now to Him who is able to do immeasurably more than all we ask or imagine, according to His power that is at work within us, to Him be glory in the church and in Christ Jesus throughout all generations, forever and ever." It is a gift that we are called and empowered by His Spirit to accomplish things of kingdom significance.

Do not sell your mission short. Len, a retired participant traced the theme of fishing through his life, from the time his grandparents took him fishing as a child through his adulthood and into retirement, saying, "Now I take some of the neighborhood kids fishing if their dads don't have time, or aren't into fishing." By the time we got to the point of crafting our mission statement Len realized God has given him a ministry of fishing. He lit up as he discovered this was a calling. This past summer Len expanded his "ministry" by renting a pontoon and giving handicapped children the opportunity to get out onto the river and experience fishing for the first time. Len realized God had taken something he loves to do and given it kingdom significance as he brings joy, builds relationships and as he spreads the love of God through fishing.

When I think of God creating the world I see a playful aspect as He created the giraffe and the octopus, the snail and the elephant. Try playing with your mission statement. Be creative. Feel free to explore. Don't get bogged down in the "right answers," or the "right way to do it." Allow the Spirit to flow through your thoughts and words.

1. Did any of your action words surprise you?
2. When you shared them with someone else were they affirmed?
3. How do you want to make a difference?
4. Who will be impacted?

24

Crafting a Vision Statement

I will pour out my Spirit on all people. Your sons and daughters will prophesy, your old men will dream dreams, your young men will see visions. Even on my servants, both men and women I will pour out my Spirit. Joel 2:28-29

"Welcome, Prince," said Aslan. "Do you feel yourself sufficient to take up the Kingship of Narnia?" " I—I don't think I do, Sir," said Caspian. "I'm only a kid. "Good," said Aslan. "If you felt yourself sufficient, it would have been proof that you were not." C.S. Lewis in Prince Caspian

Once we have developed the mission statement we need to take the next step of fleshing it out in a vision statement. For years I could not tell the difference between a mission and vision statement. When I read Laurie Beth Jones book and it became so clear. The vision statement tells you how your mission will look in a very literal sense. Where will it happen? What will you be wearing? With whom will you be doing it? And what do you want your end result to look like? Even if it may feel presumptuous to spell this out, go ahead and do it. Don't know how it will be accomplished? Don't worry about that for now.

According to Jones, "Not to have your own vision is to live somebody else's." It may be your parent's, spouse's, your children's, the culture's, or your friends', but you are living someone's vision of who you should be. The challenge is to listen to your own life, and the Spirit of God at work in you to discern your true mission and create your own vision. Hopefully that is what you have been doing throughout this book.

I encourage you to live into this verse from Scripture: "For God did not give us a spirit of timidity, but a spirit of power, of love and self-discipline." II Timothy 1:7.

Your vision statement will be longer than your mission statement, yet it needs to remain specific in order to provide a path to follow as you live into your mission. Following are some questions which will help flesh out the picture:

1. Where will it happen?
2. Who will be involved?
3. What will you be wearing?
4. How will it impact your calendar?
5. What will you be doing?
6. What do you love about this picture?
7. What do you fear?
8. On a scale of 1-10 how well does this "FIT" you?
9. What will be your first step in making this picture happen?

Until you can begin to see the answers to some of these questions your mission statement will be a nice theoretical piece of work, but nothing into which you can sink your teeth, let alone your heart and soul. For example: My mission in life is to be a person of compassion and kindness. That's a great goal, but what does it mean? What will that look like? How will you know when you are living into that mission? You need a vision.

Another way to think intentionally about living your mission is to consider how it will impact each of these areas of your life: Family and relationships, professional, health and wellness, emotional, spiritual, financial, personal development. Be honest. There will be challenges if we make significant changes. When I began this journey with Midlife Momentum I recognized that it would mean financial challenges for several years. And it has. Yet God has been faithful as we live into this mission, and we have grown as we step out in faith. The impact will include amazing blessings, but it won't always be easy. God doesn't promise easy, but he does promise a reward for our faithfulness. One night when I was so frustrated and feeling like a failure God spoke to me through these words of Isaiah:

But I said, "I have labored to no purpose; I have spent my strength in vain and for nothing. Yet what is due me is in the Lord's hand, and my reward is with my God." Isaiah 49:4

I didn't remember ever having read those words before, but that night they were exactly what I needed to hear. When I read these verses I knew again that God was the one who had called me to this mission, and I needed to trust God to work all things according to his plan. I just need to be faithful, growing and learning, seeking guidance and partners who can help me on my journey.

There is a danger throughout this process and this book that people will believe that to be a person of worth, living into God's purposes we have to do more...always. That is not the point at all. For some of us, yes, we need to get a vision for how we can live significantly by giving, investing time, energy and resources into our communities, congregations, relationships, etc. For others there is a great need to simply, intentionally, focus our lives, and it may involve "being" more and "doing" less.

1. What does it mean to BE a person of compassion? Where would God have you focus that compassion? What would that look like?
2. What does it mean to BE light in the world? Where would God have you focus your light?
3. What does it mean to BE an encourager? Who particularly tugs at your heart strings, needing encouragement?
4. What does it mean to BE in relationship with the God of the universe, the One who created you

Your vision statement forces you to think specifically so you can live intentionally, or you could say, **LIVE WITH PURPOSE ON PURPOSE in every season of our lives!**

25

Entrepreneurial Congregations

We're all entrepreneurial when we're seeing, sizing up and seizing opportunities for God. The person who pursues this life launches initiatives that respond to real needs, takes advantage of opportunities that fit the vision God gives, creates services that meet real needs, and most important, affect lives that are destined for eternity. Entrepreneurial faith, by Walt Kallestad and Kirbyjon Caldwell

Walt Kallestad and Kirbyjon Caldwell have written a book, *Entrepreneurial Faith: Launching Bold Initiatives to Expand God's Kingdom* that has transformed the way I look at the giftedness of the church, and how it connects to our communities. After reading it I could look back on the various churches we have been a part of and see several significant ways these congregations should/could have been impacting their local world, beyond what they were doing.

I have been a part of many spiritual gifts analysis, read many book on the subject, but this book gave me a new perspective on how our gifts can function in the Body and beyond.

I would encourage you to get your hands on this book. Currently it is out of print, so you may need to order it online.

It is well worth the read. In many of the same ways in which we have been looking at our individual lives it helps communities of faith look at who they have been created to be, what the passions of their people are, and how they relate to the needs evident in the world outside their doors.

I believe people who are hungry for more of God are also hungry to be a part of a fellowship with a greater purpose than maintaining a ministry. Way too often we try to convince our people to get involved in something in the church that has no relevance to who they are, or the life in which they are engaged.

A couple more quotes from this book to whet your appetite:

> Churches that refuse to become entrepreneurial by reaching beyond their sanctuary walls with the gospel will simply fade away.
>
> Entrepreneurial faith is all about confronting challenges and obstacles and believing God is bigger than anything that tries to oppose His work.
>
> We have the mind of Christ, (I Corinthians 2:16) and His mind is never contained in a box.

1. What happens when the members of your congregation believe God is calling them into mission?
2. What are the careers present in your church? What gifts are inherent in those careers?
3. How could those gifts impact the community and kingdom?

SECTION 5
Leaders Guide for Midlife or Renewing Momentum events:
Retreats
Seminars
Small groups

Midlife Momentum is all about:
Moving from Fear to Courage
Focusing on Gains Rather than Losses
Acknowledging the Pain, but Embracing the Pleasures
Refusing to Become Less and Choosing To Become More
Wrestling with Doubts While Growing in Faith

LEADERS GUIDE FOR MIDLIFE MOMENTUM EXERCISES

Throughout these exercises you are given suggested time allotments. Adjust according to the level of participation, and the time constraints of your event.

Instructions to process include recording answers and discussion, recognizing recurring themes, connecting participant's stories to the stories of God, and encouraging them to think deeper.

Throughout the experience the flow is from total group into personal work, sharing in triads, and then processing again in total group. This provides learning environments for different personalities and learning styles. It also builds community and natural support groups as the process progresses. When I have groups of both genders I normally have women share with women and men with men at least for the first several exercises.

If you have the gift of time and place incorporate activities such as taking walks, flying kites, canoeing down a stream, bird watching. These will add time and space for contemplation and listening to the Spirit and our lives.

Session 1: Introductory exercise

See Chapter 17—Becoming

This simple exercise provides a way to introduce participants to one another, while also communicating some helpful information about personalities, preferences, etc. It also leads into a deeper theological discussion about who we are becoming by the grace of God, and how we can impact that process with our decisions

1. Ask participants, "What color do you most like to wear?" Or "What color are you most often wearing if you get a compliment?" After each person has answered ask them if they remember hearing the phrase, "That color is so becoming on you" or "That hairstyle is very becoming on you" ?

Initially I thought this question would be limited to women, but as I did couples retreats I found that men had strong opinions about what they wear as well. What "becomes us" tells us what fits us well. There are colors or styles that bring out the best in us. They help us to be more fully who we are.

2. Ask participants, "What style of clothes do you most enjoy wearing?"

Answers will range from favorite old T's and sweats to crisp, clean tailored dress clothes and beyond. Early on it sets the tone for diversity and uniqueness.

Lead into a discussion: when we intentionally look at what "becomes us" we are able to make decisions based on this criterion, in areas far beyond clothing. We are called to be the representatives of Christ, continually growing into his image. We are called to become!

Midlife Questionnaire

See Chapters 4-9
Please answer the following questions

A. **What things make you realize you are in the stage of life in which you find yourself today?** This question has dozens of answers. When processed with others in the group there is much laughter, exploration, and recognition that in midlife there are many factors which determine the health, happiness and stress of this season of life.

B. **What are the best things about your present age?** Name at least 8 positive things. Again if you process this alone it is easy to focus on negative things, but when done in a group we realize there are more and more positive aspects to this stage.

C. **Okay, what are some difficult things about your current age?** Name about 6-8.

D. **When do you feel most fully alive? What do you love to do?**

E. **What unique opportunities does your present stage of life offer you?** Again, name 6-8 opportunities that you have now, which you didn't have about 10, 20 years ago.

This exercise is important in helping participants realize that we have freedom to decide how we will approach midlife and retirement. Are we:

Moving with courage and rejecting fear.
Focusing on gains rather than losses.
Embracing pleasures while acknowledging pain.
Growing in faith while wrestling with doubts.
Becoming more and refusing to be less.

As people enter a Midlife Momentum event they often see the negative aspects of getting older. By the time we finish this simple exercise they recognize so many of the positives.

Session 2: River of Life

See Chapter 18—Tracing Grace

To begin this exercise, ask participants to engage their imaginations, close their eyes, relax their bodies and breathe deeply.

Say: Imagine that you are walking through a forest. What kind of day is it? Are you following a path? Etc. You come to a stream and find Jesus (Your Creator, God, or another name you choose to use for God) waiting there, with a canoe. He invites you to get into the front of the canoe, while he takes his place behind you. He tells you that this is your river of life, and he wants to show to you. You push off from shore and Jesus guides you down the river.

As you go he calls your attention to different things in the river. Look for boulders.....rapids.....low hanging branches. Where are the whirlpools.... the deep quiet places...places where the river flows swiftly.....dams....sandbars....places you need to portage, etc? Do other streams feed into your stream? Are there places where water is siphoned off your river to feed into other streams, to irrigate?

What kind of countryside do you pass through: woods, meadows, canyons? Do you see any life in or around your river? What does the Jesus say to you about your river?

(As you are leading this meditation images will come to you, feel free to incorporate them into the river, as long as you are not manipulating the images, trying to get people to see a particular thing with which you feel they need to deal.)

You come to a sandbar. Up ahead the river disappears around a bend. Jesus brings the canoe up on the sandbar and reaches out to help you out, onto the sand bar. He gives you a hug, and as he hugs you, you realize that he melts right into you.

Whenever you are ready you may open your eyes and return to the room.

Now take time to capture the river on paper.

1. Allow the participants 15-20 minutes (or until you sense that most of the participants have finished) to make a representation of the river on paper. Some may be more comfortable writing a story or poem about the river.

2. Ask the participants to gather in groups of 3 to share as much of their river as they are comfortable sharing. The processing of this river is important in building community for the rest of the experience. Depending on your schedule you might give them this schedule:
   A. The first person shares their river (5 minutes). During this time the others in the triad listen in silence. There will be time for questions and

comments later.

B. The facilitator rings a bell 1 minute before time is up.

C. The facilitator rings the bell after the last minute.

D. The triad observes one minute of silence, during which they may jot a few notes, or questions they want to come back to, or places where they felt identification with the storyteller's experience. (Ring bell again)

E. The one who has shared stays sitting while the other 2 gather around her/him, lay hands on her/him and silently prays. (For some reason having the other 2 stand over them seems to be significant.)

F. Repeat the process for each one in the triad.

G. After everyone has had their opportunity to share allow time for conversation about where they found identifying themes, and time for asking clarifying questions, etc.

3. Now call the triads back into total group to process what they have learned through this exercise.

The flow of silence and prayer honors each one's story and acknowledges the presence of God on our journey. Setting the time limits assures that each person will have the time and attention they deserve. No one will be able to dominate the conversation, or one-up the other's story, etc.

(You will need to provide paper and crayons or colored pencils, and a bell.)

This exercise was adapted from the River of Life Exercise in Richard L. Morgan's book, *Remembering Your Story: Creating Your Own Spiritual Autobiography*. He provides many additional insights and exercises for making meaning of the life we have lived.

Session 3: Timeline of the Positive

See Chapter 18—Tracing Grace

Make a timeline representing your life beginning with your birth, and indicating that it goes beyond the present. For instance, if you are relatively healthy at 65 you can statistically expect to live until you are 85. Divide the time line into 5-year segments 0-5, 5-10, etc.

For each segment note at least one positive memory, something you loved to do, a success, an accomplishment, etc. This timeline only deals with positive things. It may reflect overcoming something hard, such as, "Survived a job loss and found something I liked better."

Part of the purpose in this is to recognize who you have been at various stages of life, and to rediscover parts of yourself that you have put on a shelf. For example: you may have loved to ride horse when you were young, but have not had the opportunity to ride since high school.

Introduce this exercise by asking, "What did you love to do when you were 11?"

At about this age we begin to shelve aspects of ourselves because they don't "fit in" with life. As we grow and get involved in more and more things the shelf often gets crowded. In midlife we have the opportunity to explore what is on the shelf, see what we would like to take back off the shelf, dust it off and reclaim it.

1. Allow about 15-20 minutes for participants to work on their timeline.
2. Participants again gather in triads to share their

story. Even though they have just worked on the positive aspects it is still important to make sure they focus on these accomplishments and positive memories. For some reason it is easier to share negative or difficult aspects of life, rather than talking about the successes.

3. For this experience give them each 5 minutes to share, ringing the bell with a 1 minute warning, but then have them move on to the next person. (During the river exercise they often share painful, difficult times and the silence and prayer seem to be more important before transitioning to the next story.)

4. After each has had time to share their timeline allow for 10 minutes of discussion.

5. Pull the group back together to process what they have learned.

6. At the end of the processing time have participants; look back at their timeline, consider what the group has processed and write one sentence that begins, "I have discovered that I......"

This exercise usually creates joy and surprise as people focus on the positive memories, and reclaim who they were at different ages.

Session 4: Biblical Mentors

See Chapter 20—Mentors Who Have Come Before Us

Distribute the accompanying sheet with biblical characters, texts and wonderings.

During this exercise we will invite a person from Scripture

to be our mentor. If this person were sitting at the table with us today, what would he or she want to say to us?

One of the most powerful aspects of this exercise is to have participants recognize how their story connects with the great stories of God, and also with the less known stories of Scripture. We are the people of God.

How you divide the participants into groups will depend on the biblical background they have. If you are working with people familiar with Scripture you may want them to work independently. If many of the people are unfamiliar with the stories of Scripture you may ask them to partner up, or get into groups of three. You will also want to point out which of the suggested people and Scriptures will be self-explanatory, and can be studied in a short amount of time. If few of the participants are biblically literate you can pre-select one or two people, tell their story to the total group, and then have them proceed to their triads.

Ask participants to choose a person from the list provided, or if they prefer, they can elect to study a person not on the list. Read the passages that apply to their person, or in the case of longer stories review the story; for example Jonah or Esther.

After reading or reviewing the story consider the wondering questions at the bottom of the page. Answer whichever wonderings most apply to your chosen person. However, do not be limited by these wonderings as they are merely a beginning place. There may be many more things you wonder about in this story. Since some of the wonderings are more related to one person's experience than another do not be worried about using all of the wonderings provided. **THE GOAL IS TO ENGAGE WITH THIS PERSON FROM SCRIPTURE, and allow the Holy Spirit to speak to your life through their experiences.** Remember, we want to imagine what this person would want to say to us, teach us, etc. if they were at the table with us right now.

1. Ask participants to choose their mentor for the day.
2. Allow time for individuals or partners to read/review the stories and work with some of the wonderings. (20 minutes)
3. Come back to total group to introduce your mentor, share what you believe they would want to say today. (More than one person or group may have chosen the same mentor.)
4. Open the conversation up to invite others to share insights from this mentor.
5. Move on to the next mentor

(For more information on the power and process of wondering read Jerome Berryman, *Godly Play: A Way of Religious Education*)

Session 5: Scriptural Identity

See Chapter 10-12

Exercise 1

If you send out information in advance of the MM/RM event you may want to include some readings, and exercises for them to do in preparation. This exercise works well. Ask participants to choose a scripture and a song that have been formative in their faith journey.

The sharing of their choices works well as devotional times during the event.

As the group gathers for each session, or for morning or

evening devotions, have someone share their scripture passage, and have the group sing the first verse of the song if it is well known to several of the participants. Allow people to share briefly why these have been important for them. If the group is over 8 people have them share this in groups of 4-5 people, depending on your time constraints.

Exercise 2: Who is our God?

See Chapter 10—God is Good, But is He Safe?

1. Ask each participant to read the texts on the accompanying sheet and note the characteristics, passions, or core values of God in each passage. (15 Minutes, or give this as part of the homework assignment.)

2. In total group process by asking: What is God passionate about? What do we learn about God in this passage?

Exercise 3: Who are we called to be as the People of God?

3. Repeat the process above with the texts chosen to help us understand who we are called to be as the people of God. In the processing ask, "How does God see us, his people?"

Session 6: Core Values

See Chapter 21—Exploring Our Core Values

This is the most difficult concept to articulate and help participants process, but it is critically important if we want to live intentional lives. Recognizing the values in our "default mode" often surprises us, leading to an awareness of areas we need to address. Below you will find several options for getting at our core values. Feel free to choose whichever you think would be the most helpful for your group.

Definitions

CORE Values: those values that drive our lives. They are embedded in all aspects of our lives in such a way that they impact decisions, actions, relationships, and time and money management.

ACTUAL Values: those values which we live out on a consistent basis. These values are evidenced when we need to resort to our default mode.

PREFERRED Values: those values we desire to grow into living out more faithfully. We want them to be core values, but we are not there yet.

DITCH'EM Values: those values with which we may have grown up, assimilated from our culture, families, friends, etc. without ever evaluating whether they are good or bad, and now we realize we do not hold them (or want them to hold us) and need to leave them behind.

Exercise 1: Proverbs

This is another exercise that can be given out before hand to save time.

On newsprint or whiteboard have the group brainstorm as many proverbs as they can come up with in 10 minutes. EX: A bird in the hand is worth two in the bush. Waste not, want not. The early bird catches the worm.

After the list is complied look at what values are reflected in each proverb and determine if this is truly a value you want to embrace, or if it needs to be "ditched."

Ask this question: Which proverbs did you most hear as a child? How was it lived out in your family/culture?

SECTION 5

This exercise helps us recognize the values that have a hold on us without our knowledge, and gives us the opportunity to decide if we want to hang on to it, or not.

Exercise 2: Cultural vs. God's Values

Based in part on previous work, generate two lists of values, one list reflecting the values of the culture, and a list reflecting values God holds. This can be done in total group if the group is under 20, or divide into groups of 6-8.

Cultural Values (Ex. are American)	God's Values
Individualism	Community
Protect our way of life	Justice for all
Independence	Caring for each other

Exercise 3: Core Values Worksheet

On this sheet life is divided into 7 categories. This breakdown was found helpful in enabling participants to name several key values for their lives, particularly for those unfamiliar with this kind of exercise.

While certain values are easier to identify when applied to a particular aspect of life, you will see that if they are core values they will impact other areas as well. For instance: Integrity in your professional life will mean that your employer/employees, business partners and colleagues, parishioners and community will know that you are trustworthy, that your word is good, that what you say and do line up. And in your family, the same will be true if this is a core value.

1. Allow participants 15 minutes to work on their Values Worksheet. It is not necessary to fill in every slot. Encourage them to have one value for each category.

2. Have participants share their values in triads.
3. Process as total group asking if they discovered any-thing new about themselves. Were there values they found were common to all in the group? Are there val-ues you realized you will need to ditch, if in fact you have preferred values you want to move into the realm of actual values?

Exercise 4: On My Tombstone

On some tombstones there is a word or phrase that de-scribes the person lying beneath it. What one word or phrase do you most wish people would choose to describe you?

Exercise 5: Key Characteristics

We all have people we admire; people who model a lifestyle that we recognize is worthy of respect and honor. What do they teach us about how to live well?

1. Distribute Key Characteristics worksheet: Allow 15 minutes for them to work individually.
2. In triads have them share who was on their list and why, and the three characteristics they would most like to have chosen to described themselves.
3. Call them back to total group and have them generate a list of all of their top three characteristics. See how they reflect back on God's characteristics, and God's desires for who we are called to be.

Choose as many or as few values exercises as is helpful and practical in your situation.

SECTION 5

Session 7: Defining Your Passion

See Chapter 22—Discerning Your Passions

This simple exercise is an effective tool for awakening people to the passions that God has built into them. It generally takes the conversation to a much deeper level.

1. Participants work on the passion sheet for 15 minutes.
2. If the group is smaller than 10 process in total group, inviting them to share their answers to each of the questions. It is helpful for them to hear the passions, joys and fears of others, as well as discover others with whom they can partner and build a support system. When working with large numbers have them share in groups of 6-8.

This is a critical exercise. One of the results is that for some, their world view is opened up as they hear the passions of others and recognize their world is too small.

Session 8: Creating Your Mission Statement for the Next Season of Life

See Chapter 23—Crafting a Mission Statement

By this point participants have spent time in life reflection, discovering streams of themes that have run through their lives, recognizing aspects of themselves which they have shelved, but value, reclaimed and reframed because they are a part of who they have been created to be. They have named and evaluated their core values and discovered things about which they are passionate. All of this has been done on a foundation of who God is, who God has created and called them to be, and the power of the Spirit at work within them. Based on this work they are prepared to begin the process of developing a mission and vision statement for the next season of life.

While this work has been started, it is critical to remember this is an ongoing process. Creating mission and vision statements for the next season of life is exciting work that can be started in this retreat or small group setting, but needs continuing support and refinement to truly implement them into our lives.

Laurie Beth Jones in her book, *The Path: Creating Your Mission Statement For Work And For Life*, has designed a process for developing mission and vision statements for individuals and corporations. The following exercise has been adapted from her work. For continued exploration and more exercises I recommend you obtain and work through this book.

Step 1: Summary sheet

Distribute the Summary Mission Statement Worksheet. Review the first 4 sections as a total group, having participants fill in their responses as you go. For section 5 they will work independently to arrive at their 3 key action words. Allow about 15 minutes for section 5.

Step 2: Putting it all together

Instruct participants to take the responses from the summary worksheet and transfer them to the Preliminary Mission Statement worksheet. At this point they will try to draw them together into a one sentence mission statement. Remind them that this is not a finished product. Feel free to change words, refine, and play with different options until you find what you believe "fits well" and excites you.

Ask: On a scale of 1-10 how likely are you to live into this mission? If the response is below 8 what needs to change?

This provides a beginning place. It may take days, weeks, or months to finalize your mission statement.

After about 20 minutes, or when you sense people need to move on, ask them to share their statement in a triad.

Allow time for others to provide input and encouragement. Some will not have arrived at a sentence with which they feel comfortable. This is fine. It is presumptuous to think that we will be able to do all of this work in a retreat weekend, or even a two month small group, but it can provide a very good beginning.

The goal is to launch an intentional life, and to raise awareness that God has indeed created us for a purpose, providing us with a personality, gifts, passions and a calling. At this point you might suggest participants form accountability groups to continue their work beyond the event.

Session 9: Creating a Vision Statement

See Chapter 24—Crafting a Vision Statement

Once again, it was Laurie Beth Jones who really helped me understand the difference between a mission statement and a vision statement. Creating this vision statement provides the energy and concreteness needed to take action on making the mission statement a reality.

1. Using the vision statement worksheet have participants answer the questions individually. Allow 15 minutes, or until you sense people are ready to move on.
2. Participants share their responses in triads. Again,

use the bell timing method to make sure each one has time to share their vision. If desired allow for the one minute of prayer for each person before moving on to the next person in the group.

3. Process in total group focusing on, "What do you love about this picture? What do you fear? What is your first action step"?

It is important to have them verbalize this vision in order to give it substance, to have it affirmed, and to allow others to ask clarifying questions. Once we have verbalized our dreams they take on power and significance for living.

SECTION 6
Exercises for a Midlife or Renewing Momentum Event

The first decision we need to make is to do the work we need to do, in order to live the life we want to live. If you are willing to commit the time and emotional energy, God will honor your commitment with His guidance. God wants you to succeed in living into all He has created you to be!

Season of Life Questionnaire

Please answer the following questions.

1. What things make you realize you are in midlife?

2. What are the best things about your present age?

3. What are the most difficult things about your present age?

4. What unique opportunities does this stage of life offer you?

5. When do you feel most fully alive?

River of Life Reflections

After you have done the guided meditation and captured your river on paper the following questions may help you think more deeply about your river.

SECTION 6

1. Where did you find the boulders/waterfalls/dams/ rapids in your river?

2. Where were you living? Who were the people involved?

3. What made the current run faster or slower? Where were the deepest places?

4. How did you feel floating down the river with Jesus/ God?

5. What did he say to you about your river?

6. Were there any parts of the river you wished you could do over again?

7. What were some of you greatest learnings on this river of life?

8. What is one thing you would like to tell your family about the river?

9. What do you hope is around the next bend?

10. What would you like to say to Jesus/God about your river?

Wondering with Women in the Scriptures

Choose a woman from Scripture and imagine she is here to mentor you today. You may use one of the women below, or another of your choice. Use the wondering questions to begin to listen to what she would speak to you. Not all of the wonderings are equally applicable to each woman.

Sarah: Genesis 11:29-31, 12:5-17, 16:1-8, 17:15-21, 18:6-15, 20:1-18, 21:1-12

Rebekah: Genesis 24:15ff, 25:20-28, 26:1-8, 34-35, 27:1-46

Miriam: Ex. 2:1-10, 15:20-21, Num. 12:1-15, 20:1, 26:59, Deut. 24:9

Rahab: Joshua 2, 6:15-25, Heb. 11:31, James 2:25

Deborah: Judges 4 and 5

Ruth: The Book of Ruth

Esther: The Book of Esther

The Shunamite Woman: II Kings 4:8-37, 8:1-6

The Widow of Zarephath: I Kings 17:8-24, Luke 4:25-26

Elizabeth: Luke 1

Mary or Martha: Luke 10:38-42, John 11, 12:1-3, Mark 14:3-9

The Woman with the fever: Matt 8:14-15, Mark 1:30-31, Luke 4: 38-39

The Woman with the issue of blood: Matt 9:20-22, Mark 5:25-34, Luke 8:43-48

The Woman of Samaria: John 4:7-42

Mary Magdalene: Matt 27:55-28:10, Mark 15:40-16:11, Luke 8:2, 24:1-12, John 19:25, 20:1-18

Lydia: Acts 16:11-15, 38-40

I wonder what (Miriam) would tell me if she spoke to me today.

I wonder what prepared (Miriam) for her role in the people of
God.

I wonder what lessons she needed to learn on the journey.

I wonder what dangers she faced, and what warnings she might
give me.

I wonder what challenges she would encourage me to
embrace.

I wonder what you would like to ask her in order to learn from
her.

Mentored by Men of Scriptures

Choose a man from Scripture and imagine he is here to
mentor you today. You may use one of the men below, or another of your choice. Use the wondering questions to begin to
listen to what he would speak to you. Not all of the wonderings
are equally applicable to each man.

Joseph: Genesis 39-45
Joshua: Numbers 13-14 and Joshua 1+
Mordecai: The Book of Esther
Nicodemus: John 3, 7:50 and 19:39
Man born blind: John 9
Peter: Acts 9-11
Thomas: John 20:19-29
Stephen: Acts 6 and 7
Philip: Acts 8
John Mark: Acts 15:36-41, Col.4:10, I Peter 5:10, II Timothy
4:11

I wonder what (Joseph) would tell me if he spoke to me
today.

I wonder what prepared him for his role in the people of God.
I wonder what lessons he learned on the journey.
I wonder what dangers he faced and what warnings he might give me.
I wonder what challenges he would encourage me to embrace.
I wonder what you would like to ask him in order to learn from him.

Foundational Scriptures

Read the passages below. What insights do they give us about God's passions? What are God's purposes?

1. John 3:16
2. Genesis 12:1-3
3. Deuteronomy 6:4-9
4. Isaiah 58:6-12
5. Micah 6:6-8
6. Matthew 22:34-40
7. Matthew 28: 18-20
8. Luke 9:46-48
9. John 13:31-35
10. John 15:1-11
11. John 17:20-23
12. Acts 8:26-40
13. Romans 12:1-8
14. II Corinthians 5:16-20
15. Romans 12:1-8
16. Ephesians 2:8-10
17. Philippians 3:8-14
18. Colossians 3:2-17
19. I Peter 2:1-10

SECTION 6

20. Revelation 7:9-10

Now reflect on what these passages tell us regarding the purpose for the life of a follower of God.

Core Values

Core Values are the key, defining values in our life. They show up in all areas of our lives.

In each of the areas below identify two key values that are either actual values, (you live them out most of the time) or preferred values (you desire they be in your life and you are working toward them).

FAMILY
1.
2.
PROFESSIONAL
1.
2
HEALTH AND WELLNESS
1.
2.
RELATIONSHIPS
1.
2.
SPIRITUAL
1.
2.
FINANCIAL
1.
2.

Key Characteristics

We all have people we admire; people who model a lifestyle that we recognize is worthy of respect and honor. What do they teach us about how to live well?

1. Name three people you most admire. They can be people you know personally, from our culture, or they can be historical characters.

    _____   _____

    _____

2. Name 6 characteristics you would use to describe each of them. The same characteristic may apply to more than one of them.

    _____   _____

    _____   _____

    _____   _____

    _____   _____

    _____   _____

    _____   _____

    _____   _____

    _____   _____

3. Of those characteristics, which three do you most hope people would use to describe you?

    _____   _____

    _____

SECTION 6

Summary Work for Mission Statement

The goal of this sheet is to help pull together things you have learned about your true self in previous sessions, preparing for your work on a mission statement.

1. What word/phrase would you most like on your gravestone?

   _____

2. You chose 3 people you admire greatly. They are:

   _____   _____

   _____

3. You named 6 characteristics they have and chose three you most wanted to describe you. You may not have completely arrived here, but they are characteristics that you are pressing toward. Those characteristics or values are:

   _____   _____

   _____

4. What cause or people group are you most passionate about? Reflect on your passion sheet. Some suggestions to prompt your thinking are: _____
   Children, youth, college age, adults, midlife, elderly, the sick, poor, hungry, financially struggling, young entrepreneurs, addicted, depressed, justice in our community, Africa, Europe, disease, the arts, recreation, parenting, education, modern slavery, human rights, etc.

5. What gifts do you have? What do you most enjoy doing? Determine 15 action words with which you identify; things you love to do, are good at, use your gifts...

   _____

   _____

_____
_____
_____

What are the three words with which you most identify?

_____   _____

_____

Creating a Preliminary Mission Statement

This process, adapted from *The Path*, by Laurie Beth Jones, for developing a mission and vision statement involves the following steps:

Transfer your work from the Summary Worksheet.
Three action words chosen: _____,
_____, _____
Your passion impacted by your values:
_____
The cause or people group with whom you want to work:
_____

Shuffle these three elements around. Experiment with other words, etc. to come up with a preliminary mission statement.

Share it with you triad. Allow input, rephrasing, open questions, and fleshing out what this means. Have fun exploring it. Nothing is finalized.

Write down a statement describing where you are in the process.

Vision Statement

Imagine what living out your mission statement will look like in 6 months...1 year...5 years...

1. What will you be doing?

2. Where will it happen?
3. What will you be wearing?
4. Who will be involved?
5. How will it impact your calendar?
6. What do you love about this picture?
7. On a Scale of 1-10 how well does this fit you?
8. What do you fear about this picture?
9. What is your first step?
10. On a scale of 1-10 how likely are you to take this first step? If it is less than an eight what needs to change to make it happen?

Recommended Reading

For all those seeking to continue the journey I recommend the following:

Caldwell, Kirbyjon and Kallestad, Walt. *Entrepreneurial Faith: Launching Bold Initiatives To Expand God's Kingdom.* Colorado Springs: Waterbrook Press, 2004.

Jones, Laurie Beth. *The Path: Creating Your Mission Statement For Work and For Life.* New York: Hyperion, 1996. All books by Laurie Beth Jones I highly recommend.

Kidd, Sue Monk. *When the Heart Waits: Spiritual Direction for Life's Sacred Questions.* San Francisco: Harper, 1990. *The Mermaid's Chair* is a novel about midlife and also a great read.

Lawrence-Lightfoot, Sara. *The Third Chapter: Passion, Risk and Adventure in the 25 Years After 50.* New York: Sarah Crichton Books, 2009.

Morgan, Richard. *Remembering Your Story: Creating Your Own Spiritual Autobiography.* Nashville, TN: Upper Room, 2002.

Palmer, Parker. *Let Your Life Speak: Listening for the Voice of Vocation.* San Francisco: Jossey Bass, 2000. I recommend that every person on a journey to discover who God has truly created them to be, as well as who they have not been created to be, read this book.

Rupp, Joyce. *Dear Heart, Come Home: The Path of Midlife*

Spirituality. New York: The Crossroads Publishing Co., 1997.

Scott, Susan. *Fierce Conversations: Achieving Success at Work and in Life*, One Conversation at a Time. New York: Berkley Publishing Group, 2004.

C.S. Lewis's The Chronicles of Narnia, and The Hobbit and *Trilogy of the Ring* by J.R.R.Tolkien are wonderful reads when seeking to live with faith and courage. ENJOY!

CPSIA information can be obtained at www.ICGtesting.com
Printed in the USA
BVOW071420091212

307639BV00001B/3/P

Interaction, Feedback and Task Research in Second Language Learning

The role of interaction and corrective feedback is central to research in second language learning and teaching, and this volume is the first of its kind to explain and apply design methodologies and materials in an approachable way. Using examples from interaction, feedback, and task studies, it presents clear and practical advice on how to carry out research in these areas, providing step-by-step guides to design and methodological principles, suggestions for reading, short activities, memory aids, and an A–Z glossary for easy reference. Its informative approach to study design, and in-depth discussions of implementing research methodology, make it accessible to novice and experienced researchers alike. Commonly used tools in these paradigms are explained, including stimulated recalls, surveys, eye-tracking, meta-analysis, and research synthesis. Open research areas and gaps in the literature are also discussed, providing a point of departure for researchers making their first foray into interaction, feedback, and task-based teaching research.

Alison Mackey is a leading international expert in input, interaction, and feedback in L2 learning, and in L2 research methodology. She has published sixteen books (one of which won the Modern Language Association's Mildenburger Prize) and more than a hundred articles in these areas. At Georgetown University, where she is Professor of Linguistics, she has received both The President's Award for Distinguished Scholar–Teachers and The Provost's Career Research Award.

Interaction, Feedback and Task Research in Second Language Learning

Methods and Design

Alison Mackey

Georgetown University, Washington, D.C.

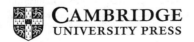
CAMBRIDGE
UNIVERSITY PRESS

CAMBRIDGE
UNIVERSITY PRESS

University Printing House, Cambridge CB2 8BS, United Kingdom

One Liberty Plaza, 20th Floor, New York, NY 10006, USA

477 Williamstown Road, Port Melbourne, VIC 3207, Australia

314–321, 3rd Floor, Plot 3, Splendor Forum, Jasola District Centre, New Delhi – 110025, India

79 Anson Road, #06–04/06, Singapore 079906

Cambridge University Press is part of the University of Cambridge.

It furthers the University's mission by disseminating knowledge in the pursuit of education, learning, and research at the highest international levels of excellence.

www.cambridge.org
Information on this title: www.cambridge.org/9781108499637
DOI: 10.1017/9781108589284

First published 2020

A catalogue record for this publication is available from the British Library.

Library of Congress Cataloging-in-Publication Data
Names: Mackey, Alison, author.
Title: Interaction, feedback and task research in second language learning : methods and
    design / Alison Mackey.
Description: 1. | New York : Cambridge University Press, 2020. | Includes bibliographical
    references and index.
Identifiers: LCCN 2020006665 (print) | LCCN 2020006666 (ebook) | ISBN 9781108499637
    (hardback) | ISBN 9781108731027 (paperback) | ISBN 9781108589284 (epub)
Subjects: LCSH: Second language acquisition–Study and teaching. | Language and
    languages–Study and teaching. | Feedback (Psychology)
Classification: LCC P118.2 .M228 2020 (print) | LCC P118.2 (ebook) | DDC 418.0071–dc23
LC record available at https://lccn.loc.gov/2020006665
LC ebook record available at https://lccn.loc.gov/2020006666

ISBN 978-1-108-49963-7 Hardback
ISBN 978-1-108-73102-7 Paperback

Cambridge University Press has no responsibility for the persistence or accuracy of URLs for external or third-party internet websites referred to in this publication and does not guarantee that any content on such websites is, or will remain, accurate or appropriate.

For my mother, Deanna Mackey. Her confidence in me is the reason I can write. And for my children, Miranda Mackey Yarowsky and William Mackey Yarowsky, whose daily interaction and feedback (along with that of their father) is a continual reminder of what's fun and important in life.

Contents

Figures

Tables

Preface

This book is designed to help those who are thinking about carrying out studies of interaction, feedback, or tasks and their role in second language learning, as well as those who want to appraise, critique, or better understand studies that they are reading in the literature in terms of the methods used. My goal in the book is to provide all the information that researchers might need to carry out a study, in a format that is as reader-friendly as possible. To aid with these goals, the book contains boxed inset "Read It!" studies to illustrate the main points, "Keep It in Mind!" bullets to summarize the gist, "Try It!" suggestions to provide opportunities for hands-on practice, and a glossary giving short definitions of all the key terms. Cartoons are included as amusing memory aids. I have also included some new findings from data that haven't been published before in two of the chapters to address topics that are currently of high interest in the area. Overall, my hope is that this book will support and inspire more research into the three closely related areas of interaction, feedback, and tasks, and how they combine to promote second language learning.

I begin in Chapter 1, with a short summary of some of the theoretical and empirical foundations for work in interaction, feedback, and tasks, including how these constructs are related, and then move on to what I hope will be of significant interest to many readers – a review and discussion of what I believe to be some timely open questions and interesting research problems in the field in these three closely related areas.

In Chapter 2, I talk about the wide range of different kinds of research designs and approaches available to further our understanding of how interaction, feedback, and tasks can drive learning.

Individual differences in interaction, feedback, and task research is the topic of Chapter 3, where I describe frequently used measures like working memory and aptitude scores, before moving on to a so far relatively under-studied area, cognitive creativity. This is a construct which is relatively new to the field of second language acquisition, and certainly, to interaction, feedback, and task research, and one that I believe has promise as we look for insights into the relationship between interaction, feedback, tasks, and L2 learning. For this reason, it is one of the chapters where I present new data and results from two previously unpublished studies of creativity, concluding with recommendations for how these cognitive-creativity measures might be used in future research.

In Chapter 4, I move in a different direction, discussing introspective methods, which are also widely used in L2 research in general, and are particularly helpful for understanding the cognitive and social processes that underlie interaction-driven learning.

I turn to survey-based research in Chapter 5, including interviews, and explaining the advantages of moving towards mixed-methods approaches in interaction, feedback, and task research. Again, I present some new findings from a survey designed to uncover information about learners' awareness of and preference for feedback and the relation of this to gender.

In Chapter 6, I talk about the importance of taking a step outwards and looking at the big picture. I describe synthetic and meta-analytic work and provide a hands-on guide for how to do it and why and when it's important to take stock in interaction, feedback, and task-based research by doing this sort of work, as well as pointing out some of the potential pitfalls.

While recognizing that instructional settings is an umbrella term that covers a huge range of different contexts and learners, from migrants to the commonly used population of college-aged adults, in Chapter 7, I cover this sort of research, finishing with a discussion particular to the research issues involving children as they interact in classrooms with tasks. There is not very much written about the logistics of carrying out research with school-aged children (and younger), and so in the second part of this chapter, I aim to raise awareness of these issues in relation to work on interaction, feedback, and tasks.

In Chapter 8, I move on to current new directions in interaction, task, and feedback research, beginning with the currently popular eye-tracking paradigm, then discussing new imaging techniques like ultrasound as articulatory mechanism feedback, and moving to the relationship between neurolinguistics and interaction, task, and feedback research, including EEGs, MEGs, and fMRIs, as well as some of the more commonly used psycholinguistic techniques used in interaction research, like priming.

In Chapter 9, I talk about coding and analysis issues particular to interaction, feedback, and task research, including information on both quantitative and qualitative/interpretivist analyses. I conclude this chapter by including information about the propensity of the field to target educated college-aged students in research, and the new moves towards targeting populations more diverse than the traditional Western, Educated, Industrialized, Rich, and Democratic (WEIRD) ones.

I conclude the book in Chapter 10, which covers pitfalls in interaction, feedback, and task research and work in related areas, by describing scenarios adapted from situations and events that have happened to me, to a few of my current and former students, and to my colleagues and friends over twenty years of carrying out research into interaction, feedback, and communicative tasks. Some of these scenarios are humorous in retrospect, and they are all derived from authentic events.

I could not have come close to finishing this book without two things. The first is my position at Georgetown University, where I have been privileged to work for more than two decades. One of Georgetown's many strengths is its adherence to the concept of *cura personalis*, or care for the whole person. In 2016, when I lost my beloved mother unexpectedly, I thought I would never be able to write another book. However, my students, colleagues, friends, and administrators at Georgetown gently helped me to remember, in multiple (implicit) ways, how lucky I am to have the academic life I do, enjoying so many freedoms and so much institutional support, together with teaching and mentoring challenges and rewards that made me want to stay current and committed. I am also fortunate to be able to spend time and summers working at Lancaster University in the U.K., where I have close friends and collaborators, and where the Department of Linguistics and English Language positively brims with research talent and opportunity.

The second is the invaluable help of my extremely talented former and current students working as research assistants. Lara Bryfonski, Ashleigh Pipes, Derek Reagan, Ayşenur Sağdıç, and Rachel Thorson Hernández have provided more assistance in multiple ways and over various time periods than I could have hoped for. They, along with Margaret Borowczyk, Erin Fell, and Yasser Teimouri, have approached the tasks I have asked them to do with a welcome combination of grit, wit, and humor as well as vision, attention to detail, and a work ethic second to none. I know that they will each produce excellent books after they do their dissertations, because they went above and beyond for me on this book, in ways that make me feel privileged to have worked with them. Although it was not by any means her only research assistant task, all the cartoons in this book were created by the multi-talented Rachel Thorson Hernández, who has a quirky sense of humor that's a good match for mine, in addition to her research skills.

Cambridge University Press enjoys, of course, a premier reputation in the field of publishing and I believe this is very deservedly so. I have worked for half a decade with the journal staff, all of whom have been careful, efficient, prompt, and talented people. This volume has been my first experience with the book branch of the press, and it has been an all-round excellent experience. Rebecca Taylor and Ishwarya Mathavan provided the perfect balance of reminders, forbearing, and support.

My family, particularly my two children, Miranda Mackey Yarowsky and William Mackey Yarowsky, put up with quite a lot of "the book" excuses for working at odd times. I have to imagine my mother, Deanna Mackey's, interaction and feedback these days, but I am getting better at doing that. I thank all of them and promise I am now free to download and watch the *Secret Life of Pets* movies whenever requested.

Any remaining mistakes in this book are, of course, entirely my own, although I do hear they say "to err is human but to really mess up, you need technology." You can read a tale about how technology can contribute to research fails in the final chapter.

CHAPTER ONE

Theory and Approaches in Research into Interaction, Corrective Feedback, and Tasks in L2 Learning

The focus of this book is explaining how to do research that examines the relationships amongst interaction, feedback, tasks, and second language learning. The book begins, in the current chapter, by talking about some of the theoretical underpinnings for this sort of research, before moving to practical considerations in the subsequent chapters, including how to design studies, the many ways of collecting, coding, and analyzing data, and what sort of issues and fixes for them can arise in research on how interaction, feedback, and task research may contribute to second language learning.

Although there are a number of different theoretical foundations for doing research in interaction, feedback, and task-based learning, this brief review begins with the paradigm that has been central to the majority of work in these areas, known as the cognitive–interactionist paradigm, or also as simply the interaction approach. This perspective posits that second language acquisition research in interaction and corrective feedback is concerned with how aspects of language can be learned through the various processes and products of interaction, including input, output, and feedback. These processes are commonly brought together through communicative tasks which are frequently used in second language research as well as in task-based instruction. The origins of this line of research into second language interaction and corrective feedback are usually traced back to Long's (1981) original interaction hypothesis, which has evolved over time to reflect a more expanded concept of interaction (see Long, 1996, 2015; Mackey, 2012a). The interaction hypothesis now encompasses how interactional processes create learning opportunities for language learners including the mechanism by which corrective feedback can be utilized to promote modification of learners' linguistic output and L2 learning. More recently, the interaction hypothesis has become known as an approach and has evolved and expanded such that in addition to the originally primarily cognitive and information-processing focus, "social factors are now regularly considered and researched as a part of the agenda" (King & Mackey, 2016, p. 211). Despite these different iterations of the definitions and scope of the interaction approach over time, the area of primary research interest remains the same – L2 learners' acquisition of language through interaction, which includes corrective feedback as well as modified input and output, and which is often realized through communicative tasks whether for research or practice.

From its roots in the 1970s, second language interaction and corrective feedback research has increased exponentially. Almost a decade ago, there were reports that the number of publications in this field had tripled since the 1980s (Plonsky & Gass, 2011), and over the last ten years this has increased even more, such that an increasing number of papers, books, and conference strands have now led to book series, special issues of journals, and even a dedicated professional organization and conference (The International Association for Task-Based Language Teaching, and its biannual conference, as just one example).

While studies in the 1980s primarily focused on whether there was a positive relationship between second language interaction and production gains, the empirical focus moved towards an emphasis on the direct assessment of learning outcomes in the mid 1990s. In the 1980s the mainstream research practice was cross-sectional investigation, with the field expanding in the 1990s to include a body of pre-test/post-test studies that directly addressed the interaction–learning relationship. Further growth of interaction–acquisition research was characterized by a move towards mainstream theoretical status (Gass, 1997; Gass & Mackey, 2006; Long, 1996; Mackey, 1999; Mackey et al., 2012; Pica, 1994). One example of its increasing reach has been the expansion of interaction work to include technology applications through computer-mediated communication (CMC) (Sachs & Suh, 2007; Smith, 2012; Ziegler, 2016).

In parallel to interaction work, task research began to take off with early definitions of task by Long (1985) and later ones by Long (2015, 2016), Long, Lee, and Hillman (2019), Skehan (1998), and Ellis (2003) as scholars and practitioners came to recognize tasks both as effective for research and as pedagogic tools within lessons and a guiding principle for developing syllabi (Long, 2015; Long & Robinson, 1998). Significantly, as compared to other approaches to language teaching that have fallen in and out of favor, task-based language teaching is distinguished by being based in syllabi grounded in the real-world (authentic) daily tasks a specific group of learners needs to accomplish in their second language. This approach to using tasks in L2 instruction has a number of theoretical underpinnings, ranging from focus on form (Long, 2000, 2015) to the cognition hypothesis (Robinson, 1995) and makes a number of specific, testable, and empirical claims, for example, in relation to task complexity (Robinson, 2007). Other approaches to tasks in instruction also exist, and full discussions can be found in excellent overviews like Bygate (2015), Bygate, Norris, and Van den Branden (2015), and Ellis, Skehan, Li, et al. (2019).

Just as tasks in language learning have been studied and used from different perspectives, interaction and feedback have also been considered in approaches other than the interactionist one. For example, sociocultural theorists (Lantolf et al., 2015) believe, based on Vygotsky's pioneering work, that developmental processes occur as a part and result of participation in cultural, linguistic, family, peer group, school, and other interactions and language learning is part of this. Studies of interaction, feedback, and tasks conducted in this paradigm use many of the same materials and methods as the ones carried out from the interactionist perspective, although the emphasis of many of them tends to be production rather than development. A number of interesting studies in this line of research have been carried out by Swain and her colleagues investigating how second language learners, often in classrooms, can progress their language learning by talking, either in the L1 or L2, about features of the new language (Swain & Lapkin, 2002; Swain et al., 2009). Other approaches include language socialization, which focuses on how learners become members of a target-language group including, for example, classroom communities or second language learner communities. Learners' and teachers' identities are increasingly a focus of studies investigating beliefs. Investigations into the role of interaction, feedback, and tasks in L2 learning from the perspective of language socialization often take ethnographic or interpretative approaches to the collection and analysis of data, but mixed methods are also sometimes seen in this sort of research, hence, some of the methodologies described here may also be of interest to researchers grounding their work in socialization approaches. Duff (2012) provides an excellent overview of work in this area.

Turning back to the approach that underpins the majority of work described in this book, the cognitive–interactionist paradigm, it is interesting to note that while interaction and feedback had been measured or valued in terms of their effectiveness on linguistic development since the mid 1990s, task-based language teaching was, until relatively recently, most frequently measured by changes to fluency, accuracy, and complexity, or simply put, production as opposed to development. However, over the last decades that has changed, with task studies, like interaction and feedback research, focusing on actual learning outcomes as well as changes in production. Currently, there are many hundreds of primary studies of interaction, corrective feedback, and tasks as well as an increasing number of syntheses and meta-analyses.

Accompanying this primary work and development of the approaches and underpinning for the theory, there have also been important innovations in research methods. Sometimes methodological advancement has driven theory and sometimes vice versa, which is quite typical in the social and psychological sciences in general. In the 1980s and 1990s traditional types of instruments and data collection methods tended to be recycled from study to study, and particular research questions and methods for addressing them showed a number of similarities across studies. This had one major advantage in that comparisons could be made of research that used similar or identical methods.

Over the last ten years in particular, though, methodologies have expanded and advanced, often driven by developments in technology and influenced by researchers who came to the area with a deeper understanding of fields like psychology, sociology, education, and even neuroscience.

With these developments, there has been a dramatic increase in the number of texts on the topic of research methodology in the general field of SLA (e.g. Mackey & Gass, 2016; Phakiti et al., 2018). Some have examined specific domains of second language research such as child language (Hoff, 2011), narratives (Barkhuizen et al., 2014), priming (McDonough & Trofimovich, 2008), replication (Porte, 2012), psycholinguistics (Jegerski & Van Patten, 2013), and qualitative methods (Zacharias, 2012). However, despite being one of the most researched areas in SLA (Plonsky & Gass, 2011), the interaction approach, including research on feedback and tasks has, until now, lacked a book specifically covering research methodology in the area.

1.1 The Scope of This Book and the Inclusion of New Data

This book fills that gap by focusing on research methods in the three distinct but inter-related areas of second language acquisition: research on interaction, corrective feedback, and task-based language learning. One of the ways it does this is to include evidence from new data taken from two different studies that illustrate and exemplify various points and trends, including (a) a quantitative, experimental study of cognitive creativity, which shows how these three areas are related while driving forward the field's understanding about individual differences in inter-action and feedback-driven learning via tasks, and (b) a qualitative, descriptive study that exemplifies how knowledge about interaction, feedback, and task-driven second language learning can be shaped by the methodology used.

The book is designed to be both a reference and a guide for students, teachers, scholars, and anyone who is interested in conducting or appraising research on interaction in second language learning contexts, corrective feedback, and tasks. Written to be reader-friendly, features include highlighted boxes asking readers to pause and consider related questions, or read an article under discussion, together with key points highlighted as memory aids, charts, and graphics. By the end of the book, readers should have a good understanding of how key findings in the separate related areas of interaction, feedback, and task research have been obtained, as well as how these areas fit together, and, most import-antly, feel confident in choosing amongst the various options and using them to carry out research in these three areas.

1.2 Theoretical Background

There are already a considerable number of published overviews of theories and research related to the topic of interaction in SLA, pub-lished in handbooks, in encyclopedias, in theories of SLA texts, and in standalone books (for just a few examples, see García Mayo & Alcón Soler, 2013; Gass, 2010; Mackey et al., 2012; Mackey, 2012a). These overviews provide comprehensive summaries of the theory in the fields of interaction, corrective feedback, and tasks, including reviews of sem-inal works in the field. Rather than repeating such efforts, the current chapter briefly outlines key aspects of the cognitive–interactionist approach that are of interest, based on the different methodologies and instruments presented in this book, and then discusses some of the many places where interaction, corrective feedback, and tasks have already been thoroughly overviewed and explained, where readers are encour-aged to go on to learn more about theory in the field of interaction, feedback, and task research. The focus of the rest of this book is on providing the information and tools needed to conduct a particular research project. Each section of the current chapter, then, concludes with open areas of research that I believe are ripe for new empirical investigations, presented to inspire new research projects for researchers to keep in mind as they read the remainder of the book.

1.3 **Interaction Research**

Research into interaction and its potential for affecting second language learning is based on investigations of the kinds of linguistic input learners receive, and the output they produce. Krashen's (1977) input hypothesis suggested that access to comprehensible input under facilitative conditions would support L2 acquisition. Swain's (1985) output hypothesis proposed that learners also needed to produce the new language in order to learn it effectively. Long's (1980) interaction hypothesis suggested that SLA is facilitated by conversational interactions where learners have to negotiate for meaning and receive corrections of their productions. Schmidt (1990) added that learners need to consciously notice linguistic features in the input in order to acquire them. Table 1.1 presents some of the seminal articles that helped define key aspects of the interaction approach.

Since the inception of this approach to SLA, hundreds of empirical investigations and several meta-analyses have connected interaction to successful L2 development (see, for example, Keck, et al., 2006; Li, 2010; Lyster & Saito, 2010; Mackey & Goo, 2007; Russell & Spada, 2006; and see Chapter 6 on meta-analysis for more details).

Overviews and reviews of work in interaction are available in a variety of handbooks and encyclopedias.

Table 1.1 Foundational articles for the interaction approach to SLA

Topic	Subtopic	Authors
Input	Input hypothesis	Krashen (1977, 1980)
	Comprehensible input	Long (1985)
Output	Output hypothesis	Swain (1985)
	Modified output	Swain (2005)
Negotiation for meaning	Corrective feedback	Carroll & Swain (1993)
	Interaction hypothesis	Long (1980, 1996)
		Gass (1997)
		Pica (1994)
		Mackey (1999)
Noticing	Noticing hypothesis	Schmidt (1990)

Read It!

García Mayo, M. D. P. & Alcón Soler, E. (2013). Negotiated input and output / interaction. In J. Herschensohn & M. Young-Scholten (Eds.), *The Cambridge Handbook of Second Language Acquisition* (pp. 209–229). Cambridge University Press.

"This chapter is organized as follows: Section 10.2 presents a historical overview of the origins of research on the role of learner interaction in language learning, where we will refer to the seminal work by Hatch (1978b) and Long (1980, 1981) and the latter's important revision of the Interaction Hypothesis (Long 1996). Section 10.3 describes the major theoretical constructs of input, output and feedback and illustrates how interaction is argued to facilitate learning by providing contexts in which learners are exposed to L2 input and are "pushed" (Swain 2005) to make their output more accurate. Interaction also provides learners with an opportunity to negotiate meaning and form with their conversational partners and to receive feedback in response to difficulties that might arise during conversational exchanges. Both negotiation and feedback have been shown to play an important facilitative role in language learning (Mackey, 2006; see also Chapters 29 and 30, this volume). Section 10.4 considers several factors that influence conversational interaction and Section 10.5 concludes the chapter, highlighting lines for further research within the IM" (p. 210).

Note that these authors refer to the theory as the "Interaction Model (IM)" rather than the "interaction approach."

Read It!

Mackey, A., Abbuhl, R., & Gass, S. M. (2012). Interactionist approach. In S. Gass & A. Mackey (Eds.), *The Routledge Handbook of Second Language Acquisition* (pp. 7–23). Routledge.

"In the 30 years since the initial formulation of the Interaction Hypothesis (Long, 1980, 1981), there has been an explosion of studies investigating the ways in which interaction can benefit second language acquisition (SLA), with the most recent work documenting its evolution from hypothesis to approach (Gass & Mackey, 2007a). This review begins with an overview of the historical background of the interactionist approach and then discusses the core issues surrounding it, examines some of the ways in which data are collected in this area of SLA, and explores the practical applications of the approach. Directions for future research will be addressed in the final section" (p. 7).

Read It!

Gass, S. M. (2010). Interactionist perspectives on second language acquisition. In R. B. Kaplan (Ed.), *The Oxford Handbook of Applied Linguistics* (2nd
ed., pp. 217–231). Oxford University Press.

"This article analyses the idea of second language acquisition from an
interactionist perspective. The field of second language acquisition has been
studied from many angles. This broad scope is due in part to the myriad
disciplinary backgrounds of scholars in the field. This article deals with the
interactionist perspective and, as such, is primarily concerned with the
environment in which second language learning takes place. It is important
to note from the outset that this perspective is by and large neutral as to the
role of innateness. In other words, it is compatible with a view of second
language acquisition that posits an innate learning mechanism; it is also
compatible with a model of learning that posits no such mechanism. This
article deals with interactionist approaches focusing on how learners use
their linguistic environment to build their knowledge of the second language. To summarize, the interaction approach considers production of
language as a construct important for understanding second language
learning" (p. 217).

Read It!

Gass, S. M. & Mackey, A. (2006). *Input, interaction, and output: An overview.*
AILA Review, 19(1), 3–17.

"This paper presents an overview of what has come to be known as the
Interaction Hypothesis, the basic tenet of which is that through input and
interaction with interlocutors, language learners have opportunities to notice
differences between their own formulations of the target language and the
language of their conversational partners. They also receive feedback which
both modifies the linguistic input they receive and pushes them to modify
their output during conversation. This paper focuses on the major constructs
of this approach to SLA, namely, input, interaction, feedback and output, and
discusses recent literature that addresses these issues" (p. 3).

You can also find shorter, more concise overviews of the interaction
approach to SLA in encyclopedias such as the *Encyclopedia of Applied
Linguistics*.

Read It!

Mackey, A. & Goo, J. (2012). Interaction approach in second language acquisition. In C. Chapelle (Ed.), *The Encyclopedia of Applied Linguistics* (pp. 2748–2758). Wiley-Blackwell.

"The interaction approach to second language acquisition posits that learners can benefit from taking part in interaction because of a variety of developmentally helpful opportunities, conditions, and processes which interaction can expose them to. These include input, negotiation, output, feedback, and attention." [Topics covered] "Input, negotiation for meaning in interaction, output in interaction, feedback in interaction, and noticing, attention, and working memory in interaction research. The entry also includes examples from data for each topic" (p. 2748).

Read It!

Abbuhl, R., Mackey, A., Ziegler, N., & Amoroso, L. (2018). Interaction and learning grammar. In J. I. Liontas (Ed.), *The TESOL Encyclopedia of English Language Teaching* (pp. 1–7). Wiley-Blackwell.

"This entry discusses the interaction hypothesis and how input, output, feedback, and attention are believed to facilitate the acquisition of second language (L2) grammar. Following a brief overview of the central tenets of the approach, the entry addresses recent research on the role of interaction, including negotiation for meaning and corrective feedback, and how empirical findings might be practically applied in the L2 grammar classroom" (p. 1).

There are also several books dedicated to the interaction approach and its implications for research in SLA, which give useful overviews.

Read It!

Mackey, A. (2012a). *Input, Interaction, and Corrective Feedback in L2 Learning*. Oxford University Press.

"The question of how interaction and corrective feedback affect second language (L2) learning has increasingly attracted the interest of researchers in recent years. This book describes the processes involved in interaction-driven second language learning and presents a methodological framework for studying them. A substantial amount of research on interaction has been carried out over the past two decades; the author provides a timely, comprehensive, and up-to-date survey of this significant body of work. In particular, she explores the recent growth in research into the role of cognitive and social factors in evaluating how interaction works. Researchers, research students, and all those working within the field of second language acquisition will find this book an authoritative and valuable resource" (Back matter).

Read It!

Gass, S. M. (2017). *Input, Interaction, and the Second Language Learner* (2nd ed.). Routledge.

"The volume provides an important view of the relationship between input, interaction, and SLA. In so doing, it should prove useful to those whose major concern is with the acquisition of a second or foreign language, as well as those who are primarily interested in these issues from a pedagogical perspective. The book does not explicate or advocate a particular teaching methodology but does attempt to lay out some of the underpinnings of what is involved in interaction – what interaction is and what purpose it serves. Research in SLA is concerned with the knowledge that second language learners do and do not acquire, and how that knowledge comes about. This book ties these issues together from three perspectives: the input/interaction framework, information-processing, and learnability" (p. i).

Other volumes explore specific interlocutors for interaction such as peer-to-peer interactions and the potential benefits for SLA.

Read It!

Philp, J., Adams, R., & Iwashita, N. (2013). *Peer Interaction and Second Language Learning*. Routledge.

"*Peer Interaction and Second Language Learning* synthesizes the existing body of research on the role of peer interaction in second language learning in one comprehensive volume. In spite of the many hours that language learners spend interacting with peers in the classroom, there is a tendency to evaluate the usefulness of this time by comparison to whole class interaction with the teacher. Yet teachers are teachers and peers are peers – as partners in interaction, they are likely to offer very different kinds of learning opportunities. This book encourages researchers and instructors alike to take a new look at the potential of peer interaction to foster second language development. Acknowledging the context of peer interaction as highly dynamic and complex, the book considers the strengths and limitations of peer work from a range of theoretical perspectives. In doing so, *Peer Interaction and Second Language Learning* clarifies features of effective peer interaction for second language learning across a range of educational contexts, age spans, proficiency levels, and classroom tasks and settings" (p. i).

1.4 Open Research Areas in Interaction

One place to look for more ideas is the end of published research articles in the section called "future directions." Often, authors will provide ideas for follow-up studies or identify gaps still existing in the line of research. Here are a few ideas from recently published articles:

- Longitudinal studies of L2 development. The majority of experimental studies of interaction examine development via pre-, post- and (sometimes) short-term delayed post-tests. More studies could follow up with learners using longer delayed post-tests to identify the durability of treatments and quite a few articles finish with statements like "more longer-term research is needed."
- Studies of interaction in non-laboratory, non-classroom settings, such as in informal conversation groups, study-abroad interactions, or other non-traditional contexts and with learners who are more diverse than the typical college-aged educated young adults. For more information on this, see the discussion in Chapter 9. In a book called *Second Language Interaction in Diverse Educational Contexts* (2013), Kim McDonough and I included work in laboratory, classroom, and computer-mediated settings, but pointed out at the end that non-traditional settings such as conversation groups (e.g. Bryfonski & Sanz, 2018; Ziegler et al., 2013) could still yield many important and interesting new insights.

- Studies of interaction with nontraditional learners like refugee populations. These are important because they get beyond the classic tertiary education settings. Tarone (2010) for example has studied low-literacy learners, and King and Bigelow (2018) conducted SLA research with East African transnational adolescents.
- Aptitude-treatment interaction (ATI) studies. This type of study examines the relationships between the effectiveness of instructional treatments and the unique characteristics, or individual differences such as in working memory, motivation, or aptitude, of the language learners. ATI studies often use mixed methods in classroom or experimental contexts. While research is increasingly taking these individual differences into account, the research presented in the current book on cognitive creativity represents one important avenue (Mackey et al., 2015; Mackey et al., 2014; Pipes, 2019) and other aspects, such as shame and guilt (Teimouri, 2018) should be considered.
- Action research conducted by classroom teachers for authentic learning purposes. These are very beneficial to other practicing language teachers and promote generalizability of findings by examining learning in diverse contexts with diverse groups of students.

1.5 Corrective Feedback Research

The provision and potential use of oral corrective feedback during interactions is both an element of the interaction approach described above, as well as a strand of research in second language acquisition that, in the context of instruction, is often discussed independently of interaction. In interaction, feedback typically occurs during instances of negotiation for meaning in which the learner's interlocutor indicates in some way that an error or misunderstanding has occurred. Corrective feedback is frequently discussed in terms of its relative explicitness or implicitness. An example of an explicit form of corrective feedback is metalinguistic explanation in which the interlocutor points out the learners' error and provides some explication of the problem, for example, a grammar rule to correct the error (e.g., *You said "He walk." You're missing the 3rd person plural –s on the verb.*) An example of more implicit feedback is a recast. Recasts are typically understood as when an interlocutor simply repeats back what a learner said, but with some or all of the learner's errors corrected (e.g., *"He walk" or "He walks"?)* There are other types of feedback as well. Some examples are clarification requests (e.g., *Sorry, what was that?)*, and simple repetitions of the error, but with rising intonation (e.g., *He walk?*). All vary in the degree to which they are explicit or implicit (or in some researchers' terms direct or indirect, most often described so in the case of written corrective feedback; see Ellis, 2008 for an overview) depending on how the error is pointed out, how it is corrected, and the context of the interaction. As with work on interaction, there are original research papers, meta-analytic works, and handbooks and encyclopedia entries on this topic, where these concepts are concisely defined and described. Some examples are given in Table 1.2.

Table 1.2 Foundational articles and empirical examples of research on corrective feedback

Topic	Subtopic	Authors
Foundations	Feedback and focus on form	Gass & Varonis (1989)
		Lightbown & Spada (1990)
		Doughty & Varela (1998)
	Implicit versus explicit	Long (1996)
	Negotiation for meaning	Pica (1994)
Theoretical issues	Learner uptake	Lyster & Ranta (1997)
		Ellis, Basturkmen, & Loewen (2001)
		Sheen (2004)
	Noticing of feedback	Mackey, Gass, & McDonough (2000)
		Egi (2010)
	Types of feedback	Mackey & Philp (1998)
		Lyster (1998a, 1998b)
		Leeman (2003)
		Ammar & Spada (2006)
Contexts of feedback	Laboratory	McDonough & Mackey (2006)
	Computer-mediated	Sachs & Suh (2007)
	Classroom	Lyster (2004)
		Mackey (2006)

The relationship between corrective feedback and L2 development has been investigated in classroom and laboratory settings (there are several meta-analyses on the topic as well, e.g., Brown, 2016; Li, 2010; Lyster & Saito, 2010; Russell & Spada, 2006; and see below), with the majority reporting positive effects for development following receiving corrective feedback, although some studies, particularly in the Canadian classroom context did not find this trend (e.g., Lyster, 2004). Corrective feedback is a relatively high-frequency topic in SLA research with studies investigating how different variables such as the target of the feedback (e.g. phonological versus morphosyntactic feedback), how salient or explicit it is in terms of type, the interlocutor (e.g., a peer versus a teacher), and other learner individual differences (e.g., age, proficiency) affect how feedback is interpreted and the extent to which feedback promotes L2 development. The interaction approach and research on corrective feedback are closely intertwined in SLA research, meaning there are also a number of reviews of the interaction approach that include sections dedicated to corrective feedback and vice versa (see the reviews of interaction above, e.g., Gass & Mackey, 2006). These reviews provide more thorough explanations of the different types of feedback and the ways in which they have been defined and studied in prior literature. Meta-analyses on the topic of corrective feedback can be helpful to read to obtain overviews of the many ways in which corrective feedback is operationalized and studied.

1.5.1 Meta-Analyses of Corrective Feedback Research

Read It!

Russell, J. & Spada, N. (2006). The effectiveness of corrective feedback for the acquisition of L2 grammar: A meta-analysis of the research. In J. M. Norris & L. Ortega (Eds.), *Synthesizing Research on Language Learning and Teaching* (pp. 133–164). John Benjamins.

"In this chapter, we report on a meta-analysis of research that investigated the effects of corrective feedback (CF) on second language (L2) grammar learning. We describe the rationale for undertaking this research and the steps taken in the collection and coding of 56 primary studies in preparation for the meta-analysis. Of these 56 studies, 31 were considered suitable for the meta-analysis and 15 provided sufficient data to calculate effect sizes. Due to this small number, a broadly inclusive approach was taken in meta-analyzing their findings. We report the results in terms of the overall effectiveness of corrective feedback for L2 learning" (p. 133).

Read It!

Li, S. (2010). The effectiveness of corrective feedback in SLA: A meta-analysis. *Language Learning, 60*(2), 309–365.

"This study reports on a meta-analysis on the effectiveness of corrective feedback in second language acquisition. By establishing a different set of inclusion/exclusion criteria than previous meta-analyses and performing a series of methodological moves, it is intended to be an update and complement to previous meta-analyses. Altogether 33 primary studies were retrieved, including 22 published studies and 11 Ph.D. dissertations. These studies were coded for 17 substantive and methodological features, 14 of which were identified as independent and moderator variables. It was found that (a) there was a medium overall effect for corrective feedback and the effect was maintained over time, (b) the effect of implicit feedback was better maintained than that of explicit feedback, (c) published studies did not show larger effects than dissertations, (d) lab-based studies showed a larger effect than classroom-based studies, (e) shorter treatments generated a larger effect size than longer treatments, and (f) studies conducted in foreign language contexts produced larger effect sizes than those in second language contexts. Possible explanations for the results were sought through data cross-tabulation and with reference to the theoretical constructs of SLA" (p. 309).

Read It!

Brown, D. (2016). The type and linguistic foci of oral corrective feedback in the L2 classroom: A meta-analysis. *Language Teaching Research, 20*(4), 436–458.

"Research on corrective feedback (CF), a central focus of second language acquisition (SLA), has increasingly examined how teachers employ CF in second language classrooms. Lyster and Ranta's (1997) seminal study identified six types of CF that teachers use in response to students' errors (recast, explicit correction, elicitation, clarification request, metalinguistic cue, and repetition) as well as target linguistic foci (lexical, phonological, and grammatical errors). These taxonomies have remained dominant in observational studies conducted in a growing range of second language teaching contexts. Several studies have acknowledged that contextual factors may influence how teachers provide CF (e.g. Mori, 2002; Sheen, 2004) with few generalizable conclusions. The present study brings together research in this area in the first comprehensive synthesis of classroom CF research seeking to aggregate proportions of CF types teachers provide, as well as their target linguistic foci. Findings reveal that recasts account for 57% of all CF while prompts comprise 30%, and grammar errors received the greatest proportion of CF (43%). The study further identifies a range of contextual and methodological factors (i.e. moderators) that may influence CF choices across teaching contexts, such as student proficiency, teacher experience, and second/foreign language context. A clearer picture of the patterns of CF that teachers provide and the variables that influence these choices serves to complement the growing body of research investigating the efficacy of CF in second language pedagogy" (p. 436).

Articles in special editions of journals and encyclopedia entries also provide concise overviews of common operationalizations of corrective feedback variables and overviews of research questions.

Read It!

Sheen, Y. (2010). Introduction: The role of oral and written corrective feedback in SLA. *Studies in Second Language Acquisition*, *32*(2), 169–179.

"Oral CF research has been largely grounded in SLA theories and hypotheses, whereas written CF research has drawn on L1 and L2 writing composition theories. These differences notwithstanding, there are a number of issues common to the study of oral and written CF: (a) whether oral and written CF works, (b) what constitutes the most effective approach for implementing CF, (c) what contextual and individual learner factors contribute to the effectiveness of oral and written CF, and (d) whether it is possible to develop a common methodology for investigating the effectiveness of oral and written CF. I will briefly consider these key issues and pinpoint articles in the special issue that address them" (p. 169).

Read It!

Nassaji, H. (2016). Anniversary article: Interactional feedback in second language teaching and learning: A synthesis and analysis of current research. *Language Teaching Research*, *20*(4), 535–562.

"The role of interactional feedback has long been of interest to both second language acquisition researchers and teachers and has continued to be the object of intensive empirical and theoretical inquiry. In this article, I provide a synthesis and analysis of recent research and developments in this area and their contributions to second language acquisition (SLA). I begin by discussing the theoretical underpinnings of interactional feedback and then review studies that have investigated the provision and effectiveness of feedback for language learning in various settings. I also examine research in a number of other key areas that have been the focus of current research including feedback timing, feedback training, learner–learner interaction, and computer-assisted feedback. The article concludes with a discussion of the implications of the issues examined with regard to classroom instruction" (p. 535).

Read It!

Lyster, R. (2019). Roles for corrective feedback in second language instruction. In C. A. Chapelle (Ed.), *The Encyclopedia of Applied Linguistics*. Wiley-Blackwell.

"This entry addresses the roles of oral corrective feedback in classroom settings in terms of its various types, functions, and effects. It concludes with suggestions for future classroom-based research on corrective feedback."

[Topics covered] "Types of corrective feedback, functions of corrective feedback, effects of corrective feedback, future directions" (Wiley-Blackwell, 2019).

Suggestions for further reading also include chapters from two handbooks dedicated to corrective feedback research.

Read It!

Nassaji, H. & Kartchava, E. (Eds.) (2017). *Corrective Feedback in Second Language Teaching and Learning: Research, Theory, Applications, Implications*. Taylor and Francis.

"Bringing together current research, analysis, and discussion of the role of corrective feedback in second language teaching and learning, this volume bridges the gap between research and pedagogy by identifying principles of effective feedback strategies and how to use them successfully in classroom instruction. By synthesizing recent works on a range of related themes and topics in this area and integrating them into a single volume, it provides a valuable resource for researchers, graduate students, teachers, and teacher educators in various contexts who seek to enhance their skills and to further their understanding in this key area of second language education" (p. i).

Read It!

Nassaji, H. & Kartchava, E. (Eds.) (2019). *The Cambridge Handbook of Corrective Feedback in Language Learning and Teaching.* Cambridge University Press.

"Provides an in-depth analysis and discussion of the role of corrective feedback in second language learning and teaching. The overall aims are to synthesize recent works on a range of related themes and topics in this area and integrate them into a single volume that can serve as a comprehensive resource for those interested in error correction and feedback in various contexts. To meet these goals, the book brings together cutting-edge research and state-of-the-art articles that address recent developments in core areas of error correction and examine their implications for second language acquisition and instruction. Although many studies have investigated corrective feedback and ample evidence exists about its role in language learning, there is clearly a missing link between the findings of this research and what is actually practiced in many second language classrooms. Thus, another major aim is to help bridge this gap between research and pedagogy by identifying and discussing principles of effective feedback strategies and how to use them successfully in classroom instruction" (Cambridge University Press, 2019).

1.6 Open Research Areas in Corrective Feedback

Researchers interested in corrective feedback might consider reading some of the overview and seminal articles described above, followed by closely related meta-analyses to identify gaps in prior research that their project could address. A few potential areas for new studies include:

- Understudied targets of corrective feedback (e.g., pragmatics, phonology). Some examples of understudied targets exist such as pragmatics (e.g., Culpeper et al., 2018; Fukuya & Zhang, 2002) and phonology (e.g., Bryfonski & Ma, 2019; Parlak & Ziegler, 2017), however more work is needed.

- Less commonly taught, learned, and studied L2s (i.e., languages other than English, Spanish, Japanese, and Korean).
- Individual differences (e.g., age, proficiency) in sensitivity or receptivity to different types of corrective feedback. New data on awareness and preference for corrective feedback, and the complex issues of learner age and gender and how these play into interlocutor effects are also discussed in this book.
- Timing of corrective feedback (immediate versus short term versus delayed).
- Modality of corrective feedback (e.g., CALL, written versus oral).
- Contexts for corrective feedback (classrooms, labs versus naturalistic environments), including more variety in socioeconomic contexts.
- Effects of opportunities and expectations to modify output following corrective feedback. Again, a small dataset of new data is presented to address this issue, but in general, research seems somewhat divided as to the benefits of participating in and observing feedback episodes. In other words, there is still a limited understanding of the benefits of self-correction following the various forms of corrective feedback.

1.7 Task-Based Research

Task-based language teaching (TBLT) is generally understood as an approach to language pedagogy that centers around authentic tasks, as opposed to grammar points, as the main focus of language instruction. Developed by Long and his colleagues (particularly in a 2015 book, described below) in response to traditional approaches to language teaching that did not take SLA research findings into account, most approaches to TBLT take cognitive–interactionist theories about SLA as a theoretical orientation. In this approach to teaching, the needs of learners (what they need to *do* with the second language) are evaluated and the curriculum is designed to prepare these learners to accomplish tasks matched to their authentic needs. In a task-based language classroom, learners interact with each other, hear corrective feedback from the teacher and their peers, while carrying out a target task (e.g., giving directions on a map, or in a more advanced class, critiquing each other's conference abstracts, for example). Many studies of TBLT have investigated the ways tasks can be manipulated to promote different aspects of

Table 1.3 Foundational articles for research on task-based language teaching

Topic	Subtopic	Authors
Foundations of TBLT	Theory	Long (1980, 1985)
	Empirical beginnings	Beretta & Davies (1985)
	Task-based syllabus design	Long & Crookes (1992)
	Task-based instruction	Skehan (1996)
	Pedagogy	Ellis (2000)
Teaching TBLT	Needs analysis	Van Avermaet & Gysen (2006)
	Task types	Pica, et al. (1993)
	Task complexity and sequencing	Robinson (2001)
	Task cycles	Willis (1996)
	Assessment	Norris, et al. (2002)
Task variables	Task repetition	Bygate (2001)
	Pre-task planning	Foster & Skehan (1996)
Teachers	Role of the teacher	Samuda (2001)
	Teacher training	Van den Branden (2006)

L2 development. Reading the foundational works (see Table 1.3) can be helpful in understanding the implications of the empirical work described below.

Tasks and the resulting outcomes have been meta-analyzed by several researchers (e.g., Cobb, 2010; Keck et al., 2006) finding positive trends in favor of the TBLT approach. Other work has investigated specific features of tasks such as task complexity (Jackson & Suethanapornkul, 2013; Sasayama et al., 2015), methods of TBLT research (Plonsky & Kim, 2016), and contexts of TBLT interactions and programs (Bryfonski & McKay, 2017; Ziegler, 2016).

Read more about some foundational meta-analyses in the following Read It! boxes.

Read It!

Keck, C. M., Iberri-Shea, G., Tracy-Ventura, N., & Wa-Mbaleka, S. (2006). Investigating the empirical link between task-based interaction and acquisition: A meta-analysis. In J. M. Norris & L. Ortega (Eds.), *Synthesizing Research on Language Learning and Teaching* (pp. 91–131). John Benjamins.

"Despite the seemingly rich context that task-based interaction provides for acquisition and the large amounts of research fueled by the Interaction Hypothesis (Long, 1996), oft-cited findings to date appear to be conflicting. While some studies (e.g. Ellis, Tanaka & Yamazaki, 1995; Mackey, 1999) demonstrate that task-based interaction can facilitate acquisition of specific linguistic features, others (e.g. Loschky, 1994) support no such relationship. This has promoted a variety of SLA researchers to question whether interaction can be empirically linked to acquisition. Over the past decade, however, and perhaps motivated by this criticism, the study of direct links between interaction and acquisition has gained momentum. The present meta-analysis was undertaken to synthesize the findings of all experimental, task-based interaction studies published between 1980 and 2003 which aimed to investigate the link between interaction and the acquisition of specific grammatical and lexical features. Results from 14 unique sample studies that satisfied stringent inclusion and exclusion criteria show that experimental groups substantially outperformed control and comparison groups in both grammar and lexis on immediate and delayed posttests. In addition, consistent with Loschky and Bley-Broman's (1993) proposal, tasks in which use of the target feature was essential yielded larger effects over time than tasks in which use of the target form was useful, but not required. Initial support was also found for Swain's (1985, 2000) arguments that opportunities for pushed output play a crucial role in the acquisition process. Drawing upon these findings, and the synthesis of study design features, we propose specific recommendations for future interaction research" (p. 91).

Read It!

Cobb, M. (2010). *Meta-analysis of the effectiveness of task-based interaction in form-focused instruction of adult learners in foreign and second language teaching* [Unpublished doctoral dissertation]. University of San Francisco.

"Research into the effectiveness of task-based interaction in acquisition of specific grammatical structures of the target language has been scarce and sometimes has presented conflicting findings. Task-based interaction engages learners in focused face-to-face oral-communication tasks that predispose them to repeated use of the target structure in meaningful contexts. This meta-analysis synthesized the results of 15 primary studies. On average, learners who received task-based interaction treatments through completing focused oral-communication tasks with native or non-native interlocutors performed better than learners who received no focused instruction in the target structure and somewhat better than learners who received other types of instruction such as traditional grammar instruction, input processing activities, and so forth. The effect sizes were medium and small, respectively. Both the learners who received task-based interaction and those who received other instruction showed large within-group gains, whereas the gains demonstrated by the learners who received no instruction in the targeted form were insignificant or small based on Cohen's 1977 classification. The effects of task-based instruction were durable" (p. ii–iii).

For an overview of the theoretical orientation and pedagogical implications of TBLT, read the short and clear encyclopedia entries cited below.

Read It!

Robinson, P. & Gilabert, R. (2012). Task-based learning: Cognitive underpinnings. In C. Chapelle (Ed.), *The Encyclopedia of Applied Linguistics*. Wiley-Blackwell.

"Over the past thirty years, proposals for task-based language teaching (TBLT) have drawn on a variety of claims about, and research into, the cognitive processes thought to promote successful second language acquisition (SLA)."

[Topics covered] "Cognitive processes in task-based learning, design characteristics affecting the cognitive processing demands of tasks (planning time, single/dual tasks, intentional reasoning, spatial reasoning, here-and-now/there-and-then), effects of cumulative increases in the cognitive demands of tasks (output, uptake, memory, automaticity, aptitudes)" (Wiley-Blackwell, 2012).

Read It!

Bygate, M., Norris, J., & Van den Branden, K. (2015). Task-based language teaching. In C. Chapelle (Ed.), *The Encyclopedia of Applied Linguistics*. Wiley-Blackwell.

"Task-based language teaching (TBLT) is an approach to pedagogy in which communication tasks are fundamental to language learning. In TBLT, the notion of task indicates language-learning activities in which students are required to use language with a primary focus on meaning, in order to achieve some communicative outcome. They range in scope from brief spoken exchanges to extended written performances to integrated, multi-modal language use in face-to-face or virtual environments."

[Topics covered] "Tasks as educational constructs, tasks and language, tasks and learning, tasks and teaching, tasks and assessment, the future of TBLT" (Wiley-Blackwell, 2015).

There are several books that provide overviews of the TBLT pedagogy and its theoretical underpinnings.

Read It!

Long, M. H. (2015). *Second Language Acquisition and Task-Based Language Teaching*. Wiley-Blackwell.

"This book offers an in-depth explanation of Task-Based Language Teaching (TBLT) and the methods necessary to implement it in the language classroom successfully

- Combines a survey of theory and research in instructed second language acquisition (ISLA) with insights from language teaching and the philosophy of education
- Details best practice for TBLT programs, including discussion of learner needs and means analysis; syllabus design; materials writing; choice of methodological principles and pedagogic procedures; criterion-referenced, task-based performance assessment; and program evaluation
- Is written by an esteemed scholar of second language acquisition with over 30 years of research and classroom experience
- Considers diffusion of innovation in education and the potential impact of TBLT on foreign and second language learning" (Wiley-Blackwell, 2015).

Read It!

Ellis, R. (2003). *Task-Based Language Learning and Teaching*. Oxford University Press.

"This book explores the relationship between research, teaching, and tasks, and seeks to clarify the issues raised by recent work in this field. The book shows how research and task-based teaching can mutually inform each other and illuminate the areas of task-based course design, methodology, and assessment" (Oxford University Press).

As mentioned earlier, there is also a dedicated book series on topics in TBLT published by John Benjamins. In particular, the volume summarized in the Read It! box below provides a good overview of the field of TBLT and its history, and provides re-prints of seminal articles.

Read It!

Van den Branden, K., Bygate, M., & Norris, J. (Eds.). (2009). *Task-Based Language Teaching: A Reader*. John Benjamins.

"Over the past two decades, task-based language teaching (TBLT) has gained considerable momentum in the field of language education. This volume presents a collection of 20 reprinted articles and chapters representative of work that appeared during that period. It introduces readers – graduate students, researchers, teachers – to foundational ideas and themes that have marked the emergence of TBLT. The editors provide a first chapter that locates TBLT within broader discourses of educational practice and research on language learning and teaching. The book then features four sections consisting of important, often difficult to find, writings on major themes: fundamental ideas, approaches, and definitions in TBLT; curriculum, syllabus, and task design; variables affecting task-based language learning and performance; and task-based assessment. In a concluding chapter, the editors challenge simplistic notions of TBLT by reflecting on how this body of work has initiated the possibility of a truly researched language pedagogy, and they highlight critical directions in TBLT research and practice for the future" (John Benjamins, 2009).

Task-based language teaching represents the pedagogical classroom implications of the interaction approach to SLA described above and tests out the theories laid out in the interaction hypothesis (and other related hypotheses), along with negotiation for meaning and corrective feedback in educational settings. Therefore, this line of research is both important in terms of its implications for classroom teachers, administrators, and learners and is also ripe for further investigation.

1.8 Open Research Areas in TBLT

As a relatively new and still emerging area of research in the field of SLA, there are a number of interesting and open or understudied areas of research still to be investigated, as well as a few areas where a number of interesting studies have been carried out, but where the results are contradictory or not conclusive. A few possibilities include:

- Effects of tasks when task variables are measured in terms of linguistic production and development (using traditional measures like complexity, accuracy, lexis, and fluency). For example, studies that investigate how different tasks encourage fluency at the expense of accuracy or complexity, and vice versa.
- Outcomes of implementing TBLT in diverse language-teaching environments (i.e., contexts outside of the U.S. and Western Europe) in terms of school and student buy-in.
- The role of teachers, their perceptions, individual differences like teacher anxiety (Goetze, 2018), and teaching practices on TBLT implementation, syllabus, and task design.
- The role of individual learner differences in task performance (e.g., aptitude, proficiency, cognitive creativity, personality traits such as introversion/extroversion, etc.)
- The role of teacher education and training programs for TBLT programs (e.g., Bryfonski, 2019b).
- Program evaluations of TBLT in classrooms and schools to determine authentic learning outcomes of the pedagogy.
- Case studies of TBLT and task implementations in worldwide contexts.

1.9 Conclusions

The goal of this chapter has been to provide a brief overview of the main theoretical and pedagogical approaches that provide the foundation for the studies and methodologies you will read about in the rest of this book. If you are a researcher looking for a topic, it may be helpful to read some of the suggested foundational work, or overviews and seminal articles referenced in this chapter before continuing on to read the rest of this book. This should help you find an area, perhaps using one of the "open research areas" sections, as a point of departure to orient your thinking as you progress throughout the rest of this book. For more experienced researchers who already have a study or research program in mind, this chapter has intended to provide a review, and illustrate how the three areas – interaction, feedback, and tasks – can be seen as related yet distinct. The remainder of the book provides detailed descriptions of the various steps involved in successfully completing an interaction, corrective feedback, and/or TBLT research project, including tips, tricks, and common pitfalls along the way.

CHAPTER TWO

Designing Studies of the Roles of Interaction, Feedback, and Tasks in Second Language Learning

2.1 Introduction

Now that we've had a brief look at the theoretical background in Chapter 1 and reviewed some potentially open research areas and questions, what I will focus on next is how to *design* research to answer questions about interaction, feedback, and communicative tasks and their role and relationship to second language learning. As I said before, this book is designed to be practical in nature, aimed at people who are thinking about carrying out studies on these topics, or who want to appraise, critique, or better understand studies that they are reading in the literature in terms of the methods used. The present chapter provides a starting point for this venture.

2.2 Research Questions

We ask research questions all the time. At the back of a slow-moving line in a coffee shop we wonder why it's going slowly, and we often come up with a hypothesis (e.g., because the person at the front of the line has given a long and complicated order, or because it is 12:30 pm and there is a lot of lunchtime traffic, or perhaps that the barista is short-handed, or new, or chatty). If we aren't too busy looking down at our phones, we usually then (unconsciously) test our hypothesis by watching and/or listening. If we see the person at the front of the line engaged in an extended interaction, we might confirm or at least strengthen our hypothesis that their order might be complicated in some way. If that person moves quickly, we might look harder at the barista, are they working alone? Asking questions about human behavior, coming up with hypotheses, and seeking evidence that helps us support one hypothesis over another are all part of life. For some of us, it's easier to be in a line that's moving more slowly if we understand why it is that way. In this chapter, I discuss what research questions are and how to develop them, what hypotheses are, and how to come up with them in the context of interaction, feedback, and task research, finishing off with issues like feasibility (how easy or not it is to answer a question) and replication (testing whether a previous study's results will hold). I'll begin by discussing a range of approaches to research, and then turn to how we move from our natural curiosity and real-life hypotheses about slow moving lines to applying the same principles of questions and predictions to research in interaction, feedback, tasks, and second language learning.

2.3 Different Approaches in Interaction, Feedback, and Task Research

Research in interaction, feedback, and tasks and how they may (or may not) link to second language learning is done in a wide range of paradigms, using quantitative, qualitative, interpretive, descriptive, and mixed methods, although these distinctions are increasingly seen as somewhat simplistic and reductive. There is also "big picture" work, usually known as synthetic and meta-analytic research. Mixed-methods research, involving a range of approaches, is becoming more common, and there is some overlap between approaches. For example, researchers working in interpretative paradigms do work which is sometimes conflated with qualitative approaches, but which can involve a different set of goals. We're going to look at each of these different approaches through examples of how they have been used in interaction, feedback, and/or task-based research, to illustrate the very wide range of approaches that are in use.

Quantitative research generally starts with an experimental design in which a hypothesis is followed by the collection and then coding and quantification of data with numerical analysis being carried out. An example of a quantitative study would be the comparison of three groups of learners' test results before and after engaging in two different treatments involving communicative tasks (and for the control groups, only the tests without the treatments). *Qualitative* studies, however, are most often not set up as experiments and are usually not intended to produce results than can be generalized. Qualitative data are not always easily quantified. An example of a qualitative study would be research in which a student keeps track of her attitudes to her interlocutors and her thoughts and beliefs about their interactions in different sorts of contexts, during a year-long study abroad period in Japan. The analysis in this sort of study would be interpretive or descriptive rather than statistical. *Interpretive* research emphasizes the interrelatedness of communication that is to be studied and acknowledges the role of co-construction of meaning in data collection. An example of this kind of research is co-constructed interviews, in other words a dynamic interview that doesn't stick to a list of pre-determined questions. *Descriptive* research, on the other hand, relies on observation of an interaction by the researcher. Surveys of participant interpretations and preferences would be an example of descriptive research. Finally, another kind of research is *synthesis*, sometimes called meta-analysis research. This kind of research takes a bird's-eye view of the field in order to draw connections and conclusions about topics of research. Studies that analyze multiple datasets across other studies is a common way that researchers perform synthesis research.

There are lots of different variations on these themes and it bears keeping in mind that, although the relationship between quantitative and qualitative research was traditionally thought of as dichotomous, or involving completely different mindsets, it is increasingly thought of as a continuum. In fact, many studies incorporate elements of both types of research, a methodology known as mixed methods. *Mixed-methods research*, also known as combined, multiple, mixed, or triangulated methods, is based on collecting and analyzing data from both quantitative and qualitative approaches. Further explained by Creswell and Creswell (2018), mixed-methods research takes as its core assumption that "the integration of qualitative and quantitative data yields additional insight beyond the information provided by either quantitative or qualitative data alone" (p. 4). One advantage of carrying out mixed-methods research is triangulation, or multiple sources and types of data being brought to bear on the same question. Labov, for example, made this point as long ago as 1972:

> Current difficulties in achieving intersubjective agreement in linguistics require attention to principles of methodology which consider sources of error and ways to eliminate them ... Intersubjective agreement is best reached by convergence of several kinds of data with complementary sources of error (p. 97).

Keep It in Mind!

Table 2.1 provides a quick reminder of what is entailed by each of the main types of research discussed above.

Table 2.1 Major methodological approaches

Type of research	Focus	Examples
Quantitative	The relationship between different variables, like a type of interaction and a type of learning	Study of the effect of clarification questions on learner perception of English tense/lax vowels
Qualitative	Naturalistic data from participants' everyday lives that involves interaction	Learner diary about language use; learner narratives about native speakers correcting their errors
Mixed Methods	Use of both quantitative and qualitative data to provide deeper, richer answers to research questions	Asking learners who have taken part in a pre-test, post-test study to introspect about their results and the interaction
Descriptive	Use of observation to report on the status of naturally occurring data Describes a phenomenon and its characteristics Can be quantitative or qualitative	Giving language students a survey about their preferences for oral corrective feedback from their classroom teachers
Interpretivist	Acknowledges social reality is dynamically shaped by human experiences and contexts, studies situated language, (e.g. the co-construction of interviews or ethnographies.).	Interviews with migrant learners, where data collection and analysis proceeds simultaneously and iteratively (e.g., carry out an interview and analyze it for insights, which may change how the next interview goes).
Synthesis/ Meta-analysis	Systematically reviews prior literature with the goal of drawing larger conclusions based on findings from separate investigations of the same topic	Examining the average effects of all prior studies of oral corrective feedback for L2 grammatical development

To further understand how studies can be categorized according to these various characteristics, let's take a look at the following abstracts from three research reports.

The first study uses quantitative data: It analyzes the data and provides results based on statistical analysis, with the data being collected experimentally.

Read It!

Dewey, D., Belnap, R., & Steffen, P. (2018). Anxiety: Stress, foreign language classroom anxiety, and enjoyment during study abroad in Amman, Jordan. *Annual Review of Applied Linguistics, 38*, 140–161.

"Anxiety is among the most frequently studied emotions in second language acquisition (SLA). Study abroad (SA) researchers have examined its effects on SLA in that setting in a number of studies. The current study goes beyond previous SA research by examining how anxiety develops and connects with language proficiency development over SA. Specifically, it uses anxiety-related measures of foreign language classroom anxiety (FLCA), foreign language enjoyment (FLE), and a physiological manifestation of anxiety (hair cortisol). As far as the classroom is concerned, learners grew more comfortable, experiencing less anxiety and more enjoyment over the period of SA. However, learners showed physiological signs of overall elevated anxiety despite these increasing classroom comfort levels. Two key factors that may have influenced their anxiety levels abroad were tendency toward anxiety prior to SA and language proficiency upon departure for SA. The latter provides support for having students more proficient prior to SA, since doing so may lead to less anxiety during SA" (p. 140).

The next paper uses naturalistic data (conversational interactive data), provides an interpretative rather than a statistical analysis, and uses a non-experimental design.

Read It!

Kinginger, C. & Wu, Q. (2018). Learning Chinese through contextualized language practices in study abroad residence halls: Two case studies. *Annual Review of Applied Linguistics, 38*, 102–121.

"A key question about study abroad concerns the relative benefits and qualities of various living arrangements as sites for learning language and culture. A widely shared assumption seems to be that students choosing homestays enjoy more opportunities for engagement in high-quality conversationally interactive settings than those who opt for residence halls. However, research on outcomes has to date produced only weak evidence for a homestay advantage, suggesting a need to understand the nature of language socialization practices in various living situations. While a number of studies have examined the nature of homestay interaction, only a few have focused on language use in residence halls or other settings where students may interact with peers who are expert second language users. Informed by a Vygotskian approach to the study of development, this article examines the specific qualities of contextualized language practices through two case studies of U.S.-based learners of Mandarin in Shanghai and their Chinese roommates. In the first case, a friendly relationship emerged from routine participation in emotionally charged conversational narrative. In the second, both participants' interest in verbal play and humor led to enjoyment as well as profoundly intercultural dialogue. In each case, there is evidence to show that all parties enjoyed opportunities to learn. These findings suggest that residence halls can be very significant contexts for learning in study abroad settings" (p. 102).

The final study uses both quantitative and qualitative methods to look at corrective feedback and negotiation for meaning in a study-abroad context in relation to recall on tailor-made quizzes after the students returned from their time abroad.

Read It!

Bryfonski, L. & Sanz, C. (2018). Opportunities for corrective feedback during study abroad: A mixed-methods approach. *Annual Review of Applied Linguistics, 38*, 1–32.

"The provision of corrective feedback during oral interaction has been deemed an essential element for successful second language acquisition (Gass & Mackey, 2015). However, corrective feedback – especially corrective feedback provided by peer interlocutors – remains understudied in naturalistic settings. This mixed-methods study aimed to identify the target and type of corrective feedback provided by both native-speaker and peer interlocutors during conversation groups while abroad. U.S. study abroad students ($N = 19$) recorded group conversations with native speakers ($N = 10$) at the beginning, middle, and end of a 6-week stay in Barcelona, Spain. Results indicate a significant decrease in the provision of corrective feedback by both native speakers and peer learners over the course of the program. Qualitative analyses revealed that both learners and natives alike engage in negotiations for meaning throughout the program, which for learners resulted in success-ful recall on tailor-made quizzes. The use of the first language by both the study abroad students and the native speakers promoted these opportunities in some instances. Results are discussed in terms of their contribution to the study abroad literature as well as to research into the effects of feedback on second language development" (p. 1).

2.4 How Do We Come Up with Research Questions and Hypotheses in Interaction, Feedback, and Task Research?

Figuring out what we want to know or understand is an integral part of research. In qualitative/interpretive studies, in keeping with the goals of such approaches, questions often emerge from the data, starting with broad topics and areas of interest, as opposed to quantitative approaches, where questions are usually quite narrowly constrained. Qualitative questions sometimes emerge from data collected, as opposed to guiding the data collection. In other words, the context comes first. A researcher finds a setting to be of interest, records or collects data, and then analyzes it to see what sort of patterns or interesting features emerge, and then develops a question. This question may be addressed by more qualitative data, or sometimes by a more quantitative study. This is a cyclical approach to research. An example of a study like this might be an examination of teachers' beliefs and classroom interaction. A researcher may have a sense that the beliefs of teachers were interest-ing, and on collecting observational, sometimes ethnographic, data, might come to the conclusion that questions that might be interesting to address in the data focused on the efficacy of feedback and the need (or not) to provide learners with opportunities to talk freely, and opportunities to be corrected and self-correct would shape the learning opportunities through interaction in their classroom. The initial context, the classroom, and the teacher and their beliefs would inter-actively drive the research such that questions and patterns emerged from the data.

In quantitative research, the questions typically guide and dictate the design of the research and are focused as narrowly as possible. We often talk about trying to make research questions "elegant" and warn about putting too much detail in the question that should really be relegated to the methodology section. For example, "How do ESL learners who are between the ages of 18 and 24 respond to picture-difference task-based interaction in terms of their development of English past tense and relative clauses?" might be unnecessarily detailed. A simpler, easier to process question might say "How do ESL learners develop in terms of grammar following tasks?" The information about age, the type of tasks, and the type of grammatical development are specifics which can be placed in hypotheses, tested, and explained in the operationalization section of the methodology. ESL learners, for example, have many more characteristics than just age, and it would be important to specify as many as possible, for example, L1, gender, prior knowledge, education, and so on. Of course, a study can also include questions that are more quantitatively oriented, or questions that are framed in a more open-ended way, representing a mixed design.

Research questions need to be interesting in the sense that they address topical issues. They should also be timely; in other words, researchers, practitioners, and others should be interested in the answers at the time the study is being carried out. Finally, they also need to be phrased in such a way that they can be answered. Put another way, the study should be feasible.

Another common problem is that the initial questions people think of are sometimes too wide. It is much easier to address wide questions if they are broken into more constrained and easily answerable questions. For example, a fairly general research question such as "What is the relationship between the native language and interaction-driven L2 learning?" is interesting, but difficult to answer. This is because the notion of exactly what interaction-driven L2 learning is needs to be operationalized or explained in such a way that it can be measured. For example, are we talking about interaction in the sense of tasks? Two or more interlocutors? Classroom, naturalistic, or experimental? Interaction in the sense of some very specific feature like a recast, or just in general? You would also need a lot of learners, given how many native languages there are. But all of this doesn't mean it's not an interesting question. To begin to break it down into a more researchable topic, we might want to think about investigating the relationship between native language and a specific aspect of interaction-driven learning (e.g., phonology or syntax). We can also pose and constrain wide general questions by asking about learning a second language that has an aspect of language that is not the same in the first language. Narrowing this down to a more specific question, we might ask, for example, "How do online clarification requests in gaming chats affect the use of definite articles by L1 Russian learners of English?" This is one specific angle on the original, broad topic, but one where we could actually start to investigate this question. We make a comparison between L1 speakers of another language and Russian, for example, Chinese, since Mandarin L1 speakers often have issues with English articles too. We would then move along to wondering whether to examine production or comprehension in order to come up with specific hypotheses and a design.

2.5 Where Do Research Questions Come From?

Above, I say that research investigations should be current or timely. By this, I mean that questions should not have already been answered by existing studies, or if addressed by previous research, should have only partially been answered, leaving space for the new study. This should be considered along with evidence that people are interested in the answer at the time you do the study. You can check this by looking at the conclusion and future work sections in recent journal articles and book chapters on similar or related, or peruse conferences for paper titles and abstracts that relate to the topic. Obviously, if your research idea is mentioned in recent books, and has not been addressed, these are all good signs that people are still interested in the answers.

Research questions also need to be theoretically or methodologically interesting in some way. Again, we get ideas about this from our reading of the literature as well as from classes, courses, or conference presentations, or from actual teaching or learning contexts in which we are involved. To help with this, below are some examples of questions emerging from journal articles. The first is a study of pragmatic development during study abroad that specifically focuses on Spanish teenagers' request strategies in English emails. The second focuses on the use of models as corrective feedback in English as a Foreign Language writing.

Read It!

Alcón-Soler, E. (2017). Pragmatic development during study abroad: An analysis of Spanish teenagers' request strategies in English emails. *Annual Review of Applied Linguistics*, *37*, 77–92.

"Further research should examine learners' pragmatic development holistically rather than with a focus on specific pragmatic features. Second, the qualitative analysis was relatively small, as this study focused on the detailed development of two learners. While enlightening, this narrow focus makes it difficult to generalize to other learners. More case studies should be added to future analyses. In addition, our data suggest that changes in the teacher–student relationship during study abroad may also influence performance and patterns of pragmatic change. This could be assessed systematically in future work.

Further studies are also needed to understand young learners' pragmatic development across language learning contexts. This study explored the effects of pragmatic instruction in the production and perception of email requests during study abroad. Another interesting setting in which to explore young learners' pragmatic gains beyond the classroom is in lingua franca (House, 2010) and multilingual contexts. As reported by Safont and Portolés, (2015, 2016) and Martín-Laguna (2016), younger learners' pragmatic production and awareness may benefit from proficiency and competence in multiple languages and cultural contexts" (p. 89).

Read It!

García Mayo, M. D. P. & Labandibar, U. (2017). The use of models as written corrective feedback in English as a foreign language (EFL) writing. *Annual Review of Applied Linguistics, 37*, 110–127.

"Third, the future research agenda should investigate learners' beliefs by using more sophisticated questionnaires, interviews, observations, or diaries, since these individual differences seem to have a great influence on the relationship between noticing and language learning. It should also consider whether more detailed guidance than the one provided in this study would lead to higher noticing quality. Finally, the results of the study may be regarded as evidence of uptake rather than acquisition. Future studies should use longitudinal designs to investigate the long-term effects of modeling as well as the evolution in learners' beliefs as they become more familiar with the feedback technique" (p. 123).

The questions raised by these two research articles are based on critical topics like how findings might be affected by using different methods, how recruiting more participants in different contexts might contribute to findings, and how tracking development longitudinally may impact findings. These are all quite common ways for research articles to end. Particularly in the case of longitudinal development, it has been quite popular in the last three decades for researchers to call for more of it. Regretfully, most of us are not doing anything that involves more than a three-month delayed post-test. There is still a significant need in the interaction, feedback, and task area, as with many areas of L2 research, for serious longitudinal research with learners. I believe Ph.D. students who take this sort of work on will be well rewarded in the future in the form of citations.

2.6 Longitudinal Research

It is possible that the need for longitudinal research may be met along with the need for more situated and interpretative research in this area. This is because most of the longitudinal studies in our field are case studies, which might lend themselves well to qualitative and interpretive analysis. For example, in a synthesis of research on the so-called critical period in second language acquisition, Hyltenstam and Abrahamsson (2003) argued in favor of more longitudinal work, including in-depth individual case studies of so-called black swans, or exceptional late-onset second language learners who achieve equivalent to native speaker like levels of ultimate attainment in their second language. Although started many years before the Hyltenstam and Abrahamsson call, Donna Lardiere's (2007) *Ultimate Attainment in Second Language Acquisition: A Case Study* describes her two-decade-long work with an adult immigrant learner of English. Patty, a Chinese-American, earned introductory and advanced degrees at U.S. institutions, has a native English speaking spouse, and many native English speaker friends with whom she socializes as well as a challenging managerial job. However, Patty's speech is not "nativelike" even after more than two decades of daily interaction with native speakers. This has important theoretical implications for linguistics, and Lardiere's careful analysis of linguistic features is fascinating. However, Lardiere is interested in questions of a theory other than the cognitive-interactionist one, and thus this case study is as interesting for the questions it raises (What does Patty notice about her interactions, her own and others' productions? Do her interlocutors ever correct her? How? Is she aware of her own patterns of errors, like omitting past-tense markers? Does she care, having achieved communication?) as the questions it answers.

2.7 Looking for Gaps in the Literature

Another way we find questions in the existing literature involves looking for gaps. Most research methods texts mention this as a source of questions. For example, we might notice that something has not been controlled for in a study that we otherwise enjoyed, or we might wonder if different settings like classrooms or labs would lead to learners responding differently. Also, a contradiction may remain. In any case, this information may turn out to form the basis of a follow-up study. For example, in their call for future research in the second example above, García Mayo and Labandibar argue that their results indicate uptake, but not acquisition, and rightly call for longitudinal studies investigating the long-term effects of modeling. This is a great example of a gap in the interaction literature that needs to be filled, and it's good to keep in mind that studies will often end with this type of suggestion for ways to carry the field forward.

It's important though, to make sure that no one else has carried out a study. Often when a researcher makes a suggestion in their conclusions section about follow-on work, they decide to do this work themselves. Because papers are published later than conference presentations and work actually being done, you need to find out if someone else got there first, particularly the original author. Authors will often raise a question in their conclusion that their current work is investigating. So, a good next step, if you see an interesting suggestion, is to try to contact the author to make sure they aren't already working on their own follow-up and if not, whether they know if anyone else is.

Another helpful step in this process is to do a comprehensive Google search, or consult a citation index (librarians can help with these) to locate work that has cited the paper on which you will be basing your study.

Try It!

How to do a comprehensive Google search.

- Choose your database wisely. Google will give the most comprehensive results but may produce an overwhelming amount of data, including many unrelated articles. Google Scholar (https://scholar.google.com/), will produce only academic articles, which may be more manageable. There are also databases that will only query linguistics articles such as the LLBA (Linguistics and Language Behavior Abstracts – visit www.proquest.com for more information) and other websites like ResearchGate.

- Carefully choose search terms. Make sure to include common synonyms for your key words. For example, you might want to search for task-based language teaching, AND task-based language learning AND communicative language teaching. Depending on the database you can also use search terms like AND, OR, + to combine searches, the minus sign (–) to exclude words, and quotation marks (" ...") for exact matches.
- Keep track of where you have already searched and which search terms you used to avoid missing any key work or searching through the same material multiple times.
- Once you have found relevant articles, examine the articles the authors have cited to find more sources. Most scholars also have their own pages on Google Scholar where they list all of their publications. These can also be helpful to examine to make sure all work from a particular author is covered. ResearchGate and Orchid are other searchable sites where authors list their work.

Try It!

How to consult citation indices and conduct backward citation searches.

- Choose a database that links all articles referenced to the source articles. Common ones to choose from are Web of Science (www.webofknowledge .com) or Scopus (www.scopus.com).
- From within the database choose to conduct a "cited reference search" and enter information about a relevant article (authors, title, year, or some combination), confirm the article and click "search."
- The database will produce all the references of work that has previously cited the work you searched for. These articles may provide more relevant work for your current project.
- Web of Science will also tell you how many times each of the referenced articles have been cited so that you can be sure to start from the most influential articles to speed up your search.

2.8 Finding Questions in Your Own Contexts

Ideas for interaction and task-based research also often stem from observing learners either in or out of a classroom context, from being a learner or an instructor, or from some curiosity having observed a certain type of non-native speaker linguistic behavior or participated in it. The study that was published as Mackey, Gass, and McDonough (2000), "How do learners perceive interactional feedback?" emerged from the work I did for my dissertation. During my Ph.D. dissertation research, I was sitting in a room in a private English-speaking school, collecting data. The room had windows that partially looked out over Bondi beach in Sydney, Australia. My participants had to keep their minds and eyes on the tasks, and I made sure they did that, rather than looking out of the window. I had already modified the task so even if they weren't talking, they were just watching, they still had to draw a picture or supply a piece of information at the end that they could only give if they paid (some) attention to the task. I did the same, or similar, tasks across five different sessions with my participants, and by the fifth session I kept finding myself wondering what they were thinking, literally what was going through their minds as they looked at the pictures, and either put them in order, or asked each other questions to follow a map, or spotted the differences, and so on. I was trying to get them to produce questions in English and sometimes they did, sometimes they didn't. By the end of the study, in the final post-test, that question just would not go away for me. One time I involuntarily interrupted a participant who had just corrected himself. First, he said something like "You go up?" and then he said, "Do you go straight?" and I just asked him: "What were you thinking just then, when you said that?" This question wasn't part of my dissertation study. I had not thought about it ahead of time. I was just wondering, and I did not want to mess up my data, so as soon as I realized it, I said: "Sorry, don't answer that, just ignore me!" He did. But it made me think – what if I had a different group, and I asked them that question?

A few months later, I found myself in my first job at Michigan State University with Susan M. Gass, who became my great friend and frequent co-author, and I said to her, "Don't you ever wonder, we get learners to move objects, talk about pictures, draw things, all to manipulate what they say, and we're so interested in what they're saying, but we never ask them what they're actually thinking when they produce language. What's going through their minds. Are they thinking about the grammar? What parts of it?" Sue was right on it, as always. She said, "OK, let's do it." Sue was also interested in Italian and suggested a different dimension, the second versus foreign language angle, would that make a difference? We started talking about whether asking them in their L1 or their L2 would make a difference.

And so, the basic research question was formed in Bondi, the method we were just shooting in the dark with. I began talking to a master's student I had then, who was very productive and enthusiastic and one of those people who makes things happen. She had already been at MSU for a semester before I got there, so she knew how things worked, and how to get participants, and so we began to plan it out. Her name is Kim McDonough, and she is now an extremely successful and productive interaction researcher and professor. At that point, I started reading to try to make sure we didn't mess the data collection up. We piloted. Once, I went completely off script and the participant was obviously not talking about what they were thinking about at the time of the original interaction but had instead moved into the here and now. Through trial and error, we realized we didn't want the here and now processing, we wanted there and then processing. We worked out the connection to Schmidt's Noticing Hypothesis and in the literature I found to my complete surprise there was already a name for this "ask them what they were thinking" technique, as well as the fact that we'd been showing them videos to jog their memories (we started with transcripts), and it was "stimulated recall."

This study led to a book (Gass & Mackey, 2005), and to the importation and use of the method in SLA research, where, other than in a few writing studies, it had not been used at all before. Now, of course, it is a relatively mainstream method, and, as we show in the revised and much expanded edition of the book (Gass & Mackey, 2017), stimulated recall is now used in an increasing number of sub-areas of the L2 research field. This is just one example of how research context can lead to a study and contribute to the body of research and methodology in SLA as a whole. For more stories like this, see the final chapter of the book.

2.9 Online Contexts and Social Media

Increasingly, scholars also publish, promote, and discuss their research online via sites such as ResearchGate, Academia.edu and on social media like Twitter or Facebook, where researchers will often point to their blogs on places like Wordpress and their Google Scholar profiles. If you're curious about what a researcher is working on or who they're working with, these sites can help you keep up with or even keep in touch with researchers whose studies interest you. For example, Luke Plonsky, a highly prolific scholar currently at Northern Arizona University, who published one of the first investigations into quality in interaction research (Plonsky & Gass, 2011), maintains a Wordpress site (https://lukeplonsky.wordpress.com/) with resources like helpful bibliographies, as well as a Facebook page (https://bit.ly/35C12YU), focusing on research methodology.

Another prolific researcher, Andrea Révész, who publishes on task-based language teaching often through integrating new technologies such as eye-tracking (e.g., Révész & Gurzynski-Weiss, 2016), has offered MOOC (Massive Open Online Courses) on websites such as Coursera (www.coursera.org) on topics relevant to researchers and language teachers such as "Teaching EFL/ESL Reading: A Task-Based Approach" (www.coursera.org/learn/esl-reading). These courses can also be excellent sources for research questions, as can what is often referred to as "academic Twitter."

Try It!

Go to the latest issue of the *Annual Review of Applied Linguistics*, *Applied Linguistics*, or *The Journal of Second Language Writing*. Find an article on an interaction topic that interests you and go to the end of the article and note the suggestions for future research given by the author. Write down at least three possible studies you would like to carry out based on the author's suggestions. Then, go to ResearchGate, Academia.edu, Twitter, and Google Scholar, and see (1) if the author(s) of the study you chose have recently published any research updates in the area of the article you read, and (2) what are the three most recent publications in that area, by any author. Having done this, (3) reflect on whether you would then go forward and carry out one of the three possible studies you came up with.

2.10 How Do We Know If Our Studies Are Feasible?

The feasibility of a research question in the area of interaction, feedback, or tasks will be based on a range of issues, some of which I have discussed (e.g. how answerable a research question is depending on the scope). We also need to think about whether we can get the right type of data to answer a question, when considering feasibility. Think about a study where you decide to conduct a survey on the individual identities of learners, and how it might impact their responses to feedback in interaction. In order to do this, it's important to define what you mean by identity and also to decide if you want the participants in your study to share the same identity markers. For example, you might ask how people who self-identify as introverts, extroverts, or introverted extroverts (and vice versa) report responding to feedback from their fellow students in a language classroom. If this was your question, you would need to choose participants who meet your definition of identity in a number reasonable enough to make the study interesting and/or statistically significant, if that interests you. How many people do you think you would need? That would depend on what you want to do with the study – present it in an end of semester project or at a conference, or publish it in a tier-one or tier-two journal or as a book chapter.

Another relevant study might seek to compare the linguistic development of learners, measured by changes in performance (improvements in accuracy, for example), on different communication task types. As will become clear throughout this book, there are multiple important dimensions on which communicative tasks can differ. However, asking participants to do ten different tasks is probably not feasible. Participants might get bored, hungry, tired, or annoyed, and the results would not provide reliable data on which to base the answer to the questions, especially if exhaustion, drift, and boredom set in, and the researcher would not know how to interpret the results. This doesn't mean a study looking at ten different tasks couldn't be done; it just means it has to involve participants who are up for taking part in the multiple rounds of data collection such a study would entail. In summary then, as we say in Mackey and Gass (2005, p. 19) "any study should be designed with a full understanding of the fact that the limitations of the setting and the population might constrain the research."

2.11 Thinking about Interaction, Feedback, and Task-Based Research: What Are Hypotheses? What Are Predictions?

In primarily quantitative, experimental, or quasi-experimental research, the ways we address a research problem usually focus on stating a problem, which is motivated by a literature review, and which logically leads to research questions which are often followed by hypotheses or predictions. As I have written elsewhere (e.g., Mackey & Gass, 2016), and as most research methodology texts point out, both hypotheses and predictions are how we, as researchers, expect the answers to the questions we asked in the research to look. Hypotheses are usually formulated quite precisely, sometimes as "null" hypotheses that we would look to reject by using inferential statistical analyses. If we can't make a clear hypothesis based in the literature because perhaps there isn't enough prior research, or perhaps what exists is contradictory, and we aren't able to clearly estimate what will happen, prediction is often a less firm notion of what might happen, based on patterns we've observed, in other data, for example. In a recent study by Nassaji (2019) that compared the effects of prompts versus recasts for the acquisition of English relative clauses by ESL learners, the author noted that the results of many prior studies comparing these structures found conflicting results. The author noted that the difficulty of the target structure and the proficiency level of the learners can play a role and therefore included these features as variables in the study.

2.12 Open Science: Materials and Data in the Interaction, Feedback, and Task Areas

A typical sort of phrasing when writing up research in our field is something along the following lines: "taken together, these results suggest the following..." For example, in a study by Li, Zhu, and Ellis (2016) "a closer look at the results suggests that the immediate feedback was superior" (p. 34). What we need to remember is that it is important that we don't only read articles like this, but that we also read the primary sources that the author is referring to, because if we don't, all we have is the author's interpretation of the literature and/or their own results.

With the advent of open science practices, it will be increasingly important for us to look at the instruments, and how the data were collected, as well as the original data, to see if we would interpret it the same way the researcher has. The *Annual Review of Applied Linguistics* in its 2020 issue presents an article by Nicklin and Plonsky (2020) which will be among the first articles in the L2 research field to present open access to the materials, methods, data, and sample analyses so that readers can re-analyze the data for themselves. Another study by Saito, Macmillan, Mai, et al. (2020) from the same issue will share their data in the same way. It is likely that other journals and authors will follow suit. Interaction, feedback, and task research is, in general, well-suited to open science practices, given its reliance on tasks, which can easily be stored in repositories like the IRIS database (www.iris-database.org) and clear coding practices. Such open science practices and articles can also be used to generate research questions. For example, the IRIS database is searchable by population, task type, linguistic feature (and a range of others), and also contains some datasets, searchable by data, so that identifying potential gaps, which can then be checked against the literature, is easy.

2.13 Examples of Research Questions and Hypotheses

I am going to illustrate both research questions and hypotheses by talking about a comprehensive study by Zalbidea (2017). Her study explored the independent and interactive effects of task complexity and modality on L2 Spanish performance, as mediated by working memory capacity (WMC). Below are two research questions from this study (p. 339):

RQ 1   How do task complexity and task modality affect global and task-specific measures of L2 output?

RQ 2   How does WMC relate to measures of L2 output in more or less complex tasks? Are relationships different based on task modality?

These research questions are expressed as explorations of relationships. Zalbidea formulated hypotheses too. Examples of hypotheses stemming from these research questions are given next (p. 339):

Hypothesis 1   Task complexity will affect the complexity and accuracy of L2 output.

Hypothesis 2   Modality is predicted to differentially affect dimensions of complexity and accuracy among L2 learners in response to task complexity.

Hypothesis 3   WMC will be related to dimensions of L2 output to a greater extent on more complex tasks.

Hypothesis 4   WMC can be expected to relate to different output dimensions across modalities.

When developing research questions, it's important to keep in mind that having too many research questions in a study can make it overly long and possibly too complicated. Researchers often take one dataset, and produce two or more studies from it, each focusing on different aspects. In doing that, good judgment is important. Too much use of the same data without complete differentiation of research questions may be problematic. An interesting short paper on this, from a different field, is entitled "Salami slicing of datasets: What the young researcher needs to know" (Menon & Muraleedharan, 2016). The authors argue that "[e]-xpert consensus is that if the 'slice' of the study in question tests a different hypothesis as opposed to the larger study or has a distinct methodology or populations being studied, then it is acceptable to publish it separately" (p. 577) but go on to warn (amongst other things) that "salami slicing of data may do more harm than good to a researcher's career over time because it significantly reduces their chances of publishing in high impact journals, thereby lending lesser weight to their accrued body of work" (p. 577).

However, it is important to note that the paper is from the medical field, and therefore patterns may be somewhat field-specific. In some pscholinguistics research, three or four experiments are often reported in one paper, but using different data and methods. In this case, there is no slicing. For example, a study by Rebuschat and Williams (2012) investigated whether second language acquisition can also result in implicit or unconscious knowledge in two different experiments reported in the same article published in *Applied Psycholinguistics*.

Read It!

Rebuschat, P. & Williams, J. N. (2012). Implicit and explicit knowledge in second language acquisition. *Applied Psycholinguistics*, *33*(4), 829–856.

Experiment 1
In experiment 1, thirty-five English speakers learned an artificial language based on German syntax. They were split into an experimental group and a control group. The participants in the experimental group were exposed to this semiartificial language through incidental learning conditions by means of plausibility judgments (i.e. after exposure to the new language, they were asked whether some sentences seemed plausible in this new language or not). Then all the participants completed a grammaticality judgment task where they were instructed to endorse sentences that obeyed the rules as grammatical and reject ones that did not as ungrammatical. Results from experiment 1 found a learning effect in the experimental group but only for participants that developed conscious knowledge of the new rules.

Experiment 2
The second experiment had a different methodology. In this experiment there were new rules for the artificial language and experimental group participants received training via elicited imitations and plausibility judgements. In the testing phase participants were allowed to guess at their confidence in their answers. Experiment 2 recruited a new group of 30 participants. Results from Experiment 2 found that the experimental group statistically outperformed the control group. The experimental participants also rated themselves as more confident in their correct answers. Participants also performed significantly above chance when they reported they based their decisions on rule knowledge or on intuition suggesting they had acquired some unconscious structural knowledge.

> **Keep It in Mind!**
>
> Studies with many research questions and varying methods are often broken up and published as different papers. However, authors should take care not to republish the exact same data and analyses. In some psycholinguistic studies, multiple related experiments are often reported on together in the same article.

So far, I've talked about designing a study from scratch, where research questions come from and the importance of hypotheses and predictions, along with feasibility. But there is also another way to do research into interaction, feedback, and tasks, and that involves replication. In other words, we can look at what's already been done and verify the results by repeating it. The repetition can be done the same way or changing some small aspect of it. Compared to other fields, applied linguistics and second language acquisition in general hasn't done too much in the way of replication, although this is certainly changing. There are now replication sections in some of our journals (e.g. *Studies in Second Language Acquisition*), and book length treatments of the topic exist (e.g. Porte, 2012; Porte & McManus, 2019). General methods textbooks usually include a chapter on replication too, for example a chapter by Rebekha Abbuhl in Phakiti, De Costa, Plonsky, et al.'s (2018) *The Palgrave Handbook of Applied Linguistics Research Methodology* as well as my own chapter "Why (or why not), when and how to replicate research" (Mackey, 2012b) in Porte's earlier book.

2.14 Replication Studies in Research on Interaction, Feedback, and Tasks in Language Learning

Many researchers are now aware of the controversy within the field of social psychology, which, like the second language research field, was an area where few replications had been published until relatively recently, and where, unfortunately, some of the landmark studies failed to replicate. For more information, see, for example, the special issue of *Social Psychology* edited by Nosek and Lakens (2014), where the Registered Reports replications failed to confirm the results in ten of thirteen studies. The larger scale ManyLabs project (Laws, 2016) though, involved thirty-six research groups across twelve different countries who replicated thirteen psychological studies with more than 6,000 participants. Interestingly, ten of the thirteen effects replicated consistently across thirty-six different samples (there was variability in the effect size reported compared to the primary studies). This effect is not restricted to social psychology, as other areas of psychology also have failed to replicate. Stanley, Carter and Doucouliagos' 2018 survey of 200 meta-analyses, found "psychological research is, on average, afflicted with low statistical power."

The most recent findings based on the Center for Open Science's ManyLabs 2 report (Klein, 2018) involved 186 researchers from sixty different laboratories (representing thirty-six different nationalities from six different continents) and their replications of twenty-eight classic and contemporary findings in psychology in general studied (a) whether or not the findings from the original papers replicated, and (b) how much findings varied as a function of variations in samples and contexts. Of the twenty-eight findings, fourteen failed to replicate despite very large sample sizes. Interestingly, though, if a finding did replicate, that result held true across most other samples, while if a finding did not replicate, that finding was also true with little variation across samples and contexts.

Replication studies are done much more typically in other fields than in the L2 research area, although things are changing (for more information on this, see the discussion of registered replications and diversity of participants in Chapter 9). In other fields, findings may not be considered to be part of knowledge until they have been through a careful process of replication. As Graeme Porte points out, though, in his introduction to his edited collection *Replication Research in Applied Linguistics* (2012), in the social sciences, "undertaking replication studies has acquired negative connotations" (p. 4). Porte also notes, like others have, that replication research is less prestigious than "original" research in its status in professional journals and in the academic community in general. Likewise, original research has traditionally been considered more important by tenure and promotion processes, by committees that determine awards, and even by journal editors. In many university settings, students are discouraged from replicating a previous study in choosing their dissertation topics, with advisors and supervisors encouraging them to be original. However, many other researchers have said that doing replication research can be a very valuable learning tool, providing important opportunities for novice researchers and graduate students to follow in the footprints of others, learning as they go, as noted by Abbuhl (2018), amongst others. In *Doing Replication Research in Applied Linguistics*, Graeme Porte and Kevin McManus (2019) walk researchers through the steps involved in replication. In summary then, as replication and open science practices expand in all sorts of different fields, it seems safe to conclude we should be directing our energies to replications in interaction, feedback, and task research too.

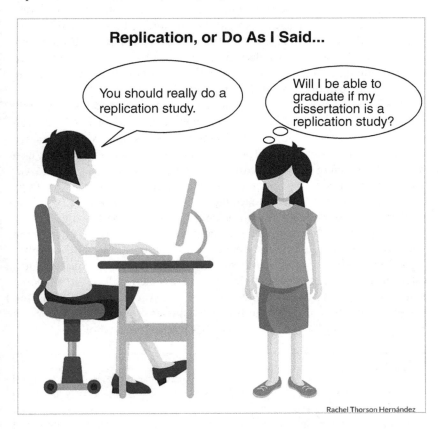

Figure 2.1 On replications

2.15 IRIS: A Source of Instruments for Interaction, Feedback, and Task Research

As I mentioned earlier in this chapter, the Instruments for Research into Second Languages (IRIS) project (www.iris-database.org) is a free uploadable and downloadable database of instruments for second language research. As part of the early movement in second language research, Emma Marsden, at the University of York, and I co-founded

IRIS. The database serves as a repository for elicitation tools and was established in 2010. IRIS holds almost 4,000 different sorts of tools, all of which can be used for replication and some datasets. Our purpose was to promote open science practices in second language research, as we discuss in articles like Marsden and Mackey (2014) and Marsden, Mackey, and Plonsky (2016). The Open Science Framework (https://osf.io) was also established in 2011 and this important initiative provides guidance and support on a wide range of open science practices including, for example, open data repositories.

IRIS is particularly helpful for interaction, feedback, and task research. For example, it can be searched by terms like, "Type of Materials" and it can display coding sheets, communicative/interactive tasks, tests, introspective techniques, interview protocols, questionnaires, and much more. It is also possible to search by linguistic feature under investigation (e.g., morphosyntax, phonetics, phonology, pragmatics, syntax), general research area (e.g., error correction, motivation, teaching methods) the L1(s) or L2(s) of the participants, and the types and proficiency levels of the participants.

If you are interested in finding the materials from a particular publication you have read, it is also searchable by author, publication date, or other identifying features. After identifying the publication that you are interested in, you are able to freely download a zip file of all of the available materials. In this way, IRIS enables researchers to stop reinventing the wheel for materials on a new study, which enables replication and supports more generalizability in applied linguistics research as a whole.

> **Try It!**
>
> Go to www.iris-database.org and click "Search and Download." Type keywords that relate to your research interests or click "see everything in IRIS" to see the filters available. Find an article you have read or that seems related to your area and download the instruments. Would you be able to replicate the study with the information provided? Why or why not? Would you be able to use these materials in a study of your own? Why or why not?

2.16 What Are the Difficult Parts about Doing Replications in SLA/Interaction?

Not all researchers agree you can do replications easily. In a topical and comprehensive paper, Marsden, Morgan-Short, Thompson, et al. (2018) provide a narrative review of challenges related to replication. They go on to report a study of sixty-seven L2 replication studies from twenty-six journals, finding a mean rate of one published replication study for every 400 articles. They note that replication studies were cited with a mean of 7.3 times per year and note that this is a higher rate than mean citations in linguistics and education. Additional interesting findings were that where there was some authorship overlap between the original study and the replication or where the original materials were used, the chance of a replication supporting the initial findings was improved. They finished their article by making sixteen recommendations relating to rationale, naming, design, infrastructure, and incentivization in relation to replications.

Another helpful paper in the area of not underestimating the difficulty of replication work is by Numa Markee, "Are replication studies possible in qualitative second/foreign language classroom research? A call for comparative re-production research" (2017). Markee makes a case that all replications are not created equal. As he notes, before replicating a study, we first need to explain why it should be replicated. We might pick a study that is exciting and fascinating, but it might not be feasible to replicate without making multiple methodological changes which could mean that the new study is different from the primary study. If we pick a study to replicate, we need to be sure that the primary study is clearly reported. Often, critical details that would allow replication are missing from the report. Problems with lack of information concern things like language proficiency, so finding an equivalent is difficult to determine in replication studies. This sort of thing can sometimes be sorted out by an email to the primary study's author(s) but authors are not always happy to hear that there are plans to replicate their work, sometimes due to the way the social science replication "crisis" has been reported in the media, and so they might not respond to potential replicators. This under-specification in papers is not always or even often the fault of the primary study author(s). Many journals don't have enough space for detailed information regarding participant descriptions, settings, contexts of experimental conditions, and coding systems. This is why open science movements are so exciting and relevant. Repositories like IRIS hold instruments and there are moves towards open data too.

Try It!

Take a look through three of the latest issues of the journals listed below, search on keywords of interaction, or corrective feedback, or tasks, according to your interests, and answer the following questions:

1. Were any of the articles you found replication studies? How many?
2. If so, in what sense of the word were they replications?
3. How many of the articles published in the latest issue of the three journals you looked at included commentary on the *need* for replication studies?
4. Does the trend of asking for replications, but not publishing them appear to continue?

Annual Review of Applied Linguistics
Applied Linguistics
The Journal of Second Language Writing
Language Teaching Research
Modern Language Journal
TESOL Quarterly
Studies in Second Language Acquisition
System

2.17 What Are the Areas of Interaction, Feedback, and Task Research Where Replication Studies Would Be Helpful?

In general, we only want to replicate research where we believe the study is sound to begin with. So, as we have discussed in this chapter, a study should have theoretically interesting and currently relevant research questions. If gaps or shortcomings in existing studies exist, and you have a sense they could be repaired with replications, that would also be a good sign. For example, if an initial study of tasks and planning failed to control for an important variable, or omitted a control group for tests only, then a replication study that identified a problem and controlled that variable would be interesting. You can also choose studies to look at in terms of generalizability. For example, would the results be the same if the setting were changed (e.g., laboratory results extending to the classroom or classrooms that were differently focused in nature) or different languages studied, or with learners of different ages (younger versus older children)? People often point to problems with participant numbers, their L1 backgrounds, or other individual difference variables, and express interest about whether their results would hold if the study was carried out with these different variables. All these are essentially invitations to researchers to do replications.

Some of the interesting controversies in the field can be addressed by adding replications to the mix. For example, some researchers have suggested that more studies on the effects of feedback in laboratory settings seem to have positive outcomes than classroom contexts. Not all classroom contexts, where multiple participants and usually only one instructor participate in feedback episodes, show positive results, but then again, not all classrooms are equal, and some do, while some don't (for example, see Goo & Mackey, 2013a, Lyster & Ranta, 2013, and Goo & Mackey, 2013b for both sides of a debate on the effectiveness of recasts).

Keep It in Mind!

- The development process for research questions in qualitative research is often quite different than for quantitative research.
- A study should be designed with a full understanding of the fact that the limitations of the setting and the population might constrain the research.
- Research questions are the questions for which answers are being sought, whereas hypotheses and predictions can be used to express what the researcher expects the results of the investigation to be.
- Replication is an important part of research, but replication studies are often overlooked in the world of publishing due to their lack of a "wow" factor.
- Open Science is an important and increasing trend in applied linguistics and second language research.

CHAPTER THREE

Investigating Individual Differences in Interaction, Feedback, and Task Studies: Aptitude, Working Memory, Cognitive Creativity, and New Findings in L2 Learning

Interaction, feedback, and task researchers often want to know more about the nature of the cognitive processes that occur while language learners are being exposed to second or foreign languages. This applies when learners are hearing (or sometimes reading) or producing language that occurs in interaction and the feedback that results, and often tasks are part of their experiences. In other words, we want to know what is going on inside learners' heads because we believe this might help us understand more about language learning. We differentiate between learners' minds (cognition tools) and their brains, where we focus on imaging. I discuss imaging in the next chapter because importantly (and perhaps strangely), the mind and brain are not usually considered to be isomorphic. Interaction, feedback and task researchers typically turn to cognitive and psycholinguistics-based research tools to help us uncover information about individual differences and their relation to learning.

In the current chapter, I describe tools and techniques for researching the increasingly popular area of individual differences, specifically constructs like aptitude, working memory, and cognitive creativity. I ask how these tools might be used to help answer relevant research questions about their relationship to learning through interaction, feedback, and tasks. Because cognitive creativity, in particular, is a relatively understudied construct to date in this research area, I also provide data from two new studies, published for the first time in this book.

For researchers studying how learners' interaction, feedback, or task performance in a second language relates to their linguistic development, the mediating factor played by their individual differences can be extremely interesting. Some examples include interaction-driven learning, and whether or not learners benefit from recasts if they have more, less, or different types of aptitude, or working memory scores, or both. Although there are several individual differences that are interesting and relevant in this line of research, here we will focus on aptitude and working memory, where there have been a good number of studies to date, after which we will move on to the relatively understudied area of cognitive creativity, finishing by presenting the new data from two studies in this area.

3.1 Aptitude

The construct of aptitude covers a variety of cognitive differences that have been argued by some researchers to be reliable predictors of certain types of subsequent language learning achievement (Abrahamsson & Hyltenstam, 2008; Robinson, 2005). It's certainly worthwhile, then, for interaction, feedback, and task researchers to be aware of how this construct has been operationalized and measured, particularly since quite a few studies in the interaction, feedback, and task areas have discussed or measured aptitude in some way (for example, Yilmaz, 2013; Yilmaz & Granena, 2016; see overviews in Dörnyei & Skehan, 2005; Skehan, 2015; Wen et al., 2017) and have raised interesting ongoing questions that should be addressed by more research in this area.

Aptitude first came to the attention of second language researchers with Carroll and Sapon's (1959) Modern Language Aptitude Test (MLAT), which was followed shortly afterwards by Pimsleur's Language Aptitude Battery (1966). Today, variations on the MLAT are available for different populations of learners (https://bit.ly/2NvRg4v). The most current version of the MLAT has five basic sections. They gauge skills such as L2 phonetic coding ability, rote learning ability, grammatical sensitivity, and inductive language learning ability. For example, the Modern Language Aptitude Test – Elementary (MLAT–E) version for younger children (ages 8–11) also created by Carroll and Sapon, is described here: https://bit.ly/35LTVNw, and there is a version for L1 Spanish speakers (the MLAT–ES). Both of these are held by the Language Learning and Testing Foundation, Inc. (https://lltf.net). The MLAT is only available through this non-profit foundation, which usually only sells the test to clinical psychologists, missionary organizations, and government entities, as noted on their website, so researchers need to contact them if they are interested in using a version of the MLAT for research purposes. However, helpful examples of research studies that have used the MLAT appear in *Exploring Language Aptitude: Views from Psychology, the Language Sciences, and Cognitive Neuroscience*, edited by Susanne M. Reiterer (2018). This collection spans related factors ranging from music to vocabulary acquisition and phonology that might be relevant for specific types of interaction, corrective feedback and task studies.

Read It!

Winke, P. (2013). An investigation into second language aptitude for advanced Chinese language learning. *The Modern Language Journal*, *97*(1), 109–130.

"In this study I examine the construct of aptitude in learning Chinese as a second language (L2) to an advanced level. I test 2 hypotheses: first, that L2 aptitude comprises 4 components – working memory, rote memory, grammatical sensitivity, and phonemic coding ability – and second, that L2 aptitude affects learning both directly and indirectly (mediated by strategy use and motivation). Native speakers of English (*n* = 96) studying advanced Chinese took the Modern Language Aptitude Test and a phonological working memory test and responded to motivation and strategy use questionnaires. Using end-of-course listening, reading, and speaking proficiency test results as measures of Chinese learning, I constructed a structural equation model to test the hypotheses. The model fit the observed data. Of the 4 components foreseen to comprise L2 aptitude, rote memory contributed the most and working memory the least. Aptitude, strategy use, and motivation had about the same impact on learning but varied in how well they predicted the individual skills of listening, reading, and speaking. The results shed light on L2 aptitude in the particular context of an advanced L2 Chinese course" (p. 109).

Try It!

Even if you can't purchase the MLAT, you can try out sample questions on your own at the Language Learning and Testing Foundation website: http://lltf.net/mlat-sample-items/. There you will find questions and answers for each of the five parts of the test. Since some parts of the test are administered aurally, consider trying it out with a friend, so that you can read parts to each other aloud for a more authentic experience.

Although widely used, the MLAT is focused on a person's potential for language learning results at a basic level. Winke (2018) points out that despite its broad use, the MLAT is not effective at predicting language learning success at advanced levels. As a reaction to the need for more proficient speakers of languages relevant to military efforts following the attacks of September 11, 2001, the Department of Defense funded the University of Maryland with a Center then known as the Center for the Advanced Study of Language (CASL) to develop a new aptitude test that would predict an adult's ability to learn a language to a high degree of proficiency in a short amount of time (Erard, 2014). The High-Level Language Aptitude Battery (Hi-LAB) (Doughty et al., 2007) tests working memory, associative memory, long-term memory retrieval, implicit learning, processing speed, and auditory perceptual acuity (phonemic discrimination) (Wen et al., 2017) to provide reports that predict which learners will be able to achieve near-native proficiency as adults. The test is also being used to develop platforms for customized language learning that tailor programs for students based on their profiles (see Figure 3.1). Doughty (2018) describes the development process and provides empirical data, further explaining what MLAT and Hi-LAB can test, with the latter being better at predicting success in what Doughty calls "super-hard" languages (p. 7).

There has been considerable discussion in the literature of the nuances of whether aptitude measures can really predict rate of learning or ultimate success. Interestingly, despite the available tests, the relationship between aptitude test scores and the construct of aptitude, or whatever is meant by "aptitude" has not always been clear. Some other ideas that have been put forward in relation to aptitude and second language learning include the fact that aptitude might be related to skill development. For example, the Cognitive Ability for Novelty in Acquisition of Language as Applied to Foreign Language Testing (CANAL-FT) was developed by Grigorenko, Sternberg, and Ehrman (2000) and emphasizes how people cope with ambiguity and novelty in language learning. It has been used occasionally, for example by Thompson (2013) who used the CANAL-FT to show that language aptitude scores can be affected by previous language experience. In other words, participants who had bilingual or multilingual experience had higher language aptitude in that study.

While there have been some interesting initial studies, the question of how aptitude might be related to interaction, feedback, and task-based learning especially remains largely open, and seems likely to lead to many interesting studies in the future. For example, individuals who score highly on aspects like grammatical sensitivity might be better able to learn from recasts, which provide feedback in a usually implicit form, where the learner needs to make a cognitive comparison between what they said and what their interlocutor said, and remember the difference. This aspect of remembering brings us to another data collection tool from cognitive science: the measurement of memory.

The results of the Hi-LAB are reported in a 9-page aptitude profile. In addition to a general assessment of the Hi-LAB taker's overall strengths and weaknesses, individual scores are presented in comparison with similar individuals in the database (percentiles).

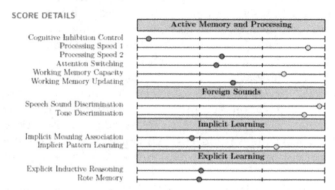

In order to help with application of the above results in pedagogy or self-study, the individual scores are grouped according to their aptitude contributions as noted in the aptitude battery test specifications. In other words, aptitude components which research evidence shows are relevant to key SLA processes are compiled as shown below (currently unweighted). The aptitude profile report provides prose explanations of the SLA processes themselves and describes learning at the ends of the continua, and subsequent pages offer examples of what learners and teachers can do in light of aptitude strengths and weaknesses revealed by the Hi-LAB results.

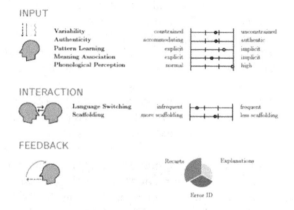

Figure 3.1 Hi-LAB profile (Doughty, personal communication)

3.2 Working Memory

There are many aspects of memory that are interesting to task and feedback researchers who are studying a potential relationship between aptitude, interaction, feedback, and other task-relevant constructs in a second language, either separately or in combination. Perhaps one of the most promising is working memory; a number of studies in the interaction and feedback area have successfully addressed the relationship between working memory and success in second language acquisition. Working memory involves not only storage capacity (what we usually think of when we hear the term "memory"), but also processing, which is what is meant by the word "working," in other words, doing something.

A number of early SLA studies investigated associations between scores on Phonological Short-Term Memory (PSTM) tests with outcomes in second language learning. These include Daneman and Case's (1981) early study from which work increased exponentially, for example, the book-length treatments edited by Wen (2016). In an early study employing artificial microlanguages, Williams and Lovatt (2003) found that PSTM was related to the learning of grammar rules. Some researchers, notably Miyake and Friedman (1998), have argued that word-span tasks and other measures of short-term storage capacity (e.g., digit span) are inappropriate for testing L2 learners' operational abilities because they do not involve dynamic, simultaneous processing and storage. Other studies (e.g., Harrington & Sawyer, 1992) show that measures of learners' abilities to both maintain and manipulate information (as in sentence-span tasks) correlate better with L2 comprehension skills than do the more passive digit- and word-span measures. In a study reported in Mackey, Adams, Stafford, et al. (2010), we looked at the relationship between working memory and output, concluding that individuals with greater working memory capacity produced more modified output in L2 Spanish interaction. We did some of the early studies in this general area too, for example, Mackey, Philp, Egi, et al. (2002). Working-memory tests were increasingly adopted into research in the interaction, feedback, and tasks area, for example by Mackey and Sachs (2012), Révész (2012), Sagarra (2007), and Trofimovich, Ammar, and Gatbonton (2007).

Another construct related to working memory is inhibitory control, that is, the ability to attend selectively to relevant input by blocking out irrelevant input. Based on Baddeley's (1986) working memory model, inhibitory control may play a mediating role in processing corrective feedback that is provided during a communicative task. Gass, Behney, and Uzum (2013) investigated the role of inhibition in processing oral corrective feedback by L2 learners of Italian during a face-to-face (FTF) picture-description task. Using the Stroop task, Gass et al. measured learners' inhibitory control ability and found that learners with higher inhibitory control benefited more from the corrective feedback than those with lower inhibitory control. In a recent study, Yilmaz and Sağdıç (2019) extended this line of research to synchronous computer-mediated conversation (CMC) learning contexts by examining the extent to which inhibitory control affected the acquisition of Spanish noun–adjective gender agreement through immediate or delayed reformulations, during a one-way information-gap picture description task. The researchers measured learners' inhibition with the non-verbal Flanker task and, unlike Gass et al.'s (2013) findings, they found no significant interaction between inhibitory control and learning outcomes under different feedback timing conditions, suggesting that task modality (i.e., CMC versus face-to-face communication) might moderate learners' executive function abilities and therefore their outcomes as well.

Read It!

Kim, Y., Payant, C., & Pearson, P. (2015). The intersection of task-based interaction, task complexity, and working memory: L2 question development through recasts in a laboratory setting. *Studies in Second Language Acquisition*, *37*, 549–581.

"The extent to which individual differences in cognitive abilities affect the relationship among task complexity, attention to form, and second language development has been addressed only minimally in the cognition hypothesis literature. The present study explores how reasoning demands in tasks and working memory (WM) capacity predict learners' ability to notice English question structures provided in the form of recasts and how this contributes to subsequent development of English question formation. Eighty-one nonnative speakers of English completed three interactive tasks with a native speaker interlocutor, one WM task, and three oral production tests. Prior to the first interactive task, participants were randomly assigned to a task group (simple or complex). During task performance, all learners were provided with recasts targeting errors in question formation. The results showed that learners' cognitive processes during tasks were in line with the cognitive demands of the tasks, at two complexity levels. The findings suggest that WM was the only significant predictor of the amount of noticing of recasts as well as of learners' question development. With regard to interaction effects between WM and task complexity, high WM learners who carried out a complex version of the tasks benefitted the most from task-based interaction" (p. 549).

In Chapter 6 we turn to a discussion of meta-analysis in interaction, feedback, and task studies of second language learning. Meta-analytic work considers the results of many studies on a particular topic. Linck, Osthus, Koeth, et al. (2014) conducted a meta-analysis to study the effects of working memory on second language learning. Using seventy-nine studies, they argued their findings show consistent positive relationships between working memory and L2 processing, and between working memory and proficiency outcomes. They looked at additional covariates such as participant characteristics and publication status and revealed even more impact from executive control than storage components of working memory and verbal working memory measures. There was only minimal publication bias detected.

Many researchers believe working memory is also related to attention, a concept we discussed in an overview for a handbook in Robinson, Mackey, Gass, et al. (2012). More recently, acknowledgment of links between aptitude and working memory is gaining traction, with Wen, Biedroń, and Skehan (2017) proposing a reconceptualization of aptitude from the perspective of working memory, with support from the meta-analyses by Li (2015) and Linck, Osthus, Koethe, et al. (2014). They carefully distinguish between the many components of working memory that have been shown to influence L2 acquisition in different ways. Phonological working memory seems to be more salient to young learners and beginner learners. Executive working memory plays more of a role for adult and more advanced learners. Using a model of testing, theory construction, and pedagogical execution, they contend that working memory is essential to aptitude theory. With working memory motivating aptitude testing, they believe aptitude measurements will be able to predict success, explain the process of language learning, and provide guidance for classroom instruction.

Read It!

Yilmaz, Y. (2013). Relative effects of explicit and implicit feedback: The role of working memory capacity and language analytic ability. *Applied Linguistics*, *34*, 344–368.

"The purpose of this study is to investigate the role of two cognitive factors (i.e. working memory capacity [WMC] and language analytic ability [LAA]) in the extent to which L2 learners benefit from two different types of feedback (i.e. explicit correction and recasts). Forty-eight adult native speakers of English, who had no previous exposure to the target language (i.e. Turkish), were randomly assigned into explicit correction, recast, and control (no feedback) groups. Learners performed two tasks with a native speaker of Turkish where their errors on two Turkish target structures (i.e. locative and plural) were treated according to their group assignment. Oral production, comprehension, and recognition tests were used to measure learners' resulting performance. Learners' WMC and LAA were measured with the operation span task (Turner and Engle 1989) and a subtest of the LLAMA Aptitude Tests (Meara 2005), respectively. Results showed that WMC and LAA moderated the effect of feedback group on both structures. Moreover, follow-up analyses revealed that explicit correction worked better than recasts only when the learners in the compared groups had high cognitive ability (high WMC or high LAA)" (p. 344).

Juffs (2004), on the other hand, contends that the role of working memory in second language acquisition may be questionable, and Juffs and Harrington (2011) note:

> It is clear from the literature that 'WM' is not a unitary construct. Rather, it is a set of processes that underpin the learning and use of a second or additional languages. The dual functions of WM (storage and processing) vary in importance according to the L2 domain, and it is clear that the various WM subsystems (PM and/or RST) may change in their importance over time and domain. How these subsystems interact, and the role they play in constraining L2 performance, remains to be answered. It is important to emphasize that the effect of WMC as a constraint on L2 performance will differ by L2 domain, and evidence for its presence or absence in an area (e.g. sentence processing) may tell us little of the role it plays in other, arguably more important, domains (discourse comprehension) (p. 159).

In terms of how we test working memory, most tests originate from research in cognitive psychology and three that are commonly used in SLA are operation span, counting span, and sentence span. In each test, learners have to do a task and then remember some information later on:

- *Operation-span tasks* require that participants solve mathematical operations while they are trying to remember words. A mathematical operation is presented (sometimes a correct equation [e.g. $(9/3)-2=1$] and sometimes an incorrect one [e.g. $(9/2)-2=1$]), where participants are required to read the equation and state whether or not it is correct. A word following the operation is then recalled by the participants after they have read through a set of operations (generally increasing two, three, four, or five operations). In a study of working memory in the interaction, feedback, and task area of research, Goo (2012) used this type of data collection tool in a study of feedback and working memory. He found that the executive attention component of working memory helped predict which participants noticed recasts but not metalinguistic feedback.

- *Counting-span tasks*, such as the one used by Baralt (2015) in her interesting exploration of working memory, computerized feedback, and task complexity, involve counting shapes and remembering the total number of shapes in the order presented for later recall. As Cowan, Towse, Hamilton, et al. (2003) point out, the visual displays can be made more complex by placing shapes against a backdrop of distractors that share the same shape or color.
- *Sequence-span tasks* are perhaps the most frequently used of the three in SLA research (see Li, 2013 in the Read It! box below). They can be performed as either auditory listening-span tests or written reading-span tests, and within each of these categories there are numerous variations. A typical reading-span task presents sentences visually in groups ranging from two to six sentences. The groups can be presented in ascending order or arranged randomly. Participants are generally asked to state whether each sentence is true or false, plausible or implausible, or syntactically/ semantically correct or incorrect. Then they are asked to remember something. There are numerous variations on what is to be remembered. Sometimes it is the last word of each sentence, sometimes a letter following the sentence, or sometimes an unrelated word following the sentence.

Try It!

Although you will want to carefully select which working memory tests you use in your own studies based on your research questions, check out these sites for quick, simple examples of working memory tests: http://opencoglab .org/memtest1/ or www.memorylosstest.com/digit-span/.

When working with language learners, it is important to consider what language is used in administering a working memory test because we want to be sure the results are due to memory, not understanding instructions, or being slower/faster because of any L1/L2 issues.

> ## Read It!
>
> Li, S. (2013). The interactions between the effects of implicit and explicit feedback and individual differences in language analytic ability and working memory. *The Modern Language Journal*, *97*(3), 634–654.
>
> "This study investigated the interactions between two types of feedback (implicit vs. explicit) and two aptitude components (language analytic ability and working memory) in second language Chinese learning. Seventy-eight L2 Chinese learners from two large U.S. universities were assigned to three dyadic NS–NNS interaction conditions and received implicit (recasts), explicit (metalinguistic correction), or no feedback (control) in response to their non-target-like oral production of Chinese classifiers. The treatment effects were measured by a grammaticality judgment test and an elicited imitation test. The Words in Sentences subtest of the MLAT was used to measure language analytic ability; a listening span test was utilized as the measure of working memory. A principal components analysis and a structural equation modeling analysis established that working memory was an aptitude component. Multiple regression analyses showed that language analytic ability was predictive of the effects of implicit feedback, and working memory mediated the effects of explicit feedback; all the statistically significant results involved delayed posttest scores. Interpretations were sought with recourse to the mechanisms of the cognitive constructs and the processing demands imposed by the different learning conditions" (p. 634).

In summary then, working memory in the interaction, feedback, and task research line of studies has made great strides in the last decade in terms of results and methodology. Findings of basic, broad relationships have grown into detailed understanding of how facets of working memory interact with specific types of feedback, interaction, and tasks. There is great promise and potential for future study in Wen, Biedroń, and Skehan's (2017) working-memory based model of aptitude. Integration of multiple individual differences is also addressed in new work on working memory and creativity in second language acquisition.

3.3 Cognitive Creativity

Promising results of demonstrated relationships between working memory, creativity, and task performance in interdisciplinary fields (See, for example, the work by Suß et al., 2002) have highlighted the need for research investigating creativity and its effects on learner outcomes in second language learning. Only a few published studies have attempted to address this potential relationship so far. Ottó (1998) found evidence of a link between creativity and English language course grades; Albert and Kormos (2004, 2011) demonstrated a relationship between creativity and performance on an L2 narrative task; and McDonough, Crawford, and Mackey (2015) showed that creativity is associated with the use of questions and coordination in a group problem-solving task. As shown in Table 3.1, along with various collaborators, I have been working on two additional studies focusing on cognitive creativity.

Using data being described here in a publication for the first time my Georgetown University collaborators, Hae-In Park, Yuka Akiyama, Ashleigh Pipes, and I investigated the relationship between learners' production in an oral interaction task and their cognitive creativity (Mackey et al., 2014). We looked at college-aged L2 Japanese language learners ($N = 20$) and assessed them on (a) linguistic production during a group oral interaction task, (b) the Torrance Test of Creative Thinking (TTCT) figural version and an alternative creativity test, and (c) working memory, anxiety, and personality indicators. The TTCT we used is commercially available in both figural and verbal versions to provide an overall creativity index and subscores on particular creative strengths of originality, elaboration, flexibility, and others depending on the version of the test. They are easy to administer, taking just thirty to thirty-five minutes in total. Professional scoring services are available, or researchers can use the scoring manual to score their own tests. Of course, there is a fee for both the tests and the scoring, which can be cost-prohibitive for some research budgets.

An alternative is to use an adaptation of Guilford's (1967) alternative uses task. We gave participants in our creativity study five minutes to write down possible uses for a paperclip, with the following instructions: *Take five minutes to write down as many possible uses as you can think of for a paperclip in English. Feel free to suggest unconventional uses and provide as much detail as you would like. You may begin now.* Responses can be scored on typical creativity measures such as fluency, originality, flexibility, and elaboration. For example, one participant wrote that the paperclip could be used for "An hors d'oeuvres skewer (also yuck)," where the evaluation "(also yuck)" might be interpreted as an elaboration of the skewer idea. Another participant suggested "doll glasses," which exhibited originality because no other participants gave that response. Other than not costing anything to administer, this type of test is useful in that it provides an additional measure of creativity that is expressed in words, whereas the more commonly used figural version of the TTCT doesn't. When administering an alternative-uses task, it is helpful to provide participants with a real paper clip (or whatever object you choose) to see and hold, rather than an image on paper. An object that they can manipulate may be more conducive to idea generation for some types of learners. Also, it is best to provide completely blank paper for the responses. Lines or bullet points might influence the number of responses participants generate by suggesting they should stop when the blanks are full, thus decreasing the variation in the number of responses participants generated.

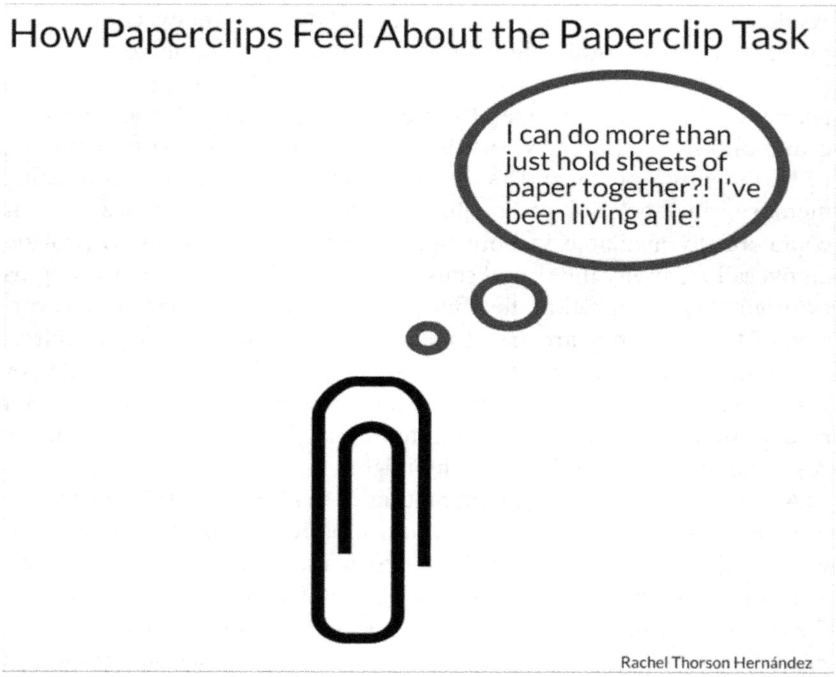

How Paperclips Feel About the Paperclip Task

Rachel Thorson Hernández

Figure 3.2 Paperclip existential crisis

Our analyses revealed relationships between creativity and measures of linguistic output, most notably conjunctions produced during the interaction task. Our results, although modest by the criteria suggested by Plonsky and Oswald (2014), suggest that participants who scored higher

---

Table 3.1 Two studies of cognitive creativity

(a) Georgetown Research Project:

"The role of cognitive creativity in L2 learning processes" (Paper presented at GURT, 2014) Alison Mackey, Hae-In Park, Yuka Akiyama and Ashleigh Pipes.

(b) Lancaster Research Project:

"The relationships amongst working memory, cognitive creativity and second language production during communicative tasks" (Paper presented at TBLT, 2015) Alison Mackey, Jenefer Philp, Yasser Teimouri, Abdullah Alroumi, Ting Zhou, Wenjing Li, Sam Kirkham, and Patrick Rebuschat

---

on various measures of creativity were also those more likely to use speech connected by conjunctions in their L2 Japanese.

We also found associations between other variables. For example, good conversant and total paperclip responses (one of our measures of creative fluency) appear to be related as did interactivity with questions and subject pronouns and total paperclip responses. Relationships between the creativity measures and other individual difference measures were less consistent. However, some associations did emerge. Out-of-box ideas and phonological short-term memory (as measured by the non-word repetition task) showed a positive relationship. Number of syllables and overall average anxiety were negatively associated. Anxiety seems likely to cause a decrease in a participant's production, so a negative relationship makes sense. Overall, this study further supported the idea that creativity is a factor that affects L2 interaction. As the first creativity study we were aware of to look at an L2 other than English, this is especially important as interest in the topic continues to grow.

In a follow-up study, again where data have not yet been described in a publication, my Lancaster University collaborators and I also found interesting relationships involving creativity along with other individual differences in a study of interaction, feedback, and tasks. In a design similar to the previous research, sixty-four Chinese students enrolled in graduate programs who were speakers of English as a foreign language completed two different interactive tasks: a decision-making task (the "lifeboat" task) and a story task. Participants reflected on their performance one to two days later during a stimulated recall interview. Students also completed two tests of creativity and two tests of working memory in addition to background surveys. Results showed several interesting patterns. Specifically, cluster analyses indicated three distinct groups with statistically significant differences between them in terms of task measures; more creative students outperformed less creative students in all task outcomes, suggesting that the measures and the topic merit further research. Working memory (operationalized as phonological short-term memory) was positively associated with L2 learners' total turns and interactivity in storytelling tasks. Examples of interactivity coding from the data can be seen in Excerpts 1 and 2 from the lifeboat task.

Excerpt 1

Weather Forecaster:	But but but if a typhoon comes, we can prepare for it.
Science Researcher:	**Why prepare?**
Weather Forecaster:	I mean, we prepare ...
Science Researcher:	**What kind of preparation?**

Excerpt 2

Weather Forecaster:	**So which elements do you think it's the most important, when you are in the sea?**
Kung Fu Master:	To be survive. [Laughs].
Weather Forecaster:	**No, I mean, like** the relevant elements, like the weather ...

There was also a positive relationship between cognitive creativity and linguistic ability in the generation of new ideas. For example, the data included the following quotes from participants (Excerpt 3), also during the lifeboat task.

Excerpt 3

Weather Forecaster:	Okay, how about thinking about this way: nothing about who should go onto the boat instead of that we should think about who can survive on an island. Because we don't know how long it will take ...
	[...]

| Science Researcher: | Maybe we can just ... build another boat. uh, you know, that would be [unclear], and we can just walk into the jungle and try to, you know, then, you [don't worry]. |

[All laugh].

In Excerpt 3, the weather forecaster changes the framing of the problem learners were tasked to solve, namely, not who could best enable survival on the lifeboat, but instead who could best survive on the island. The science researcher came up with the idea of simply building another boat!

Creativity was also positively related to both L2 learners' willingness to participate (a measure of involvement in interaction) in story-telling tasks and to how many turns learners took in problem-solving tasks, suggesting a creativity–learning opportunities relationship. Additionally, creativity was positively associated with usage of pronouns in linguistic tasks, suggesting greater inclusivity in the way creative learners approached tasks, communication, and therefore learning opportunities. Dynamic anxiety fluctuations in tasks were associated with changes in linguistic performance. Levels of anxiety (which introspective measures suggested were related to tasks and interlocutors) were noted to be low in this particular population. This may have pedagogical implications for instruction (curriculum and setting/contextual variables within the control of the instructor or language program). In sum, our results showed that high working memory and highly creative learners with relatively low levels of anxiety had the most learning opportunities. A study using the gold standard of a pre-test, post-test design and longitudinal methods, to empirically test this proposition would be another logical approach in this research trajectory.

A comprehensive new study by Ashleigh Pipes (2019) has furthered this endeavor by considering the role of creativity in relation to English language learners' communication strategy use, the effects of creativity on narrative structure, and outcomes in terms of English course grades. Pipes reported that creativity accounted for 13.6 percent of variation in participants' direct and indirect communication strategy use in an interactive speaking task even when controlling for proficiency. Creativity did not play a role in a monologic narrative task or course grade outcomes, which is consistent with findings in psychology that interaction is conducive to creative outcomes (Katz & Hussey, 2011; Torrance, 1970).

Taken together, the relatively few existing studies of creativity and second language learning, for example Ottó (1998), Álbert and Kormos (2004, 2011), McDonough, Crawford, and Mackey (2015), and Pipes (2019), together with the data described here for the first time suggest that further exploration of the role of cognitive creativity in L2 interaction-driven and task-based learning is a very potentially very interesting and fruitful line of enquiry.

Keep It in Mind!

- Research shows that aptitude can affect language learning success in various ways, which are frequently assessed using the MLAT and CANAL-FT. The LLAMA Language Aptitude Tests are another option, more readily available to students and independent researchers (Meara, 2005).
- Working memory is well established as another individual difference that influences uptake of corrective feedback, interaction, and task-based activities. New frameworks suggest a tight relationship between working memory and aptitude.
- Cognitive creativity is a budding area of research that has shown some associations with interaction-based L2 tasks. The TTCT and alternative uses tasks are simple and accessible ways to assess a learner's creative potential.

CHAPTER FOUR

Collecting Introspective Data in Interaction, Feedback, and Task Research

In this chapter, I talk about how we can uncover introspective information, and by this I mean data shedding light on learners' mental processes during interactions while they are receiving feedback and carrying out tasks. I describe a range of commonly used tools for obtaining introspections, including stimulated recalls, think-alouds, interviews, discourse completion tasks, and self-reports on social media, all in the context of research on interaction, feedback, and tasks.

4.1 Introspections in Interaction, Feedback, and Task Research

Commonly used in psychology, education, sociology, and cognitive science research, introspections are also popular in current SLA research and have been used in a wide range of studies to collect information on language learners' perceptions about their own, internal language learning processes (Gass & Mackey, 2015). Introspections, sometimes also known as verbal reports, are particularly helpful for interaction, feedback, and task research as they allow us to supplement what's often termed *observational data* (linguistic and non-linguistic) with information gained from our participants' self-reflections. In other words, we are able to gather information about their cognitive processes that are otherwise not visible to us. By analyzing introspective data, researchers can triangulate or validate, for example, ensuring that the tasks we have used in our study have been effective in collecting the type of data that we intended to elicit, meaning that the learners understand what we intend them to understand in the tasks. Of the various introspective methods used, stimulated recalls and think-aloud protocols are the most frequently used introspective data collection methodologies in second language research so we will start with them. Figure 4.1 shows the different factors to be considered when using introspective methods.

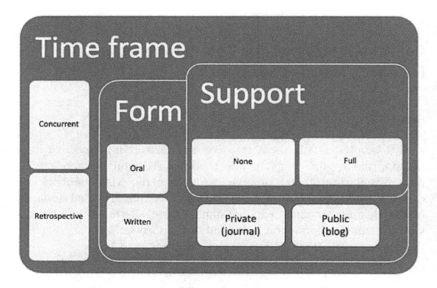

Figure 4.1 Factors to consider in introspective methods

4.2 Stimulated Recalls in Interaction, Feedback, and Task Research

Stimulated recall, as a type of introspection, makes a basic assumption that what goes on in consciousness can be observed and reported. Verbal reporting is a special type of introspection where we ask learners to verbalize what was going through their minds as they were solving a problem or completing a task. It is important to pay attention to the accuracy of the reporting in self-report and self-observational data, meaning that the time between the event being reported and the reporting itself should be as short as possible to avoid memory delay and ensure the reporting is as accurate as possible.

Stimulated recalls use stimuli to help learners to recall and report thoughts they had during the process of performing a task or participating in an event. In Gass and Mackey (2015), we provided extensive descriptions of stimulated recall, together with examples of how they can be carried out (see Mackey et al., 2000, for an example of stimulated recall in an experimental context, and Smith (2012), for an example of stimulated recall in a synchronous computer-mediated communication [SCMC] context). The degree of support in stimulated recalls can vary; for example, learners may be given the pictures of the task or material from the activity they were doing, or they might watch themselves carrying out the task on video, as they did in Smith's (2012) study. If they were writing, they may be given their essay or journal, so that they can follow the changes they made, commenting on their motivations and thought processes while looking at the writing. Sometimes they might have several recall supports at the same time, for example, a video and the materials from a task. The main thing is to help them remember what they were thinking at the original time, not what is going through their heads at the time of the retrospective interview, so balance is important in terms of support. They should be using the support as a memory aid, not to distract them or bring them into here-and-now processing.

We can see from the large number of studies using stimulated recalls in interaction, feedback, and task research, as well as from a similarly high number of papers outlining the various issues with verbal report methodologies, that stimulated recall should take place with trained and experienced researchers. As well as participants' memories, other potential problems can arise from the instructions for the recalls.

Despite the need for care, stimulated recall is an extremely popular means of collecting and supplementing data for interaction, feedback, and task research, and as part of the research for our 2015 book, we documented hundreds of such studies (Gass & Mackey, 2015). Egi's (2010) research provides a classic example of the use of stimulated recall in interaction, feedback, and task research.

Read It!

Egi, T. (2010). Uptake, modified output, and learner perceptions of recasts: Learner responses as language awareness. *The Modern Language Journal, 94*, 1–21.

"Recent research has shown that certain learners' responses to feedback, specifically repair and modified output, are predictive of subsequent second language (L2) development. Yet, little is understood about why these responses are associated with second language acquisition (SLA). The current study investigated this question by exploring the cognitive processes underlying learner responses. Learners of Japanese (*N* = 24) engaged in task-based interactions during which they received recasts of their errors. Each learner then watched video clips of the recast episodes and commented on them. The learners' stimulated recall reports were analyzed in relation to their responses to the recasts: uptake, repair, and modified output. In recast episodes where they produced uptake, their reports indicated that they perceived the recasts as corrective feedback significantly more frequently compared to cases where they did not produce uptake. In episodes where learners correctly repaired their errors, they were significantly more likely to report not only recognizing corrective recasts but also noticing the interlanguage–L2 mismatch. Modified output was also significantly related both to learners' recognition of corrective recasts and to their noticing of the gap (Schmidt & Frota, 1986). Given the developmental benefits commonly associated with noticing the gap, these findings may partly explain why repair and modified output have been found to be predictive of SLA" (p. 1).

4.3 Think-Aloud Protocols in Interaction, Feedback, and Task Research

As the name suggests, in think-aloud protocols we ask learners to express what they are thinking as they are completing a task. Again, these data can shed light on the cognitive (and sometimes physical) steps that learners go through and provide first-hand information on how learners describe and experience the event. Think-aloud protocols elicit real-time (sometimes referred to as *online*) information regarding learners' thought processes as they are doing a task or activity. Think-alouds have the advantage of not being subject to memory decay. However, they have the potential disadvantage that learners' performances during the task might be impacted by the need to vocalize about it (and vice versa). Like stimulated recalls, think-alouds often provide supplementary or triangulation data, and sometimes primary data. In the study that follows, Révész and Gurzynski-Weiss (2016) used think-aloud data to help address questions about how difficult teachers perceived certain tasks to be. They used think-alouds and eye-tracking in order to better understand the data from each. This study also appeared in the chapter on eye-tracking, since it's an excellent example of the well-rounded use of each measure and triangulation.

Read It!

Révész, A., & Gurzynski-Weiss, L. (2016). Teachers' perspectives on second language task difficulty: Insights from think-alouds and eye tracking. *Annual Review of Applied Linguistics, 36*, 182–204.

"The majority of empirical studies that have so far investigated task features in order to inform task grading and sequencing decisions have been grounded in hypothesis-testing research. Few studies have attempted to adopt a bottom-up approach in order to explore what task factors might contribute to task difficulty. The aim of this study was to help fill this gap by eliciting teachers' perspectives on sources of task difficulty. We asked 16 English as a second language (ESL) teachers to judge the linguistic ability required to carry out four pedagogic tasks and consider how they would manipulate the tasks to suit the abilities of learners at lower and higher proficiency. While contemplating the tasks, the teachers thought aloud, and we also tracked their eye movements. The majority of teachers' think-aloud comments revealed that they were primarily concerned with linguistic factors when assessing task difficulty. Conceptual demands were most frequently proposed as a way to increase task difficulty, whereas both linguistic and conceptual factors were suggested by teachers when considering modifications to decrease task difficulty. The eye-movement data, overall, were aligned with the teachers' think-aloud comments. These findings are discussed with respect to existing task taxonomies and future research directions" (p. 182).

4.4 **Immediate Recalls in Interaction, Feedback, and Task Research**

There is one more kind of introspective measure which falls under the category of recall. This is a somewhat modified version of a think-aloud, which incorporates elements of stimulated recall. It is known as *immediate recall*, where retrospection is carried out immediately after completing part of an activity, task, or interaction. Another term for this is *immediate retrospection*. For example, during a picture-sequencing task, where learners are receiving diffuse oral feedback, the researcher can stop the task at regular intervals and ask the learner to verbalize about their perceptions of the task and the interaction up to that point. Philp's (2003) interesting study of how learners notice a gap between what they said and what the target is using immediate recall. The abstract is reproduced below.

Read It!

Philp, J. (2003). Constraints on "noticing the gap": Nonnative speakers' noticing of recasts in NS–NNS interaction. *Studies in Second Language Acquisition, 25*, 99–126.

"Interaction has been argued to promote noticing of L2 form in a context crucial to learning – when there is a mismatch between the input and the learner's interlanguage (IL) grammar (Gass & Varonis, 1994; Long, 1996; Pica, 1994). This paper investigates the extent to which learners may notice native speakers' reformulations of their IL grammar in the context of dyadic inter-action. Thirty-three adult ESL learners worked on oral communication tasks in NS-NNS pairs. During each of the five sessions of dyadic task-based inter-action, learners received recasts of their nontargetlike question forms. Accur-ate immediate recall of recasts was taken as evidence of noticing of recasts by learners. Results indicate that learners noticed over 60–70% of recasts. However, accurate recall was constrained by the level of the learner and by the length and number of changes in the recast. The effect of these variables on noticing is discussed in terms of processing biases. It is suggested that attentional resources and processing biases of the learner may modulate the extent to which learners "notice the gap" between their nontargetlike utter-ances and recasts" (p. 99).

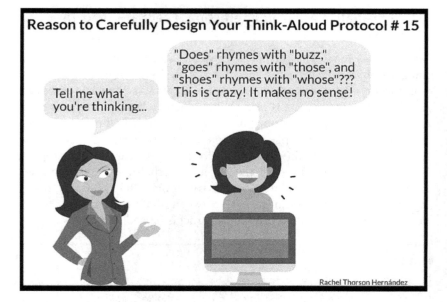

Figure 4.2 The importance of giving clear instructions for introspecting

---

Keep It in Mind!

Like any research method, introspective tools have strengths and weaknesses.

- Advantages: Introspective tools help researchers collect data on learner-internal processes that can be used to supplement observational data.
- Potential drawbacks: There may be memory-decay problems, the nature of the task may be changed as a result of verbalizing problems, and there may be individual differences associated with L2 proficiency (a participant may feel or know much more than they can express in a second language if the recall is not done in the L1).

I will now turn to interviews, discourse completion tasks, and self-reports on social media as additional forms of introspection, and their utility in interaction, feedback, and task research.

4.5 Interviews in Interaction, Feedback, and Task Research

Interviews, which are discussed more in Chapter 5, can allow researchers to ask specific questions of their participants. They can be more structured, meaning the interviewer asks the interviewees a set list of questions, or they can be less structured or semi-structured, meaning the interviewer has guide questions to ask, but depending on how the interview goes, they might also modify, remove, or add questions. Interviews can be used in interaction, feedback, and task research to find out about participants' understanding, perception, attitudes, beliefs, opinions, or behaviors. Like all introspective measures, interviews can be used to triangulate other sources of data, such as classroom observations and recordings of learners interacting.

When we use interviews as an introspective method, we need to keep in mind the relationship between the interviewer and the interviewee and how this might impact the outcomes of the interview and even, potentially, how the interview data are analyzed. As we explained in Kirkham and Mackey (2015), concepts like reflexivity and positionality/positioning can help us better understand interview data. If interviews are less structured, it's often the case that the data are co-produced by both the interviewer and interviewee. *Positionality* refers to traits associated with the interviewer and how it might impact the interview, for example, in interaction, feedback, and task research, characteristics like age, gender, race, ethnicity, languages spoken, education, and other

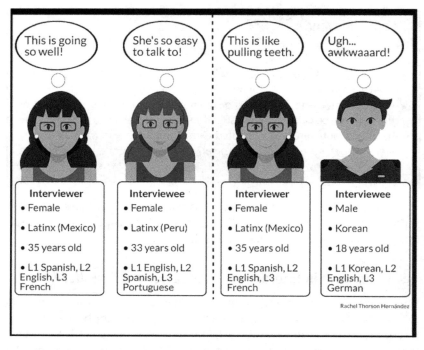

Figure 4.3 Thoughts on the effects of researcher positionality

characteristics might affect the way the interviewer and interviewee interact. Figure 4.3 provides some examples of this.

Once these have been considered, though, interviews can be very helpful data collection tools in interaction, feedback, and task research. In the abstract that appears next, the authors used interview data collected in a testing context to investigate the oral proficiency of younger Chinese learners. They also used test scores, but their detailed linguistic analysis of the interview data illustrates how helpful such data can be in assessing spoken language of the type that we often see in interaction, feedback, and task research.

Read It!

Fortune, T., & Ju, Z. (2017). Assessing and exploring the oral proficiency of young Mandarin immersion learners. *Annual Review of Applied Linguistics, 37*, 264–287.

"This article presents original empirical research carried out in the early total Mandarin language immersion context. The study involves K–5 learners from three early total Mandarin immersion programs whose home language is English. We examined students' second language (L2) oral proficiency in Mandarin in two ways: (a) a statistical comparative analysis of cross-sectional assessment data for kindergarten, Grade 2, and Grade 5 students and (b) a detailed linguistic complexity analysis comparing immersion students' speech samples (one per grade level) produced during the assessment interview. Results indicate significant differences in median scores between kindergarten and Grade 2 in all domains; however, no median score differences were found between Grades 2 and 5. An exploratory complexity analysis of three speech samples revealed increasingly higher levels of grammatical complexity across grades. Measures of lexical complexity for the Grade 5 sample, while higher than those in kindergarten, were lower than those of Grade 2. Study findings question the efficacy of existing proficiency assessments at capturing the multidimensionality of oral proficiency in the intermediate and pre-advanced range.- They also highlight the important role finely grained complexity measures can play in informing curriculum, instruction, and assessment practices" (p. 264).

4.6 Journals and Blog Entries in Interaction, Feedback, and Task Research

As introspective methods, writing, or recording journals and blogs can enable learners to reflect on a particular event and/or their perceptions about their learning in a relatively open and self-paced manner in that researchers are not usually present as they write. They can be written or oral. Researchers do not need to be present to collect the data. Journals are typically private and can be written by the learner and shared with the researcher at a later point. On the other hand, blogs are usually shared with an audience. Some learners choose to write blogs independent of research, and these can often be found on social media as another option for introspective but public data. With the permission of a participant, tracking their posts or photos related to language learning on platforms such as Facebook, Twitter, or Instagram, as the following Try it! box demonstrates, might yield fruitful data.

Try It!

Read the following abstract from Benson (2015), then look up a few YouTube videos to see if you can find evidence of interaction that might yield useful data for a study of corrective feedback. Do you see any recasts or other evidence of self-correction?

  Benson, P. (2015). Commenting to learn: Evidence of language and intercultural learning in comments on YouTube videos. *Language Learning & Technology 19*(3), 88–99.

"It is often observed that the globalization of social media has opened up new opportunities for informal intercultural communication and foreign language learning. This study aims to go beyond this general observation through a case study that explores how discourse analysis tools might be used to uncover evidence of language and intercultural learning in comments on YouTube videos involving Chinese-English translanguaging. Analysis of exchange structure – interactional acts involving information exchange and stance marking – suggests that translanguaging triggers interactionally-rich comments that are oriented towards information exchange and negotiation for meaning on topics of language and culture. It is argued that the methodologies used have good potential for use in studies that aim to investigate learning in online settings, both at the environmental level, in macroanalysis of large data sets, and at the individual/situational level, in microanalysis of shorter interactional sequences" (p. 88).

4.7 Discourse Completion Tasks in Interaction, Feedback, and Task Research

As we suggested in Culpepper, Mackey and Taguchi (2018), the learning of pragmatic ability in a second language is often studied (and taught) using methods involving interaction, feedback, and tasks. Although not a high-frequency data collection method in interaction, feedback, and task research, some applications of what are known as discourse completion tasks can be used to obtain valuable information about pragmatic abilities in using a target language in these sorts of contexts.

Discourse completion tasks (DCTs) were originally developed by Blum-Kulka (1982) to elicit data on L1 and L2 Hebrew speakers' speech-act production. DCTs typically involve a scenario where a situation is provided to learners, they read or view it, and then write or say what they would do or say if they were in that particular situation. DCTs allow researchers to control what learners see or hear, while also giving some control over the context by creating scenarios. Researchers can target certain kinds of interaction and feedback by creating task-based scenarios that might be challenging to collect data on naturalistically. Robinson's hypotheses about task complexity are the focus of the study mentioned in the next Read It! box, and DCTs are used as part of the methodology.

Read It!

Kim, Y., & Taguchi, N. (2015). Promoting task-based pragmatics instruction in EFL classroom contexts: The role of task complexity. *The Modern Language Journal, 99*(4), 656–677.

"Robinson's (2001) Cognition Hypothesis claims that more complex tasks promote interaction and language development. This study examined the effect of task complexity in the learning of request-making expressions. Task complexity was operationalized as [+/− reasoning] following Robinson's framework. The study employed a pretest–posttest research design and was conducted over 6 weeks. Korean junior high school students from 3 classes (N = 73) were assigned to one of the following groups: simple, complex, or control. Both task groups performed a pretest, 2 collaborative tasks, and 2 posttests, whereas the control group performed the pre- and posttests only. Learners' oral interaction during tasks was audio-recorded and analyzed by the number of pragmatic-related episodes (PREs). Learners' knowledge of request expressions was measured by a discourse completion test (DCT). The results indicated that task complexity levels influenced the occurrence of PREs, but no difference was found in the quality of task outcome between the simple and complex groups. In terms of learning outcomes, both task groups outperformed the control group, but no difference was found on the immediate posttest. However, the complex group maintained its gain on the delayed posttest" (p. 565).

Interaction, feedback, and task researchers using DCTs can use technology to provide paralinguistic cues and elicit oral data in research related to interaction, feedback, and tasks. Winke and Teng's (2010) study used a computer-delivered DCT, in which the L2 Chinese learners watched a video that set the scene. Their learners provided their answers orally, while Sydorenko (2015) used a computer-aided structured task (CAST) to investigate focus on form in requests. The abstract below also shows how DCTs can be used in a directly relevant interaction, feedback, and task study.

Read It!

Brunfaut, T., & Révész, A. (2015). The role of task and listener characteristics in second language listening. *TESOL Quarterly, 49*(1), 141–168.

"This study investigated the relationship between second language (L2) listening and a range of task and listener characteristics. More specifically, for a group of 93 nonnative English speakers, the researchers examined the extent to which linguistic complexity of the listening task input and response, and speed and explicitness of the input, were associated with task difficulty. In addition, the study explored the relationship between L2 listening and listeners' working memory and listening anxiety. The participants responded to 30 multiple-choice listening items and took an English proficiency test. They also completed two working memory tasks and a listening anxiety questionnaire. The researchers analysed listening input and responses in terms of a variety of measures, using Cohmetrix, WebVocabProfiler, Praat, and the PHRASE list, in combination with expert analysis. Task difficulty and participant ability were determined by means of Rasch analysis, and correlational analyses were run to investigate the task and listener variables' association with L2 listening. The study found that L2 listening task difficulty correlated significantly with indicators of phonological, discourse, and lexical complexity and with referential cohesion. Better L2 listening performances were delivered by less anxious listeners and, depending on L2 listening measure, by those with a higher working memory capacity" (p. 141).

CHAPTER FIVE

Creating and Using Surveys, Interviews, and Mixed Methods for Research into Interaction, Corrective Feedback, Tasks, and L2 Learning

5.1 Introduction

Whether doing an end-of-semester project, starting a dissertation, or undertaking a cross-sectional or longitudinal study for an organization or publication, researchers of interaction, feedback, and tasks often turn to surveys as a good way to collect data. In this chapter, I will first explore the types and purposes of survey options available for this line of research and introduce some of the advantages and disadvantages. I will discuss questionnaires and question types, and how we develop and administer surveys. Quite often, follow-up interviews are helpful following surveys; but sometimes, interviews start the process and are followed by surveys.

Integrating different sorts of methods into one research design is an increasingly common approach in current research into interaction, feedback, and tasks. In the final section of this chapter, I take a look into effective uses and designs of mixed methods when surveys are combined with other avenues of investigating interaction, feedback, and tasks in learning.

5.2 How Are Surveys and Questionnaires Defined in Interaction, Feedback, and Task Research?

The terms *survey* and *questionnaire* are often used interchangeably, so I will start by clarifying these terms. Most researchers use the term *survey* to indicate a method for collecting data. *Questionnaires* and *interviews* are typically thought of as instruments for conducting a survey. Questionnaires are the most common type of survey. Surveys typically involve obtaining reactions to questions from a representative sample of a target group, often one from which researchers hope to generalize. For example, in the general L2 research area, Teimouri (2017) used a questionnaire to examine adolescent language learners' emotional experiences and motivations using an L2 future-self theoretical approach, while Thorson Hernández and Subtirelu (2018) used interviews with high school language teachers to explore how teachers represent their agency and identity vis-à-vis their English-language learning students. In the interaction, feedback, and task area of research, Kartchava (2016) surveyed populations from both English as a second language (Canada, N = 197) and English as a foreign language (Russia, N = 224) contexts for her study "Learners' Beliefs About Corrective Feedback in the Language Classroom: Perspectives from Two International Contexts." Data elicited through surveys like these can be categorized as either qualitative/interpretive, quantitative, or somewhere on the continuum between them.

For a general introduction to questionnaires in second language research, Dörnyei's (2010) text is classic. Dörnyei argues that questionnaires (as a subset of survey research) are not easily defined, but says that the typical questionnaire "is a highly structured data collection instrument, with most items either asking about very specific pieces of information (e.g., one's address or food preference) or giving various response options for the respondent to choose from, for example by ticking a box" (p. 14). For a shorter version of a "how-to" text in terms of designing questionnaires, there is also a helpful chapter by Dörnyei and Csizér (2012) in the research methods collection edited by Mackey and Gass (2012).

Various different types of questionnaires have been used to investigate questions in interaction, feedback, and task research, with some questionnaires being written to present all learners in the study with the same questions or statements, and asking them to respond with written answers, scale-style judgments, or by option-selection. For example, Révész and Brunfaut (2013) used a questionnaire containing eight questions with a 5-point Likert scale to judge participants' perceptions about task difficulty.

5.3 How Have Questionnaires Been Used in Interaction, Feedback, and Task Research?

Questionnaires can allow researchers to gather data about learners, including their beliefs and motivations or perceptions about interaction and feedback, or their reactions to particular types of task activities – in other words, to gather information that we usually cannot figure out from observational data. Information about learners' levels of language anxiety, their motivation, and their willingness to communicate are all constructs that have been studied in interaction, feedback, and task research using questionnaires.

Biographical data are also typically obtained via questionnaires. For example, learners' L1, age, gender, socioeconomic status, language learning history, and other sorts of background information can be useful for a study. As we discussed in Mackey and Gass (2016), most studies in L2 research involve learners being given a background questionnaire like this, often administered before the study and right after the consent form is signed. Sometimes participants will be ruled out before the study starts on the basis of this questionnaire. For example, if a researcher wants to look at a learner's perceptions about the interactions they took part in during a study abroad experience, and the background questionnaire showed that they left after a very short period of time or the experience was too long ago for the researcher to have confidence in the memory of the participant, this participant might not end up being a part of the study.

Read It!

Révész, A., & Brunfaut, T. (2013). Text characteristics of task input and difficulty in second language listening comprehension. *Studies in Second Language Acquisition, 35*(1), 31–65.

"This study investigated the effects of a group of task factors on advanced English as a second language learners' actual and perceived listening performance. We examined whether the speed, linguistic complexity, and explicitness of the listening text along with characteristics of the text necessary for task completion influenced comprehension. We also explored learners' perceptions of what textual factors cause difficulty. The 68 participants performed 18 versions of a listening task, and each task was followed by a perception questionnaire. Nine additional students engaged in stimulated recall. The listening texts were analyzed in terms of a variety of measures, utilizing automatized analytical tools. We used Rasch and regression analyses to estimate task difficulty and its relationship to the text characteristics. Six measures emerged as significant predictors of task difficulty, including indicators of (a) lexical range, density, and diversity and (b) causal content. The stimulated recall comments were more reflective of these findings than the questionnaire responses" (p.31).

5.4 Interview Instruments Held in IRIS

As I mentioned in Chapter 2, IRIS is a free and downloadable database that holds instruments. IRIS includes a large number of representative

What is helpful about the conversation group for you?

What is least helpful about the conversation group for you?

What is most enjoyable about the conversation group for you?

What is least enjoyable about the conversation group for you?

Have you noticed any changes in your German since you started the conversation group?

○ Yes
○ No

Figure 5.1 IRIS search terms: "questionnaire" + "interaction" (Ziegler et al., 2013)

5. When doing speaking activities in class, do you usually give your students feedback on their language mistakes?

If you don't, what is the reason for this?

If you do, do you give them feedback during the activity, or afterwards?

Do you usually correct the students' mistakes, or do you encourage them to self-correct?

How often do you use peer correction (letting the students correct each other)? What do you think about this technique?

Do you give different kinds of feedback to different students? If yes, what do you do and why?

Figure 5.2 IRIS search terms: "questionnaire" + "feedback" (Roothooft, 2014)

1. What course are you currently teaching?

2. What was on the syllabus for the day I recorded your class?

3. Describe the first task you designed for your class in as much detail as possible. Include instructions, how students were paired, etc.

4. Describe the pre, during, and post-task phases of the first task.

5. Describe the expected task outcome(s) of the first task.

Figure 5.3 IRIS search terms: "questionnaire" + "task" (Gurzynski-Weiss, 2016b)

questionnaires and can be searched using parameters like "tasks" and "questionnaires" at the same time. Figures 5.1, 5.2, and 5.3 show screenshots of different sorts of questionnaires held in IRIS where the search terms included (a) "questionnaire" and "interaction" (Figure 5.1) (b) "questionnaire" and "feedback" (Figure 5.2), and (c) "questionnaire" and "task" (Figure 5.3).

Try It!

Think about how you would select a questionnaire for your own research on interaction. Go to https://bit.ly/35H3BJk and enter the search terms "questionnaire" and "interaction" in the search box. Browse the results and choose at least one that you think you could use or adapt for your own research purposes.

5.5 How Are Interviews Used in Interaction, Feedback, and Task Research?

Although I discussed interviews in Chapter 4 as part of introspective methods, interviews are very versatile tools and used in all sorts of paradigms. Researchers explain interviews in many different ways. For example, Dörnyei (2010) talks about them as targeting three main types of data about language learners: factual, behavioral, and attitudinal. Other perspectives that are more qualitative can be seen in Williams and Menard-Warwick (2014) and Block (2010). In the current chapter, I am focusing on interviews that come under the umbrella of survey-based methods of eliciting L2 data in interaction, feedback, and task research. As with questionnaires, there are a wide variety of different types of interviews, which range from highly structured, pre-planned data-collection sessions to ones that are closer (by design) to casual conversations, which may be used in qualitative or interpretive paradigms.

Read It!

Block, D. (2000). Problematizing interview data: Voices in the mind's machine? *TESOL Quarterly, 34*(4), 757–763.

"In recent years, there has been a noteworthy increase in the number of language education researchers publishing work that might be defined as ethnographically oriented. Although the questions being explored in this research vary greatly, there is a common tendency to use interviews as an important part of triangulated data collection, along with observation, diaries, letters, and questionnaires (e.g., recent TESOL Quarterly articles by Cox & Assis-Peterson, 1999; Flowerdew, 2000; Harklau, 2000; Ibrahim, 1999; Morita, 2000). When analyzing and discussing the data resulting from interviews, these and other researchers tend to focus on the content of the words produced by research participants, or as Freeman (1996) suggests, to take research participants "at their word." The researchers relying on interviews for data are not oblivious to the problems this stance entails. However, given the space restrictions in journals and books, there is generally very little scope for discussion of this issue. What most readers encounter, then, is presentation of data plus content analysis, but no problematization of the data themselves or the respective roles of interviewers and interviewees" (p. 757).

Other examples of interviews in the areas of tasks and technology can be found in Sykes's (2014) chapter on TBLT and synthetic immersive environments, where she discusses how "the combination of participant observations via in-game behavior observation and retrospective interviews allowed for a more complete picture of... the learners' experience" (p. 165).

Researchers sometimes use interviews to expand on particular topics or to clarify details (e.g., about the sorts of feedback learners have become aware of previously). Behavioral questions typically target data related to learners' processes, habits, and actions (e.g., their strategies for asking about vocabulary they don't understand during interaction). Questions typically classified as attitudinal or introspective elicit data about learners' perceptions, attitudes, beliefs, opinions, interests, and even values. For example, researchers may ask about learners' perceptions of corrections and whether they are aware of them in the classroom versus in conversation groups in the language they are learning, and even what their preference is in terms of such corrections.

5.6 Data on Attitudes in Feedback Research Collected Using a Questionnaire (Including New Data)

In a study I carried out with my (then) Georgetown University collaborators, Rebecca Adams, Cathy Stafford, and Paula Winke entitled "Exploring the relationship between modified output and working memory capacity" (Mackey et al., 2010), we looked at the task-based interactions of forty-two college-level, native English-speaking learners of Spanish as a foreign language. We reported on an interesting relationship between learners' WM test scores and their tendency to modify their output during interaction. In our results, greater processing capacity was related to greater production of modified output during interaction. However, what we didn't report on at the time were the answers these learners gave to some questions I included in a final questionnaire. At the time, I was becoming interested in learners' awareness of feedback and their preferences for feedback. After taking part in the task-based interactions, learners were asked three questions focused on whether they had noticed they were being corrected during the interaction (e.g., "Did you notice your interlocutor correcting you?"), whether the learners viewed the correction(s) as more or less explicit (e.g., "If you noticed any correction, please indicate how explicit it was"), and the learners' preferences in terms of how they found these corrections in general (e.g., "How do you usually like to be corrected?").

We did not report on the answers to these questions in the paper due to space constraints, the primary focus of the journal articles, and the fact that my co-authors were, at the time, more interested in working memory and output than they were in awareness and preferences for feedback, and so we considered those data to be outside the scope of the main study. Looking back on my field notes from the time, I believe an additional but still important reason that we did not report on the data was that some of the learners' answers seemed possibly flippant.

"My parents and nanny spanked me a lot so I like my feedback extremely explicit" was one example. We didn't know if this was a genuine answer, in which case it might have been potentially troubling, or a flippant answer, in keeping with the high spirits of some of the college-aged students in this study. This led me to view the data as pilot data and resolve to follow up with a better designed and targeted questionnaire at a later point. I also wanted to explore whether there were gender differences, but since the Spanish native and near-native speakers who were the task interlocutors (who delivered feedback when it was task appropriate) were all female, and the thirty-four Spanish learners in the study were not divided equally between genders (as in many college language classes), I was unable to obtain any firm information about gender patterns despite a trend towards those whose biodata identified them as males being less happy with the feedback than the ones whose biodata showed that they were female. What the questionnaire did reveal was that almost a third of the participants whose answers were clear reported noticing some form of feedback, and that when they noticed it and classified it, they tended to report it as being quite explicit. Also, the majority of participants who noticed feedback reported that they liked being explicitly corrected, which on most answers seemed to equate with receiving metalinguistic feedback, although almost a quarter of them mentioned that being corrected after they had made their point or said their piece was preferable to being corrected during the conversation.

Interestingly, more male participants said they did not like being corrected than female participants, although, again, the sample was not equal in numbers, and the interlocutors were all female. Five participants did not answer any of the questions, possibly because they were tired or rushed after completing the task-based interaction, and this too could also be responsible for the flippancy I was concerned about in the answers to some of the questions. I have reported on these data in this book, for the first time in part because (1) they are interesting, (2) they may lead others to do a study like this but with better design and execution, and (3) they show that questionnaires can be messy and that writing clear items is a critical part of the process. I turn to this next.

5.7 Writing Questions for Surveys in Interaction, Feedback, and Task Research

Closed-ended questions are typically those where participants are provided with answers that they choose or rank. Common closed-ended questions are rating scales such as Likert scales, true–false questions,

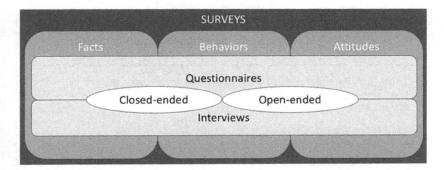

Figure 5.4 Types of data and surveys based on Dörnyei's Model

rank-order items, checklists, and multiple-choice items. Open-ended questions are those not followed by response options; they require participants to write, draw, say, etc. something. Types of open-ended questions include clarification questions, short-answer questions, and sentence-completion items. Facts are commonly gathered via closed-ended questions, while data about behaviors and attitudes may be gathered more often with open-ended questions. Surveys often use a mix of both types of items (see Figure 5.4).

5.8 What Are the Benefits of Surveys?

As we have seen, surveys have broad uses and forms in interaction, feedback, and task research. Depending on your goals, though, there will be both advantages and drawbacks to any instrument you use. Before you start designing a survey, it is helpful to think through what gains and sacrifices you will make depending on your priorities and resources. We will now work through some of the various considerations that will help you decide how to proceed, with a primary focus on questionnaires because they are the most commonly used method.

Try It!

Jot down notes about the pros and cons that are most applicable to your own current projects or ideas in the blank table provided in Table 5.1 (or on another paper, if you are using a library book!) as you read. If you don't have a specific project in mind, imagine you are creating a forty-participant study examining the effects of in-class and at-home planning time on a task-based middle school German lesson about visiting a school nurse for an injury.

Table 5.1 Pros and cons of survey research for reader's project	
Project idea:	
Data needed (circle all appropriate): Facts Behavior Attitudes	
Instruments under consideration (circle one or both): Questionnaire Interviews	
Survey pros	**Survey cons**

Depending on how they are structured, questionnaires can provide both quantifiable data as well as qualitative insights, meaning that they are suitable for a wide range of research types. These days, with the proliferation of free or low-cost survey software, such as Qualtrics and SurveyMonkey, creating a questionnaire can be relatively quick work with the software guiding you through the design process, and then the administration of a questionnaire can be quick, easy, instantly collatable and quantifiable, and can be carried out by a large number of participants in different locations at one time. It's possible to administer questionnaires to participants by email, weblinks, text, in computer labs, or on mobile devices, where a QR code can be used (see Figure 5.5).

For example, in a study reported by Pipes (2017), participants completed a biodata questionnaire on their mobile phones using a link provided by QR code while they were rotating through turns to complete a paired speaking interaction task. This minimized the amount of time asked of them to participate (since they could easily link to the questionnaire and fill it out while they were waiting) and eliminated the need for

Figure 5.5 QR code for survey participants

the researcher to manually enter any biodata. Working online also allows participants quick access to online translators or dictionaries if they are not taking the survey in their L1, which might be the case in an EFL class with learners from many countries. Furthermore, because answers are usually clicked, typed, or options chosen from drop-down menus, the data do not need to undergo the time-consuming process of discerning ambiguous results or illegible handwriting, and data entry and transcription become obsolete questionnaire tasks. Furthermore, basic frequency data are usually available immediately from the software, with data being easily imported from some survey software directly into statistical software such as SPSS or R. This ease of getting and down-loading/exporting also allows researchers to keep data in multiple secure places, thus minimizing fear of losing valuable data.

Another advantage of using questionnaires is that they can, in many cases, elicit longitudinal information from learners because they are easily repeatable and directly comparable. For example, the same survey can be administered several times in a year or over a period of years to track things like how learners' attitudes toward classroom tasks change (or don't) as their proficiency improves. Questionnaires can also elicit comparable information from a number of respondents for cross-sectional study.

Beyond electronic administration, questionnaires can be administered by phone, mail-in forms, or even in-person in places where electronic distribution is not possible. Researchers can ask learners to fill out paper-based surveys all at the same time, perhaps in class, or they can distribute the questionnaires and ask learners to bring them back a few hours or a

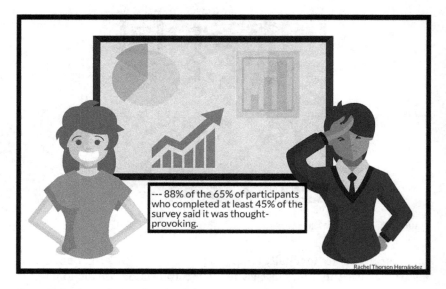

Figure 5.6 How not to analyze your survey data

few days later. The latter method allows participants more time and may possibly lead to more data; it also allows researchers a greater degree of flexibility in the data-gathering process although not as many questionnaires will be returned.

5.9 Caveats

As with any method for eliciting data, there are potential problems related to the collection and analysis of questionnaire data in relation to interaction, feedback, and task research. As discussed in Mackey and Gass (2016), an important concern is that responses may be inaccurate or incomplete, because introspecting about perceptions and attitudes, for example, can be hard to do, especially if the questionnaires are being completed in the L2, where language proficiency may constrain the responses.

Learners may find it hard to give an in-depth description of their language learning experiences, though they may be able to describe their general, main issues. It's important to keep this in mind if you choose open-ended questions in a survey, because it may make participants feel uncomfortable or self-conscious and may put an unnecessary linguistic burden on them. This can lead to short, undeveloped answers that do not truly reflect participants' thoughts or feelings. As such, every effort should be made to translate questionnaires into learners' native languages. Additionally, learners should be given as much time as they need to answer, and modalities other than writing should be an option. Children or learners with limited literacy, for example, should be given the option of answering orally, and those who speak a sign language should be given the option of signing. These responses can then be audio- or video-recorded.

Participant fatigue is another common concern that must be addressed when using questionnaires for research in interaction. In the original data I reported on for the first time in this chapter, I strongly suspect the reason some students didn't answer, and others appeared to answer flippantly was fatigue. For example, text messages and other rapid means of communication are common for the college-age students who tend to be the participants in many interaction studies (although this is being addressed as an issue; for more details, see Chapter 9). If a researcher asks these participants or, honestly, any participant at all, to complete a long, multi-screen questionnaire, it is likely that the participant will get bored and stop answering properly midway through (see Figure 5.7 for how such a bored participant might choose to begin answering).

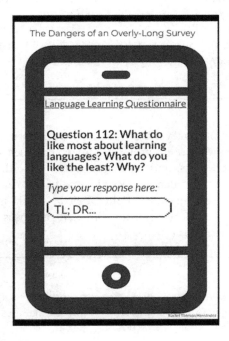

Figure 5.7 An overly-long survey

There is also the possibility that the participant won't complete the questionnaire on their own – friends may be around and influence the participant's answers or draw their attention away from the questionnaire. Fortunately, survey software such as Qualtrics provides data about how long participants spend on individual questions and the survey as a whole. This allows researchers to judge if a response should be deleted. For example, if a participant took only one minute to answer a detailed 30-item questionnaire, it's likely that the data from that participant should be thrown out. See Table 5.2 for a summary of pros and cons of questionnaire research.

Table 5.2 Pros and cons of questionnaire research

Pros of questionnaire research	Cons of questionnaire research
Fast	Impersonal
Large amounts of data	Language (L1) constraints
Wider reach/more participants	Literacy constraints
Information not available from	Shallow information
production/observation	Cannot control participant effort
Economical (usually)	Accuracy
Flexible with time	Clarity of questions
Flexible with location	Participant fatigue
Longitudinal capacity	Halo effect

Whatever form of survey administration you choose, the most important thing is to be aware of its strengths and weaknesses, capitalize on the opportunities it presents, and take precautions to address or minimize any potential issues as much as possible. As we get ready to talk about mixed methodologies in more detail below, think about how both surveys and interviews are used for different purposes in this study by Préfontaine and Kormos (2015).

Read It!

Préfontaine, Y., & Kormos, J. (2015). The relationship between task difficulty and second language fluency in French: A mixed-methods approach. *The Modern Language Journal, 99*(1), 96–112.

"While there exists a considerable body of literature on task-based difficulty and second language (L2) fluency in English as a second language (ESL), there has been little investigation with French learners. This mixed methods study examines learner appraisals of task difficulty and their relationship to automated utterance fluency measures in French under three different task conditions. Participants were 40 adult learners of French at varying levels of proficiency studying in a university immersion context in Québec. Appraisal of task difficulty was assessed quantitatively by participants' self reports in response to a five-item questionnaire and qualitatively by retrospective interviews. Utterance fluency was operationalized by four temporal variables and measured by Praat, a speech analysis software program. Across tasks, the quantitative results indicate that appraisals of lexical retrieval difficulty and fluency difficulty were most strongly related to perceived overall task difficulty. The qualitative analysis shows how L2 speakers evaluated the difficulty of each task as well as the features that either contributed to or limited their L2 fluency. Students' fluency in performing the three tasks was found to differ for articulation rate and average pause time, but not for pause frequency or phonation–time ratio" (p. 96).

5.10 How to Create and Administer Surveys for Interaction, Feedback, and Task Research

Now that you understand the types, advantages, and disadvantages of survey methods, we will turn to the specifics of creating and administering surveys. First, a look at question types will help with question formulation, then tips and hints for creating the right data-collection instrument will follow.

As we have discussed, both closed- and open-ended questions are common in surveys and the type of question asked will depend on the research questions being addressed in the study. For example, if you wanted to look at the sort of interaction that was taking place in a conversation club setting, an example of relatively unstructured research, open-ended questions that allow participant responses to guide hypothesis formation would most likely suit your needs more than closed-ended questions. You might ask a question like "What sort of conversations go on in your meetings?" Then, once hypotheses are formulated, you could develop and ask closed-item questions that allow you to focus on important concepts and themes that emerged during the course of the club. You might ask, for example, "What do you notice about errors and corrections during your conversation club?" Of course, as mentioned previously, question-naires can blend open- and closed-ended questions depending on the purpose of the research and on the outcomes of the study.

Try It!

Blending types of questions is perhaps more common than not. In a feedback focused study, Gurzynski-Weiss (2016a) used a questionnaire to inquire about facts, behaviors, and attitudes with a variety of question types in "Factors Influencing Spanish Instructors' In-Class Feedback Decisions." Using SurveyMonkey software, she administered a questionnaire including the questions shown in Figure 5.8 prior to videotaping the instructors and then having them complete a stimulated recall session concerning corrective feed-back.

8. Have you attended course(s) on language acquisition research or theory?

○ Yes

○ No

9. Please describe the course(s) in detail, including information about the topics covered, and information regarding where, when, and for how long you attended the course(s).

Figure 5.8 Sample questions from a survey (Gurzynski-Weiss, 2016a)

Label the types of questions above, based on the type of information they are collecting (fact, behavior, or attitude), and whether each is open-ended or closed-ended.

What other types of questions can you imagine that might be relevant to this study or one of your own?

5.10.1 Open-Ended Questions

Open-ended questions allow learners opportunities to respond with their thoughts and ideas in their own styles, for example, "Describe tasks that you found helpful in learning a second language." Answers to open-ended questions may be difficult to analyze but may result in richer, more complex data than closed-ended questions.

5.10.2 Closed-Ended Questions

In closed-ended items the possible range of responses is pre-determined by the researcher. Compared with open-ended, closed-item answers can usually be easily quantified and analyzed and are more consistent and reliable in terms of the data obtained. An example of a closed-item question might be: "How many times do you give oral corrective feedback to your students in a one-hour class? Circle one: 2 or fewer, 3, 4, 5, or 6 more."

Try It!

Look at Table 5.3, which compares closed- and open-ended questions for a study on oral corrective feedback of L2 pronunciation in a foreign language classroom. Make a list of advantages and disadvantages of each question in the table.

Table 5.3 Sample closed- and open-ended questions for a study on oral feedback on pronunciation in a foreign-language classroom

Closed-ended	Open-ended
Rate how helpful you find the oral feedback your teacher gives you in class on a scale of 1–5 (1=very unhelpful, 5=very helpful).	How helpful do you find the oral feedback your teacher gives you in class?
In a given class, how many times do you stop to make note of oral feedback your teacher has given you?	How often do you make note of the feedback your teacher gives you in class?
Which sort of feedback do you like best? Please circle one: Individual oral feedback given to me privately, individual oral feedback given to me in front of the class, whole-class oral feedback	Which sort of feedback do you like best?
Do you think the oral feedback your teacher gives you helps you improve your pronunciation? (Yes, No)	What things does your teacher do in class to help you improve your pronunciation?

Even when you are clear on what kinds of instruments and questions you want to use, there are still things you need to think about to ensure the success of a survey in terms of the exact wording of questions and overall survey design. For instance, it is important to avoid biasing responses through the wording of a question. If you use an older questionnaire as a model, you may find that some of the questions allude to stereotypes. Current biodata forms, for example, often don't force binary sex distinctions anymore but provide more options. Try to avoid negative questions or overly long and confusing questions. Ensure each possible response is included only once on multiple-choice items. For example, if asking learners how many conversations they have in a week outside the classroom, instead of only giving them options such as 1–2, 2–3, 3–4, also add an option for none. Don't ask double-barreled questions, for which respondents might have conflicting answers. A Likert scale rating in response to a statement such as "I like interaction and feedback" could be impossible to answer for a student who likes interacting but hates feedback during interaction. Coombe and Davidson (2015) provide more helpful suggestions.

5.10.3 How to Administer Surveys in Interaction, Feedback, and Task Research

Whether you administer a survey on a smartphone, paper, or a computer, the appearance of a questionnaire is important. Questionnaire software can help considerably. If not using software, remember not to put too much text, or too many questions on a screen or page at one time. White space is important in any medium. In the interest of credibility, Dörnyei (2003) and other methodologists have suggested researchers give their questionnaires a title and focus on providing clear instructions to answer the items. Additional information may be required by ethics boards (such as how to reach the researcher, or the general purpose of the questionnaire). You should always check with your institution's ethical review board to find out their requirements for obtaining informed consent. Finishing, of course, with a statement thanking the participants for their participation is customary.

In terms of identifying information such as age or gender, it is better to ask for this information at the end of a questionnaire, rather than at the beginning. Participants may feel that they are being identified right off the bat (even though you have assured them that their information is anonymous), or they may be uncomfortable providing demographic information. Finally, it's always best to have questionnaires reviewed by other researchers and peer-group members, and piloted with a sample similar to your participants to ensure that the format is user-friendly and the questions are clear.

Keep It in Mind!

Checklist for good survey design. Some characteristics of good surveys include:

✓ Contains a title, introduction/instructions, and concluding remarks
✓ Are visually simple and uncluttered
✓ Items only ask about one piece of information
  o Not: "I like when my teacher gives me oral feedback and it helps me improve my pronunciation: Agree or disagree?"
✓ Avoids negative wording
  o Not: "I do not like when my teacher corrects my pronunciation in class: True or false?"
✓ Only asks for information necessary to answer research questions
  o Not: "What is your favorite animal?"
✓ Only has one possible answer
  o Not: "How many times in a class does your teacher correct your pronunciation? 1–3; 3–5; 5–7"
✓ Has been pilot-tested at least once on a subset of the sample before administration.

Try It!

1. Rewrite the questions from the "Not" examples in the previous box so that they are clear and unambiguous.
2. Find a survey online or in www.iris-database.org and check it against the characteristics of a good survey in the list above. Does it have all of the suggested elements? Are the questions clear? Does it ask for personal information at the end? How could it be improved?

5.11 Using Mixed-Methods Approaches to Carrying Out Research in Interaction, Feedback, and Task-Based Learning

Quite a few interaction studies use questionnaires or interviews to triangulate production data. As I mentioned in Chapter 2, mixed-methods approaches are becoming more popular in interaction, feedback, and task research in particular, and L2 research in general (e.g., Creswell, 2015; Hashemi & Babii, 2013; Jang et al., 2014; Riazi, 2016, 2017; Tashakkori & Teddlie, 2010), and a journal dedicated to this research area, *Journal of Mixed Methods Research* (http://mmr.sagepub.com), began in 2007 and publishes helpful "how to" articles, like Fetters and Molina-Azorin's (2019) "A Checklist of Mixed Methods Elements in a Submission for Advancing the Methodology of Mixed Methods Research." Clearly, there is acceptance in the field now that quantitative and qualitative data can complement and supplement one another, leading to a richer, more complete understanding of the phenomenon under investigation. Indeed, in King and Mackey (2016), we took the concept of mixed methods further and argued that the field of second language acquisition can benefit from a layered approach, which involves "the explicit consideration of research problems from a range of distinct epistemological perspectives" (p. 210).

A very simple definition of mixed methods is "research combining quantitative and qualitative/interpretive data usually to different degrees in the same study." Some researchers, like Hashemi and Babaii (2013), believe that for authenticity, mixed-methods research should include both quantitative and qualitative data at all stages of a research project, including data collection, data analysis, and interpretation. Tashakkori and Creswell (2007, p. 4) provide the following definition: "research in which the investigator collects and analyzes data, integrates the findings, and draws inferences using both qualitative and quantitative approaches in a single study or program of inquiry," while Riazi and Candlin (2014) characterize it as research that combines quantitative and qualitative methods in the collecting and analysing of research data to provide "a more comprehensive understanding of the object of study" (p. 136).

Keep It in Mind!

Why use mixed methods? Purposes for using mixed-methods research, as discussed by Riazi and Candlin (2014, pp. 143–146) include the following:

- Triangulation: using more than one data collection method to corroborate the results obtained through each
- Complementarity: using quantitative and qualitative methods to address research questions relating to different aspects of a research phenomenon
- Development: Using one method or phase (quantitative or qualitative) to develop or refine the methods for the other phase

- Initiation: Using the results from one method to look at the questions or results of the other method in a new light; this then encourages the researcher to collect further data
- Expansion: using the two methods together (whether sequentially or concurrently, see below) to develop richer, more layered answers to the research questions

There are numerous ways to design quantitative and qualitative studies. Similarly, there are multiple ways of combining these two research traditions. Creswell et al. (2008), based on Creswell and Plano Clark (2007), present five typical research designs that are dfferent based on when data collection takes place, concurrently or sequentially; the first two (see Figure 5.9) exemplify concurrent designs, and the latter three (see Figure 5.10) are examples of sequential designs.

The important concept to mixed methods, *triangulation*, in this model (Figure 5.9) is a concurrent design that involves collecting two sets of data simultaneously and considering them in parallel as a way of conceptualizing and addressing the research question more thoroughly. In other words, the data types complement one another. They also explain and describe concurrent embedded design. In this design type, rather than both contributing equally to the interpretation, one tries to understand the impact of an intervention. Qualitative data are collected along

I. Triangulation Design

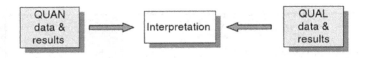

II. Concurrent Embedded Design

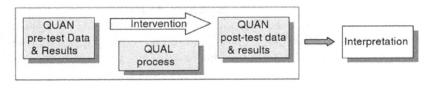

Figure 5.9 Triangulation (Creswell et al., 2008, p. 68)

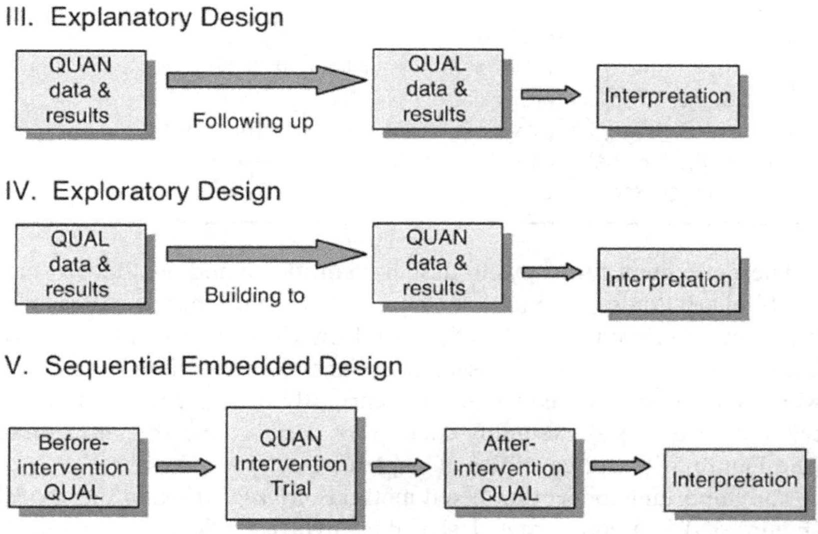

III. Explanatory Design

IV. Exploratory Design

V. Sequential Embedded Design

Figure 5.10 Mixed-methods design model (Creswell et al., 2008, p. 68)

with the intervention, for example, when one wants information on the experience of the intervention itself. Thus, the two data types are used for different purposes, quantitative data to determine the impact of the intervention and qualitative data to understand the ways in which participants relate to the intervention. Both, then, contribute to the overall understanding of the impact of the intervention.

Try It!

Draw a diagram of how you would conduct a mixed-methods study for a topic of interest to you.

It is important that, when we conduct mixed-methods studies, we have a clear rationale for collecting more than one type of data. Analysis of data from a mixed-methods study is not unlike the analysis of data from more quantitative or more qualitative studies, but writing up the research can be more complicated because the results of each have to be compiled and integrated.

Read it!

Take another look at the summary of Préfontaine and Kormos (2015) in Section 5.9. Would it be considered true mixed-methods research according to all of the definitions presented above? Find the complete study and consider how the quantitative and qualitative analyses were integrated.

Try It!

1. Use the IRIS database to go on a "scavenger hunt" for studies that have used each type of survey instrument described in this chapter.
2. You are designing a hypothetical study of an elementary school L2 Spanish program. Think about what types of survey information you might collect from students, parents, and teachers. Would it be the same or different? What different instruments would you use?

CHAPTER SIX

Doing Meta-Analytic and Synthetic Research on Interaction, Feedback, Tasks, and L2 Learning

6.1 Introduction

In this chapter we take a look at the emerging role of meta-analysis and research synthesis in interaction, feedback, and task-based research into how second languages are learned, as well as provide some instructions on how to systematically conduct a meta-analysis to achieve sound results in these areas. The chapter begins with a description of meta-analysis and research synthesis and their contributions to research in applied linguistics and second language research in general. Next, previous meta-analyses on the topics of interaction feedback, tasks and task-based language teaching (TBLT), and related methodologies are summarized. Then, clear guidelines for conducting meta-analyses are provided. The chapter ends with a discussion of how meta-analysis and replication research can help in answering essential questions in respect to interaction, feedback, and task research and also provides a few cautions, or things to look out for.

6.2 Why Carry Out Meta-Analytic Research into Interaction, Feedback, and Tasks?

Interaction, corrective feedback, and tasks are, as we have seen, some of the most frequently investigated topics in the second language research field, and, as with many areas in the field, studies sometimes result in contrastive findings. For example, there is an ongoing debate about the utility of explicit versus implicit forms of oral corrective feedback for L2 development with evidence supporting both types for various linguistic targets, often differing by setting (Goo & Mackey, 2013a, 2013b). Another example is the issue of task repetition: What sort of repetition is most helpful, and helpful in what way? We have the same questions about pre-task planning: Is it useful? How much planning is useful? For which sorts of learners? What sorts of effects does planning have on language? Different and complex sets of results sometimes result in language teaching professionals preferring to rely on their own judgment about their own settings rather than research findings. Complex results can also lead to researchers not knowing whether to consider data with reference to one paradigm or another. For example, is it worth repeatedly comparing recasts and prompts to see if results are context dependent? In other words, how can anyone make sense of their findings when there are so many studies on the same set of topics, with all sorts of outcomes?

One way to do this is by research syntheses and meta-analyses, as previously mentioned in Chapter 2. This type of research surveys, captures, and compares findings from prior studies. Such overview work can provide a more trustworthy account of what is actually going on in a given phenomenon than simply reading the primary sources alone. This type of research uses the findings from prior studies (descriptively in the case of research syntheses and quantitatively in the case of meta-analyses) to answer a research question rather than collecting original data. Meta-analyses, in particular, are able to then report the average effect of all the studies analyzed. Most commonly known from within the medical field, meta-analyses of a wide range of clinical studies carried out with different populations and strengths of drugs, can provide a simple answer to questions such as "are headaches helped by painkillers?" (Yes, but some painkillers are better than others depending on the type of person and headache).

The first meta-analyses in the second language research field emerged as recently as 1998 (Ross, 1998, on self-assessment in second language testing, according to Plonsky & Oswald, 2015), but meta-analysis has exploded in popularity in the past twenty years. Results from a Google and Google Scholar search found over 400 publications and presentations of research syntheses and meta-analytic findings on topics in applied linguistics and SLA. Findings from corrective feedback research for example, have been meta-analyzed many times (e.g., Brown, 2016; Li, 2010; Lyster & Saito, 2010; Mackey & Goo, 2007; Russell & Spada, 2006) on a variety of sub-domains ranging from a focus on written corrective feedback to oral feedback, from classroom instruction contexts to computer-mediated contexts. Interestingly, even these meta-analyses provided disparate findings leading to the meta-meta-analysis by Plonsky and Brown (2015), which examined how eighteen of those meta-analyses defined their search domains and the search techniques the researchers used to determine which studies to include. When we talk about meta-meta-analyses, we know the field has come quite a long way, especially in only a few years. Defined as a "meta-analysis of multiple meta-analyses" (Cleophas & Zwinderman, 2017), a meta-

meta-analysis allows researchers to identify problems with the methodology of the original meta-analyses. Common errors include pooling studies that are a mix of randomized and non-randomized trials and only examining published studies. The latter error can lead to people wondering if there is a publication bias, that is, journals publishing only studies with positive findings, and not publishing studies that have been done, but which have negative findings. The bilingual literature has recently seen active debate on this topic with a paper by de Bruin et al. (2015) alleging "the idea of a bilingual advantage may result from a publication bias favoring studies with positive results over studies with null or negative effects" (p. 99). I will return to this important point later in the chapter.

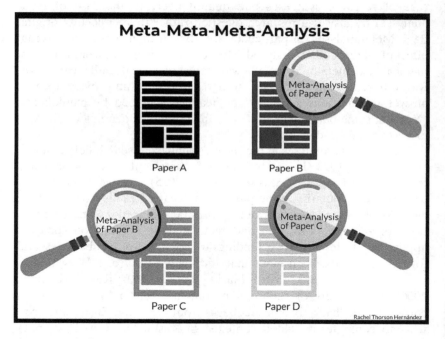

Figure 6.1 That's so meta!

6.3 What Is a Research Synthesis?

Most research papers begin with some kind of a literature review. When reporting on an original empirical study with new data, a literature review is typically narrow in scope, surveying only the previous work directly related to the new study and its variables. Literature reviews help research consumers contextualize new data in prior work. A good literature review might also criticize the weaknesses in previous studies and point out the gap the new results will fill in the body of research under investigation. For example, in a study by Parlak and Ziegler (2017) on the impact of recasts on the development of primary stress in computer-mediated versus face-to-face contexts, the authors covered the following topics in their literature review: the interactionist approach to SLA research, a review of prior studies of interaction and L2 phonology, a review of studies involving recasts and interactional tasks, and a review of the use of technology for L2 pronunciation development. These topics were all closely related to the variables the authors reported on in their own study.

Research syntheses and meta-analyses are really just more systematic, broader versions of a typical literature review. Research syntheses can be defined as reviews that "focus on empirical research findings and have the goal of integrating past research by drawing overall conclusions (generalizations) from many separate investigations that address identical or related hypotheses" (Cooper, 2017, p. 7). A research synthesis often is a narrative that describes prior related work and highlights future directions for still unresolved questions in a given domain. The review articles published by the Cambridge University Press journal, the *Annual Review of Applied Linguistics* (ARAL), to give one example, systematically review research for particular topics. These articles typically provide an historical overview of a topic and its current status, and some point out future directions. From 2016, ARAL began to add other article types to its publications, including empirical articles and position pieces. Other journals also publish reviews; for example *Language Teaching* publishes timelines which are also review articles. Reviews are often useful papers for early-career scholars to produce since they can be the published versions of the literature reviews conducted for their dissertations and other studies. An example of a review article can be found below.

Read It!

Scovel, T. (2000). A critical review of the critical period research. *Annual Review of Applied Linguistics, 20,* 213–223.

"Two decades of international research in applied linguistics provides a large number and variety of topics from which to choose for this special anniversary edition, but certainly one of the most significant among these choices is the critical period hypothesis (CPH). Few topics in applied linguistics have continued to captivate the interests of researchers and practitioners so intensively and for such a long period of time as the CPH. Indeed, one could easily go back to reviewing three, not two decades of sustained research and continuous interest in this topic (Lenneberg 1967, Scovel 1969). If the number and diversity of publications is indicative, the CPH has engendered even more interest and controversy now than in any previous decade. Why is this so?" (p. 213).

As an example of a *Language Teaching* article, consider the following review timeline.

Read It!

Leow, R., & Donatelli, L. (2017). The role of (un)awareness in SLA. *Language Teaching, 50*(2), 189–211.

"The construct 'awareness' is undoubtedly one of the more difficult constructs to operationalize and measure in both second language acquisition (SLA) and non-SLA fields of research. Indeed, the multi-faceted nature of awareness is clearly exemplified in concepts that include perception, detection, and noticing, and also in type of learning or learning conditions (implicit, explicit, incidental, subliminal), type of consciousness (autonoetic, noetic, anoetic), and type of awareness (language, phenomenal, metacognitive, situational). Given this broad perspective, this article provides, from a psycholinguistic perspective, a timeline on the research that addresses the role of awareness or lack thereof in second/foreign language (L2) learning" (p. 189).

6.4 What Is a Scoping Review?

Another type of research synthesis is a scoping review. This type of review summarizes all of the studies currently available in a domain of interest. A scoping review is usually a review undertaken when little is known about a particular topic, for example prior to starting a pilot study or larger research project. A scoping review can also help researchers identify research questions. There are even second order scoping reviews (or scoping reviews of scoping reviews, for example, see Pham et al., 2014). One example of a recent scoping review is "Look who's interacting: A scoping review of research involving non-teacher/non-peer interlocutors" by Laura Gurzynski-Weiss and Luke Plonsky (2017). This scoping review looked at several types of articles as described in the current chapter, including meta-analyses and review articles. It pointed out innovative themes or insights that emerged in order to address a gap in the literature on non-peer/non-teacher learner interlocutors and their individual differences. This provided researchers with recommendations for future research in areas ripe for conceptual development in the domain of different types of interlocutors.

State-of-the-art articles are yet another popular type of synthesis. The following synthesis discusses L2 interaction research.

Read It!

Loewen, S., & Sato, M. (2018). Interaction and instructed second language acquisition. *Language Teaching, 51*(3), 285–329.

"Interaction is an indispensable component in second language acquisition (SLA). This review surveys the instructed SLA research, both classroom and laboratory-based, that has been conducted primarily within the interactionist approach, beginning with the core constructs of interaction, namely input, negotiation for meaning, and output. The review continues with an overview of specific areas of interaction research. The first investigates interlocutor characteristics, including (a) first language (L1) status, (b) peer interaction, (c) participation structure, (d) second language (L2) proficiency, and (e) individual differences. The second topic is task characteristics, such as task conditions (e.g., information distribution, task goals), task complexity (i.e., simple or complex), and task participation structure (i.e., whole class, small groups or dyads). Next, the review considers various linguistic features that have been researched in relation to interaction and L2 learning. The review then continues with interactional contexts, focusing especially on research into computer-mediated interaction. The review ends with a consideration of methodological issues in interaction research, such as the merits of classroom and lab-based studies, and the various methods for measuring the noticing of linguistic forms during interaction. In sum, research has found interaction to be effective in promoting L2 development; however, there are numerous factors that impact its efficacy" (p. 285).

6.5 What Is a Meta-Analysis?

A meta-analysis is a type of research synthesis that only examines studies that can be synthesized quantitatively, by averaging effect sizes (or other statistics). Effect sizes (e.g., Cohen's d) are a statistical calculation that do not describe statistical significance (i.e., p-values) but rather measure the size of the difference between two groups or the strength of an effect. Effect sizes are handy for meta-analyzing data because they are independent of sample size and can be easily calculated from quantitative data (e.g., means and standard deviations). Using effect sizes to compare findings allows researchers to compare studies that have different sample sizes or measures. Researchers can also examine moderators to the main effect, or variables that mediate study results. For example, following the initial applied linguistics meta-analysis by Ross (1998) focusing on language testing, Norris and Ortega (2000) conducted another early meta-analysis. Their process began when they were graduate students in Cathy Doughty's class at the University of Hawai'i and focused on the effectiveness of L2 instruction and examined pre-, post- and delayed post-test effects as well as moderators such as the duration of treatment and type of dependent variable. They found an overall advantage for L2 instruction (as opposed to no instruction or exposure) from forty-nine studies.

From these early studies, interest in meta-analyses grew and, luckily, there were quite a few texts and "how-to" books in related fields. A 2018 article in the journal *Nature* points to 1904 as being the first year in which meta-analytic techniques were used: "The first formal attempt to combine information from multiple sources... was made in 1904 by K. Pearson" in the medical field, and the authors go on to say that meta-analytic "[m]ethodology was formalized and developed in the two decades following 1977 in multiple fields" (Gurevitch et al., 2018, p. 176). It is important to note though, that this article also sounds some warning bells: "Four decades after its introduction, we are seeing widespread mainstream acceptance of meta-analysis as a research synthesis tool, but also the signs of what may be considered a 'midlife crisis' as it has begun the transition to a mature field. While the number of published meta-analyses has continued to increase rapidly, too many meta-analyses and systematic reviews are of low quality" (p. 175). I will return to this point later in the chapter.

6.6 Why Do Meta-Analysis?

By using meta-analysis instead of traditional narrative reviews, researchers can avoid bias resulting from consciously or unconsciously giving certain studies more weight or importance than others. They can also avoid sampling error caused by smaller sample size. The use of effect sizes avoids the common problem of an overreliance on null hypothesis significance testing (NHST) which has been discussed for decades in related fields but has only recently seen attention in work in applied linguistics (notably for example, Norris, 2015; Plonsky, 2015, 2017; Plonsky & Oswald, 2014). Szucs and Ioannidis argue in their 2017 article in *Frontiers in Human Neuroscience* that the method is inappropriate for scientific research and is likely responsible in part for the replication crisis problems we discussed in Chapter 2. They go on to argue that "[t]he current statistics lite educational approach for students that has sustained the widespread, spurious use of NHST should be phased out" (para. 1). This paper quotes scholars from many decades ago pointing out the problems, for example:

> What used to be called judgment is now called prejudice and what used to be called prejudice is now called a null hypothesis. In the social sciences, particularly, it is dangerous nonsense (dressed up as the 'scientific method') and will cause much trouble before it is widely appreciated as such. (Edwards, 1972, p. 180, as quoted in Szucs & Ioannidis, 2017, para. 2).

Meta-analysis can help address issues like those mentioned above. It provides more systematic, objective answers to questions that are asked and has been profitably applied to issues in the domain of oral corrective feedback, task-based interaction and task-based language teaching, and on the methodologies used to investigate these topics, to which we turn in the next section.

Keep It in Mind!

- Effect sizes are useful for meta-analyses because they are independent of sample size and can be calculated from quantitative data.
- Using effect sizes avoids the common problem of an overreliance on null hypothesis significance testing (NHST).
- Meta-analyses can help researchers avoid bias and sampling errors.

6.7 Meta-Analyses on Oral Corrective Feedback

Early meta-analyses on the topic of oral corrective feedback have ranged from investigations of the overall effectiveness for learning (e.g., Miller, 2003; Russell & Spada, 2006), contrasting various forms of feedback (e.g., Li, 2010; Lyster & Saito, 2010), contexts of the delivery of feedback (e.g., Brown, 2016; Ziegler, 2016), and specific types of feedback (e.g., Miller & Pan, 2012). Moderating variables that have been meta-analyzed within these studies have included: study type, treatment length, instructional setting, types and timings of outcome measures, teacher experience, and individual differences such as learners' age and proficiency level. These meta-analyses (summarized in Table 6.1) have shed light on a variety of questions in the domain of corrective feedback.

Try It!

Read one of the articles in Table 6.1 and summarize (1) the researchers' main objectives for conducting your chosen meta-analysis and (2) how their research contributed to the literature on corrective feedback. Then, ask yourself how you might go about replicating (i.e. conducting a meta-meta-analysis) of the authors' work. Consider the following questions: What are the strengths of the article? What might you do differently?

Table 6.1 Sample meta-analyses of corrective feedback

Authors and year of publication	Domain	Moderators	Number of studies analyzed	Effects (d)
Russell & Spada (2006)	Oral and written feedback on grammatical form	–	15	1.16 (CF overall)
Mackey & Goo (2007)	Interaction-driven L2 development	Type of target, occurrence of feedback, timing of feedback, focus of feedback, opportunity for modified output, context, setting, post-testing	28	.71 (immediate) 1.09 (delayed) .96 (recasts) .47 (meta-linguistic)

		(immediate versus delayed), implicit (recasts) versus explicit (metalinguistic) feedback		
Li (2010)	Oral corrective feedback on grammatical form and vocabulary	Implicit versus explicit feedback, publication type, context, task type, treatment length, timing and type of outcome measures, age and proficiency	33	.64 (CF overall)
Lyster & Saito (2010)	Oral corrective feedback in classrooms	Types of feedback, outcome measures, timing of outcome measures, settings, treatment length, learner age	15	.74 (CF overall)
Miller & Pan (2012)	Oral corrective feedback focused specifically on recasts	Task type, grammatical target, L2	40	.38 (recasts)
Brown (2016)	Oral corrective feedback in L2 classrooms – descriptive studies	Types of feedback, target, student characteristics, setting, context features, teacher characteristics	28	Not reported Recasts used most often by teachers (57%)

Li (2010) looked at the effectiveness of corrective feedback in SLA by conducting a meta-analysis that included thirty-three primary studies published between 1988 and 2007. Of these thirty-three studies, twenty-two were published studies and eleven were doctoral dissertations (as discussed previously, including unpublished studies reduces the risk for a meta-analysis to suffer from publication or availability bias). The thirty-three studies included in the pool were coded for seventeen substantive and methodological features, fourteen of which were identified as independent and moderator variables. Li's meta-analysis reported findings based on two models commonly used in meta-analysis research: fixed-effect models (FE) and random-effects models (RE). FE models are "based on the assumption that the population effect size is the same in all the studies included in the meta-analysis and any variation between the studies is attributable to sampling variability" (Li, 2010, p. 326), while RE models "allow variation of the true population effect in the included studies, and the variation results from heterogeneous factors" (Li, 2010, p. 326). With outliers included, the average effect size of the overall effect of feedback on immediate post-tests was 0.70 for the FE model and 0.88 for the RE model.

Russell and Spada (2006), another of the earlier examples of a meta-analysis on the topic of corrective feedback, examined fifty-six studies of both written and oral corrective feedback in both laboratory and classroom contexts. Fifteen of the included studies were quantitatively analyzed producing an average effect of 1.16 (large) in favor of corrective feedback for both oral and written performance. However, at the time of that publication there was not a sufficient amount of prior work investigating other moderators of interest, such as the effects of implicit versus explicit feedback, to report quantitative moderating effects to the main effect.

In Mackey and Goo (2007), we expanded on Russell and Spada's findings, adding further research that enabled statistical comparisons of explicit and implicit feedback. We found that implicit feedback in the form of recasts provided higher effects than explicit (metalinguistic feedback) and negotiations. We also found that average effect sizes were larger for short-delayed post-tests than immediate post-tests and the effects were durable at long-delayed post-tests.

As noted above, Li (2010) was able to shed further light on this debate by examining even more moderators in a meta-analysis of thirty-three studies of corrective feedback. Findings confirmed a medium effect in favor of corrective feedback compared to a control group. An examination of explicit versus implicit feedback over immediate, short-delayed, and long-delayed post-testing indicated that in the immediate and short term, explicit feedback worked better than implicit feedback. However, at the long-delayed post-tests, implicit feedback produced larger effects than explicit. This added to the evidence we presented in Mackey and

Goo (2007) indicating that the effects of implicit feedback are more enduring than explicit.

6.8 Meta-Analyses on Task-Based Interaction

As I outlined in Chapter 1, along with corrective feedback, access to input, output, and negotiation for meaning together form the basis for the cognitive-interactionist approach to SLA (Gass & Mackey, 2015; Long, 1996), and this approach is one of the theoretical foundations on which task-based language teaching (TBLT) is based. The kinds of interactions that form the basis of task-based instruction have been meta-analyzed several times (Cobb, 2010; Keck et al., 2006; Mackey & Goo, 2007), robustly linking interaction processes to SLA. Task-based meta-analyses have also been extended to specific task features such as task complexity (e.g., Jackson & Suethanapornkul, 2013; Sasayama et al. 2015), contexts of interaction such as in computer-mediated settings (Ziegler, 2016), and full-scale implementations of task-based programs (Bryfonski & McKay, 2017). See Table 6.2 for a summary.

The first meta-analyses of TBLT examined the role of interaction in tasks in terms of grammar and lexis performance, opportunities for output, and the effects of corrective feedback (Cobb, 2010; Keck et al., 2006; Mackey & Goo, 2007). Mackey and Goo (2007) expanded on Keck et al.'s (2006) first meta-analysis by adding additional studies and examining methodological factors that impact interaction findings.

Since these first meta-analyses affirmed the link between task-based interaction and successful SLA, other studies have examined specific factors and approaches to TBLT. A study by Ziegler (2016), for example, compared interactions in face-to-face (FTF) and computer-mediated (CMC) contexts. Her meta-analysis of previous work found a small advantage for interaction in synchronous CMC (SCMC) on measures of overall L2 learning outcomes. However, she did not find significant differences between CMC and FTF, suggesting the mode of communication has no statistically significant impact on the positive developmental benefits associated with interaction.

Bryfonski and McKay (2017) examined the effects of TBLT when it is implemented program wide in comparison with traditional language teaching pedagogies. Prior research and meta-analysis of TBLT had focused on the effects of short-term interventions, especially in laboratory settings, because of the difficulties involved in finding good-quality longer term TBLT implementations. This timeline problem was

Table 6.2 Sample meta-analyses of task-based interaction and TBLT

Authors and year of publication	Domain	Moderators	Number of studies analyzed	Effects (d)
Keck et al. (2006)	Task-based interaction and L2 development	Target feature (grammatical versus lexical), task type, treatment length, task essentialness, opportunities for pushed output	14	.92 (task-based interaction overall)
Mackey & Goo (2007)	Task-based interaction and L2 development	Type of target, occurrence of feedback, timing of feedback, focus of feedback, opportunity for modified output, context, setting, post-testing (immediate versus delayed), implicit (recasts) versus explicit (metalinguistic) feedback.	28	.75 (task-based interaction overall)
Cobb (2010)	Task-based interaction and L2 development	Task types, target structures, treatment length, outcome measures	15	.67 (task-based interaction overall)
Jackson & Suethanapornkul (2013)	Effects of increasing task complexity and for L2 output	Resource-directing dimensions (Measure type (complexity, accuracy, lexis, fluency), task type (monologic versus interactive), task modality (spoken versus written)	9	Complexity (−.02) Accuracy (.28) Lexis (.03) Fluency (−.16)
Ziegler (2016)	Task-based interaction in computer-mediated contexts	Type of learning outcome, context, setting, interlocutor characteristics, type of target	14	.13 (computer mediated task-based interaction)
Bryfonski & McKay (2017)	Implementation of task-based programs	Program region, institution type, needs analysis, and cycles of implementation, stakeholder perceptions	52	.93 (task-based language teaching)

discussed by the authors, who reported a positive and medium effect ($d =$ 0.92) for TBLT implementation for a variety of developmental outcomes and described implications for the domain of TBLT implementation and language program evaluation in general.

6.9 Summary of Related Methodological Meta-Analyses

While meta-analyses can be useful for making sense of the vast results from empirical investigations, they can also be useful for pointing out the methodological approaches researchers use and making suggestions on where the field should go next. In the domain of tasks and corrective feedback, there have been several meta-analyses that have specifically investigated the methodological approaches researchers take to investigating interaction, corrective feedback, and tasks. Table 6.3 gives some examples of important meta-analyses.

Plonsky and Gass (2011) carried out what I believe was the first empirical assessment of study quality in SLA and they focused their investigations specifically on research in the tradition of the interaction approach to SLA. The authors specifically examined methodological features of the studies including statistical analyses and reporting practices. The authors point out strengths and weakness in current research methodology in interaction research. This is one example of how a meta-analysis can be used to inform future research.

Plonsky and Brown's (2015) methodological meta-analysis examined other meta-analyses in the domain of corrective feedback research. They looked at eighteen prior meta-analyses, the results those analyses found, and what contributed to the different outcomes observed. They found that domain definition (described more below) and search techniques contributed to variability in findings. For example, studies of written corrective feedback have found different results than those that have examined only oral feedback. The authors utilized their results to provide recommendations for future meta-analyses by L2 researchers.

The methodology utilized to examine task-based language teaching has also been meta-analyzed. Plonsky and Kim (2016) examined the range of linguistic and interactional features (e.g., accuracy, complexity, fluency, language-related episodes), task conditions (e.g., pre-task planning), modes (oral versus written, face-to-face versus computer-mediated), and settings used in TBLT studies. They uncovered that prior work has focused on analyses of grammar, vocabulary, accuracy, and different features of L2 interaction, and less on task-induced pronunciation, pragmatics, and task performance. The authors point out the need

Table 6.3 Important methodological meta-analyses of tasks and interaction

Authors and year of publication	Domain	Moderators/variables of interest	Number of studies analyzed
Bowles (2010)	Think-aloud protocols in task-based studies	Type of report, outcome measure, language or verbal report/task, type of task	9
Plonsky & Gass (2011)	Methodological quality in interaction research	Methodological features, statistical analyses, reporting practices associated with research quality and timing	174
Plonsky & Brown (2015)	Domain definition and search techniques used in corrective feedback meta-analyses	Search techniques, reported effect sizes, confidence intervals	18
Plonsky & Kim (2016)	Interests and methodological practices in task/TBLT studies	Contextual and demographic variables, methodological features related to study designs, sampling, analyses, reporting practices	85

for better reporting practices and recommendations for researchers interested in TBLT. Additionally, Plonsky states that "meta-analyses of language assessment generally lack comprehensive searches for primary studies" and "fall short in transparency surrounding the development and implementation of their data collection instruments" (Plonsky & Han, in preparation).

6.10 How Do We Do a Synthesis/Meta-Analysis?

Unlike in primary empirical investigations, syntheses utilize existing findings from selected publications as the "data" for the analysis.

However, the steps to conducting meta-analyses and research syntheses have a lot in common with primary research studies. The researcher must carefully define the research domain and operationalize the variables of interest. Researchers also "collect" data in the form of a well-specified literature search. Then, instruments must be created for analyzing the studies (usually in the form of a coding sheet) and then piloted. Data are then coded, analyzed, and interpreted, just like in primary research. This section provides some tips and tricks for performing each of these steps.

6.11 Tips for Defining the Research Domain

What will the synthesis be about? What gaps exist in prior literature? What is available to be analyzed? Answering these questions and subsequently deciding on the research domain, much like in primary research, is an important first step in a meta-analysis and one that is important to get right. Domain definition will have implications for the remainder of the process of conducting a meta-analysis and broader implications for the body of research the synthesis contributes to (Plonsky & Brown, 2015; Plonsky & Oswald, 2012). Plonsky and Brown's (2015) synthesis of fourteen meta-analyses on corrective feedback illustrates the importance of domain definition by demonstrating how eighteen meta-analyses with the same general domain (corrective feedback) yielded different results. A study with a very wide scope (e.g., written and oral corrective feedback) will produce very different results than one with a narrower scope (e.g., implicit oral corrective feedback in classroom contexts). One method is not inherently superior to the other, but each will offer different benefits and drawbacks. For example, a domain with a narrow scope might be able to answer targeted research questions, but not have very many studies available that meet the search criteria and therefore will have a limited sample. A broad research domain might be able to include many studies and therefore produce more generalizable results but may lose the targeted focus of a narrowly defined domain. In their 2015 study, Plonsky and Brown found that the varied results were related to the different ways that the authors of the earlier studies had defined their domains – ranging from broad topics like written corrective feedback for grammar in classroom contexts (Truscott, 2007) to broader domains like corrective feedback as a type of instruction (Norris & Ortega, 2000). Notably, the various domains resulted in varied effect sizes. Researchers embarking on a new meta-analysis project should keep a few key tips in mind when defining their research domain:

- The broader the topic, the greater the chance of available studies and possibly more generalizable results.
- The narrower the topic, the smaller the chance of available studies and more targeted but possibly less generalizable results.
- In order to conduct moderator analyses, there must be a sufficient number of studies included with the moderator variables under investigation.
- The scope of the research domain will have implications for all subsequent stages of the meta-analysis and for the findings. Carefully consider domain definitions before defining research questions and embarking on a full literature search.

Try It!

Conduct a broad search of a topic of interest to you in the Google Scholar database. How many relevant articles does the search produce? Now try a narrower domain within your topic of interest and search again. How many relevant articles appear now? How might the number of articles influence your decision on the scope of your meta-analysis?

6.12 How Do We Conduct a Thorough Literature Search?

After deciding on a research domain and research questions, the next step in a meta-analysis is to decide where to look for studies. It is critical to conduct a thorough search to avoid publication bias in the meta-analytic findings. Publication bias is the propensity of scientific researchers and publications to only publish findings that had statistically significant results (Rothstein et al., 2005). This phenomenon has also been referred to as the "file drawer problem" (Rosenthal, 1979), because studies that produce results that contradict researchers' hypotheses or produced null (nonsignificant) results end up in their file drawers (or maybe a dusty external hard drive as a more modern example) rather than being submitted for publication at journals.

As I mentioned earlier, in the general field of second language learning, there is a certain amount of controversy over the so-called bilingual advantage, with three researchers, de Bruin et al. (2015), questioning the reality of a bilingual advantage in executive control by arguing that the reported effects reflect a publication bias favoring positive results over null and negative results. They claimed that the publication bias invalidated the credibility of the positive published evidence. In a hard-hitting response, "Publication bias and the validity of evidence: What's the connection?" (Bialystok et al., 2015), many of the researchers who had published the original studies critiqued the methods and interpretations, concluding that the value of the critical meta-analysis was questionable, because the data analyzed did not provide adequate sensitivity to allow one to draw even tentative conclusions. This provides a cautionary tale for the use of meta-analytic research, while also making clear the importance of a thorough literature search.

A researcher might ask themselves the following questions:

- What databases should I search through?
- What keywords should I use in my searches?
- How do I avoid bias in my searches?
- How can I do more searches than reported in previous work?

Despite having the best intentions, prior investigations have found that applied linguistics researchers rely on the same three or four databases when searching for studies to include in meta-analyses and often do not employ techniques that would enable the inclusion of unpublished studies (or studies outside "mainstream" journals) (Plonsky & Brown, 2015). The most popular databases include: The Education Resources Information Center (ERIC), Linguistics and Language Behavior Abstracts (LLBA), and PsycINFO (Plonsky & Oswald, 2012). Other recommended databases include the increasingly popular Google Scholar, ProQuest Dissertations and Theses, and Web of Science. In order to increase the likelihood of finding unpublished or non-mainstream publications, researchers should also look at relevant listservs, personal websites, conference programs, and even consider what they see on social media since researchers increasingly report their work on Twitter. Many conference websites host PDFs of presentations and email addresses of presenters. Researchers who are planning on meta-analyzing a certain area might also consider reaching out to presenters or authors who have published in the area to see if (a) they can obtain the data they need to calculate effect sizes and include these studies in the analysis, and (b) to ask about any studies they might be unaware of but the person they are reaching out to might know about.

The technique of forward and backward citation searches can also be helpful: by looking through the citations relevant papers have cited, or places the relevant paper itself has been cited, more potentially includable articles might be found.

> **Try It!**
>
> Choose a meta-analysis cited in this chapter and conduct a forward and backward citation search for it. Try to identify at least one paper the authors did not include that you think it would be worthwhile to consider if you were to conduct a meta-meta-analysis of the article you chose.

6.13 How Do We Come Up with Inclusion and Exclusion Criteria?

After an exhaustive literature search that has attempted to find all relevant work, published or unpublished, the next step is to define specific criteria for inclusion (or exclusion) of each article in the synthesis. Some inclusion criteria might be simply practical: articles published in an accessible time-frame; articles published in the language(s) spoken by the synthesis authors. Other criteria will have to do with the calculations necessary to analyze results reported in each study (e.g., means, standard deviations, N sizes). Articles that fail to report the necessary information (perhaps even after the authors were contacted) will be necessarily excluded. The remainder of the inclusion and exclusion criteria will be driven by the domain and research questions. For example, a meta-analysis on interaction in classroom settings will exclude all studies that focus on interaction that takes place in labs or naturalistic settings. Many studies that seemed relevant at first will likely be excluded. It is best to keep a database of all studies for future reference and to make sure the same searches are not being repeated. If one of the criteria for inclusion is higher inference, multiple raters can be used to decide if studies should or should not be included and inter-rater reliability can be calculated. Ultimately, the inclusion and exclusion criteria should be specific and clear enough (in implementation and in the final write-up) that the search could be easily replicated producing the same set of included studies.

> **Try It!**
>
> Find a meta-analysis or research synthesis on a topic of interest to you and read the section on the study's inclusion and exclusion criteria. Were the criteria specific enough for you to replicate the author's search? Try to see if you can find the same studies that were ultimately included in your own search. Think of ways you might refine the description of the author's search criteria.

6.14 How Do We Code the Data?

Now that the studies have been collected and decisions have been made about what to include and exclude, the next step is to design the main instrument of a meta-analysis: the coding sheet. The coding sheet will need to be designed, reviewed, and piloted, just like any good data collection instrument. It is always better to code for more features of the study than may ultimately end up in the final analyses, or to include separate coding for items that ultimately may be combined. The first aspects of the coding sheet will deal with characteristics of the included articles, such as journal of publication and title of the article. Some suggestions and an example are presented in Table 6.4.

In the final analysis, it will be better to replace many words in the coding sheet with codes (e.g., 0, 1, 2...) so that totals can be more easily computed along columns and rows. For example, instead of typing "yes" for "funding" in Table 6.4, make a code for 0 for "no funding" and 1 for "funding."

Typically, in interaction, feedback, and task research, the next aspect of the coding sheet will collect information on the characteristics of the study context and participants (see Table 6.5 for an example).

The next section of the coding sheet will summarize the study's methodology and design. The parts to include will depend heavily on the

Table 6.4 Example of coding sheet for article characteristics

ID	Coder	Authors	Year	Type	Peer review	Funding	Funder
85	Mary	Doe et al.	2019	Handbook Ch.	Yes	Yes	NSF

Table 6.5 Example of coding sheet for study context and participant characteristics

Participant L1s	Target L2s	Age(s)	Proficiency level(s)	Proficiency measure	Location	Setting	Context	Institution type
Spanish	English	5–10	Beginner	Self-Assessment	Mexico	EFL	Classroom	Elementary school

Table 6.6 Example of coding sheet for study methods and design characteristics

N size	N treatment	N control	Selection criteria	Treatment length (weeks)	Pre-test	Delayed post-test	Intervention leader
60	30	30	Random assignment	3	Yes	Yes	Teacher

Table 6.7 Example of coding sheet for study outcomes

Dependent variable	Within-groups?	Reliability reported	Treatment mean	Treatment SD	Control mean	Control SD	ES (d)	F	p
Map task	Yes	No	44.14	4.93	38.55	35.24	.75	7.69	.008

domain of the synthesis. Table 6.6 shows an example for an oral correct-ive feedback study using a classic pre-, post-, delayed post-test design with two experimental groups.

Finally, the coding sheet will have a place for study outcomes and how they were measured (see Table 6.7). This is where your effect sizes will be reported and used for final effect size calculations.

You will likely refine the coding sheet several times as you go along, and you should expect that you will have to go back a few times to recode. No two coding sheets will look alike, however, and once the coding sheet has been developed you should have it reviewed, if pos-sible, by two or three experts to ensure nothing is ambiguous or forgot-ten. These people should be familiar with meta-analytic work, or familiar with the content area being analyzed (and if at all possible, both). Next, the coding sheet should be piloted and revised and possibly re-piloted and revised again. As just noted, changes are expected to be made during the coding process, even with the most carefully vetted sheets. This is the nature of meta-analytic work. New and unanticipated vari-ables or details come up as each study is added. Some areas might require more detail, while other codes may need to be combined. For example in Table 6.5, age might be collapsed into three codes: "1" for ages 5–10, "2" for ages 11–13, "3" for ages 14–16, depending on the studies included in the analysis.

If you have more than one researcher on your team, a column should always be included to indicate which rater coded which studies for inter-rater reliability checks. At least one additional rater should be trained to code a sub-sample of the included studies. In larger meta-analyses the additional rater should code somewhere between 20 and 50 percent of the studies (Lipsey & Wilson, 2001) or more, if a high level of agreement cannot be achieved. In smaller meta-analyses (which is the norm in applied linguistics and second language research), Oswald and Plonsky (2010) recommend all of the included studies be double coded. A question that emerges is how high the agreement needs to be. In Mackey and Gass (2016), we suggested, based on a review of method-ology books and articles in related fields, that 85 percent is a minimum acceptable coding agreement rate for our field.

Try It!

Pick a study in an area interesting to you and design a coding sheet that would account for all of the important characteristics and variables in that study. Would your coding sheet still work for additional studies? What areas might you have to add? What variables might you collapse?

6.15 How Do We Analyze and Interpret Findings?

The final task in a meta-analysis is calculating and reporting the mean effect of all the coded studies. There are a few aspects for consideration in this process:

- What to do when studies report multiple effect sizes for the same variables
- What to do when some studies have pre-post within-groups designs and others have between-groups designs
- What to do with missing data
- How to weight effect sizes
- How to graphically display results

Although there are no hard and fast rules for any of these questions, there are some best practices to keep in mind when analyzing the final results of a meta-analysis. These are outlined in several of the works on meta-analysis in our field (e.g., Norris, 2012; Oswald & Plonsky, 2010; Plonsky & Oswald, 2012). When multiple effect sizes are reported for the same relationships, there are a couple of options. The multiple effect sizes could be averaged together at the onset of the analysis which can be an easy fix. However, care should be taken to ensure that these effect sizes are truly compatible. In the case of within- and between-groups designs reported in the same study, it is better to keep the effect sizes separate to ensure within-groups designs are not biased (see Plonsky & Oswald, 2012, for more details). If critical data are missing, the researcher has several options, including reaching out to the original study's author(s) to ask for the missing data, estimating unreported values, or removing the study from analysis. When averaging effect sizes from included studies, we need to keep in mind that a simple average that does not take into account sample size or other factors will limit the reliability of the findings. Programs, such as CMA (Comprehensive Meta-Analysis: see Borenstein et al., 2005) and other freely available statistical packages, like R, are available to assist researchers in weighing effect sizes and other advanced decisions such as calculating the effects of moderating variables and the choice of a meta-analysis model.

When writing up the results of the meta-analysis, it can be effective to graphically display the results. There are a few graphs that are useful. One popular type is a funnel plot, which can help demonstrate the presence or absence of publication bias. A funnel plot graphs the effect size on the x-axis and (typically) the sample size of each study on the y-axis. An asymmetrical funnel plot will uncover publication bias in the sample (i.e., more points will appear on the positive effects side of the plot and fewer on the negative side of the plot as seen in the example in Figure 6.2).

Another graph that is useful for displaying the results of a meta-analysis is a forest plot (see the example in Figure 6.3). A forest plot lists all of the included studies by name on the y-axis and the effect sizes on the x-axis. Each box on the plot can be sized to represent the size of the sample and the "whiskers," or lines next to each point, represent the 95 percent confidence interval. The main effect is represented by the diamond at the bottom of the graph. This type of plot enables readers to quickly view all of the effects included in the study.

Finally, the results of the meta-analysis must be interpreted and contextualized in the literature review just like in primary research. Effect sizes can be interpreted using the benchmarks presented by Plonsky and Oswald (2014) where for between-groups studies a d value of 0.40 indicates a small effect, 0.70 a medium effect, and 1.00 a large effect. For within-groups designs, slightly different benchmarks are used to

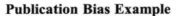

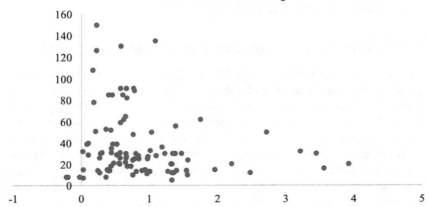

Figure 6.2 Funnel plot example

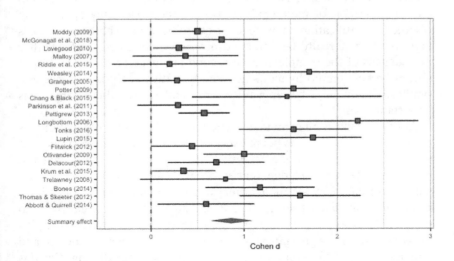

Figure 6.3 Forest plot example

account for the use of the same participants: 0.60 is a small effect, 1.00 a medium effect, and 1.40 a large effect. For *r* values, use the following benchmarks: 0.25 for a small effect, 0.40 for a medium effect, and 0.60 for a large effect. Using these benchmarks will allow readers to compare with other studies on the same topic and make sense of the meta-analysis in the domain of applied linguistic research.

6.16 Are There Any Issues with Meta-Analysis Research?

To answer the above question: Yes! Ellis (2018) points out that notwithstanding the fact that meta-analysis is increasingly popular and has provided much valuable information in second language acquisition research, there are potential dangers in doing meta-analysis research. He talks about issues of inclusiveness, the heterogeneity of language learners, definitions of variables, the need to consider alternative explanations, the critical nature of quality, and of comparing things that are not the same (apples and oranges). Ellis illustrates his discussion with examples from a number of meta-analyses from the second-language research area (e.g., Norris & Ortega, 2000; Plonsky, 2011; Qureshi, 2016; Spada & Tomita, 2010). Ellis argues that while there is a place for systematic reviews, findings may be better presented in narrative form rather than statistically. This is an important point. We should not jump on a bandwagon of meta-analytic work without carefully considering whether quantification may be over-quantification, whether variables that should not really be conflated are being conflated, and whether the nuances of the complexities in second language research might not always be best served by meta-analysis. Narrative analysis and research synthesis might be a better way forward and we shouldn't forget this important point.

Another issue is that meta-analytic work, like doing replications, is recommended by some as being excellent ways for novice researchers to start building a publication record. However, I would argue that the broad and deep knowledge that is often required to do solid meta-analytic research makes it a different undertaking from replications, where you follow a set design. For Ph.D. students in particular, who do meta-analyses as part of coursework and then seek to publish them, it's important to be cognizant of the fact that their level of detail and understanding of the scope of an area is often still developing. For this reason, partnering with a more experienced colleague or professor is often a good way to begin to publish meta-analyses.

A helpful development resulting from the increase in meta-analytic work is the understanding that doing work of sufficient quality that it might be reported in a meta-analysis (by oneself or by others) is part of being a good research citizen. We should take steps to include all the data in our work that is necessary for it to be meta-analyzed. This may mean taking advantage of open science initiatives, like the IRIS database (www.iris-database.org), and keeping our eye out for data repositories that are sure to emerge too. It is a sad fact that in meta-analyses one often has to exclude a study from consideration because the author(s) failed to include essential information. Thus, accurate reporting is particularly important when thinking about the future researchers who might conduct a meta-analysis.

CHAPTER SEVEN

Investigating Interaction, Feedback, Tasks, and L2 Learning in Instructional Settings

In this chapter I focus on research on interaction, corrective feedback, and TBLT in instructional settings. I describe this research in a wide range of classroom-based settings, including factors such as integrating observations into task studies, designing quasi-experimental studies, and carrying out action research. I talk about some of the practical considerations in classroom research into interaction, feedback, and tasks, including some of the challenges (and rewards) of carrying out research with younger learners in classrooms.

7.1 Instructional Settings for Interaction, Feedback, and Task Research

We usually distinguish classroom or instructional studies from those we carry out in a lab or as part of an experiment by acknowledging that while classroom research is much closer to the authentic practice of language teaching and learning, laboratory (or "lab") research allows us to exert control over experimental variables. In lab research, we can randomly assign learners to different types of control and treatment groups. Random assignment is typically not possible in classroom-based research contexts, due to school and student schedules and restrictions imposed by research regulatory bodies such as the IRB. Experiments without random assignment are known as quasi-experimental research, which allows us some controllable options such as selecting classes for study that are held at roughly the same time each day to avoid a situation where learners who prefer early or late classes all self-select into one group.

There are obviously advantages and disadvantages to labs and to classrooms, although it is important not to be too reductive or oversimplify them. For example, the term *instructional settings* covers a very wide range of classroom and related contexts, including "general education, professional expertise, replenishing the profession, heritage language, study abroad" and a wide range of learners, such as the "school children, university students, asylum seekers, transnationals, sojourners, returnees, seniors, multilingual learners, advanced learners, Generation 1.5 students, refugees, those with interrupted schooling, distance learners" mentioned by Larsen-Freeman and Tedick, (2016, p. 1339), who also point out that learners come from a wide range of L1 and L2 linguistic backgrounds. In other words, research can vary in terms of the studies done under the instructional setting umbrella almost as much as instructional setting varies from lab research.

Let's take as an example the sort of study which has come to be known as aptitude–treatment–interaction. Such research has a relatively high level of control, and typically tests learners for some kind of aptitude for language learning (working memory, for example, or cognitive creativity), and then assesses them, typically within an instructional setting, to see how they respond to some kind of treatment (for example, explicit versus implicit corrective feedback from instructors, or other students, as they carry out oral communicative tasks), the goal being to see if particular aptitude profiles and particular types of treatment lead to different learning outcomes. In an instructional setting, this is an example of a relatively tightly controlled quasi-experimental study.

We can contrast that sort of research with a different sort of study: a study where migrant learner children's thoughts and beliefs, expressed in their L1s, about (often unfamiliar) classroom settings and instructional techniques. Researchers in such a study could ask how data on factors like reported anxiety during classroom interaction might be used by instructors to lessen stress and increase opportunities for language learning.

These would both qualify as instruction studies but are each very different. The second study with migrant children would use relatively unstructured learner-focused oral interviews and focus groups versus the pre-test/post-test data of the first study that would focus on aptitude.

Often, instructional studies begin as an idea that gets tested in a lab, and then, moves to being suitable for testing in the classroom. Whether research carried out in the laboratory can (or cannot) be generalized to the L2 classroom is, of course, an empirical question and must be addressed by research. This chapter focuses on classrooms while also recognizing that given the wide variety inherent in interaction, feedback, and task data, instructional settings for studies involving these variables are not monolithic.

7.2 Using Observations in Interaction, Feedback, and Task Research

Observations can be used as tools in several different settings where interaction, feedback, and task research are carried out. In second language classrooms in particular, L2 researchers use observations to gather information about things like the different types of input, interaction, corrective feedback, and output in the classroom, together with information about the context, including the instructional activities, tasks, and conditions that occur in second and foreign language classrooms. The abstract in the next Read It! box is of an observational classroom study.

Read It!

Llinares, A. & Lyster, R. (2014). The influence of context on patterns of corrective feedback and learner uptake: A comparison of CLIL and immersion classrooms. *The Language Learning Journal, 42*(2), 181–194.

"This study compares the frequency and distribution of different types of corrective feedback (CF) (recasts, prompts and explicit correction) and learner uptake in 43 hours of classroom interaction at the 4th–5th grade level across three instructional settings: (1) two content and language integrated learning (CLIL) classrooms in Spain with English as the target language; (2) four French immersion (FI) classrooms in Quebec (using published data from Lyster and Ranta, 1997); and (3) three Japanese immersion (JI) classrooms in the US (using published data from Lyster and Mori, 2006). The findings revealed that teachers in all three settings used recasts, prompts and explicit correction in similar proportions, with recasts being the most frequent, followed by prompts then explicit correction. However, in the CLIL and JI classrooms, the majority of learner repair moves followed recasts, whereas the majority of repair moves in FI classrooms followed prompts. The similarities and differences across contexts are discussed in terms of the different types of recasts used by the teachers (i.e. didactic recasts in CLIL and JI; conversational recasts in FI), as well as in terms of context-specific influences and the teachers' professional trajectories" (p.181).

Being an effective observer in a classroom means two things. First, we need to be sure we collect the data we need to answer our research question or, if doing interpretive research or classroom ethnography, to be sure we gain sufficient understanding of what we are observing. Second, we need to be unobtrusive observers, taking care that our presence is not felt in the classroom to the extent that we may be influencing the class and affecting the validity of our research. In other words, we must try to avoid Labov's (1972) well known observer's paradox, although it is also worthwhile considering Gordon's (2012) argument that researchers should move beyond seeing the observer's paradox as a methodological limitation and instead investigate the opportunities it might offer researchers and study participants alike. In classrooms, for example, it often turns out that, in small group or dyadic work, having another speaker of the language of instruction is helpful and even if all the learners can see is that we know if they are interacting in the L2, it might make them try a little harder than if we weren't there. This might negatively impact our observation (we're not getting what we would get if we weren't there), but positively impact their learning in line with Gordon's arguments.

Being obtrusive could potentially risk alienating instructors and students in impacting the quality of the lesson. Children, for example, can become very easily distracted by recording equipment, even if it's just an iPhone, and may pay more attention to a new person than to their instructor. It's worth considering these things and observing the same group on a number of occasions, to get children or students used to your presence as an observer.

7.3 Interaction, Feedback, and Tasks in Action Research and Issues of Objectivity

Classroom observations are carried out by a range of people, for example researchers outside the educational environment and instructors or supervisors who may be observing for a study or for professional development. Instructors sometimes also carry out self-observations, usually by making video recordings for watching later. When classroom teachers investigate questions they have about their own students' learning using research techniques, it is sometimes known as action research (see below for more details).

We also need to think about how objective or subjective observers are. The level and impact of subjectivity on our research needs to be clearly recognized and reported in write-ups. Traditionally, objectivity is valued in second language research, particularly in experimental work. In classroom studies, it is usually important for researchers to simultaneously strive for objectivity while also taking into account that there will often be subjective elements in how they gather data, analyze data, and report the results of analyses. As I said in an article with Kendall King

(King & Mackey, 2016): "Classroom researchers are often poised (or torn or pulled) between these varied understandings of objectivity" (p. 218). On the one hand, an insider to a classroom context might be better positioned to gain rich qualitative data from participants with whom they have already established rapport. Teachers, students, and research participants in general might be wary of an outsider that they do not know and may be more reluctant to share their experiences. On the other hand, too much rapport with a participant could result in biased data, such as, for example, data obtained by asking leading questions in an interview. This may occur without the researcher even knowing they are doing it, due to a pre-established relationship with the participants. So, it is critical that researchers reflect on the many ways objectivity can come into play in collecting and analyzing data.

When observing interaction, feedback, and tasks in an instructional setting, obviously you need the permission of the instructor to observe their class and it's best to obtain this well in advance of the scheduled observation(s). This is usually a requirement in any IRB or ethics board consent process (for universities, for school districts, and so on) and it might even allow the classroom teacher to consider the observation as they plan their lessons, and help to alleviate nerves and thus impact implementation. One thing to be aware of when working with schools and language programs is that administrators can give permission, but it's best to follow up yourself with individual classroom instructors to make sure they also know and have consented, and to negotiate the schedule and observation process with them. It is also important to ask about logistics, like when to arrive. Arriving a little before the learners or when they are engaged in some activity when their attention will be focused elsewhere can all lessen the impact of the observer. You can also negotiate with the instructor where to sit in the classroom so as to be minimally intrusive while also capturing the view you need. Some instructors prefer observers to sit in the back or off to the side of the class. As I've already said, coming to class a few days before conducting the research can habituate the students to your presence. Sometimes learners are accustomed to being observed, either by supervisors or peers of the instructor, so little explanation is necessary. However, in other classes, particularly those early in a program, observation might be new for the students. In this case it is helpful if you make contact with the instructor beforehand because having more than one observer in the classroom at any time might be disruptive to instruction, and the teacher is always best placed to comment on this.

Keep It in Mind!

Review this checklist for setting up observations:

- Contact the classroom instructor (in person if possible).
- Ask about the schedule for observation and convey your preferences.
- Negotiate your observer's role in the classroom, including pre-visits, arrival time, introductions, and seating arrangements.
- Offer to debrief the instructor (either during or after the observational period) on the findings of the study.
- Clearly express appreciation to the instructor, students, and administration afterwards.

Read It!

Wang, W. & Loewen, S. (2016). Nonverbal behavior and corrective feedback in nine ESL university-level classrooms. *Language Teaching Research, 20*(4), 459–478.

"Nonverbal behavior is an area of recent interest in second language acquisition (SLA). Some researchers have found that teachers' nonverbal behavior plays a role in second language (L2) learners' learning. Furthermore, corrective feedback during L2 interaction can also be facilitative of L2 development; however, little is known about how nonverbal behavior accompanies teachers' corrective feedback. The current study investigated teachers' nonverbal behavior in corrective feedback during 48 observations (about 65 hours of recordings) of nine classrooms for English as a second language (ESL). The results indicated that teachers used a variety of nonverbal behavior in their corrective feedback, including hand gestures (specifically iconics, metaphorics, deictics, and beats), head movements, affect displays, kinetographs, and emblems. Specific nonverbal behaviors that commonly occurred in the observations were nodding, head shaking, pointing at an artifact, and pointing at a person" (p. 459).

7.4 Introspections in Classroom Research on Interaction, Feedback, and Tasks

I introduced introspections in Chapter 4, covering a range of different types, including stimulated recall, which is one of the most commonly used in second language research. There are other forms of introspections which are particularly useful in instructional settings where interaction, feedback, and task research are carried out, including uptake charts, to which I turn next.

7.5 Uptake Sheets in Classroom Research on Interaction, Feedback, and Tasks

As I have explained previously (for example, in Mackey & Gass, 2016), uptake sheets were initially developed as a method of data collection based on a Lancaster University researcher, Dick Allwright's, interest in understanding what learners were perceiving about what they learned in their language classes; his piece is memorably titled "Why don't learners learn what teachers teach?"(Allwright, 1984). Why, indeed? Allwright collected learners' reports about "whatever it is that learners get from all the language learning opportunities language lessons make available to them" (Allwright, 1987, p. 97). In classroom research into interaction, feedback, and tasks, learners can be asked to check boxes and/or write down what they are focusing on during interaction, or while receiving or hearing feedback as part of tasks. Using uptake sheets requires taking a moment away from what's going on right in front of the learner, but can provide researchers with one more source of data on learners' perspectives about interaction, feedback, and tasks while they are in process. Learners can be trained to fill out uptake sheets so they become less obtrusive for them.

An example of an uptake sheet can be found in Table 7.1. This chart focuses on the tasks that classroom learners are doing during a class, and requests information about their anxiety, motivation, and corrective feedback. Learners are asked to make note of their anxiety levels, their motivation, and the feedback they receive. To make this as quick and easy as possible, learners fill in a thermometer graphic to note their level of anxiety and circle the thumbs up or thumbs down to indicate motivation. Feedback is marked on a graphic in the form of a corrective pencil, next to which learners can jot down any feedback they receive. Responses on this sort of uptake sheet can be made on paper, online, or via an app.

In an early study of the effects of different uptake sheet formats on learner reports about their learning, we (Mackey et al., 2001) asked learners to fill out different formats of uptake sheets because we were interested in how the format of the uptake sheet shaped the quantity and quality of what learners reported. Learners were given three formats to indicate "(a) which language forms or concepts they noticed, for

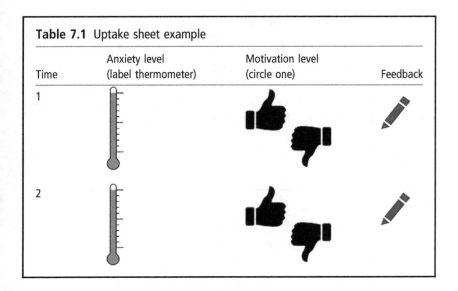

Table 7.1 Uptake sheet example

Time	Anxiety level (label thermometer)	Motivation level (circle one)	Feedback
1			
2			

example, pronunciation, grammar, vocabulary, or business; (b) who produced the reported items, for example, the learner, the instructor, or their classmates; and (c) whether the reported items were new to the learner" (Mackey et al., 2001, p. 292). We provided our classroom learners with uptake sheets at the beginning of class for each of the six consecutive classes and they wrote what they noticed about language during the class. Results indicated that the format of the uptake sheet affected both the quantity and the quality of what learners reported, for example the language-focused format encouraged greater quantity of reporting while the language- and context-focused format encouraged quality in terms of more detailed reporting. We suggested piloting and comparing multiple versions of uptake sheets before utilizing them in a study to ensure maximum effectiveness.

7.6 Stimulated Recalls in Classroom Research on Interaction, Feedback, and Tasks

As I explained in Chapter 4, a typical stimulated recall would involve making a recording of a class, or a portion of the class, for the stimulus, which would then be played to a student (or instructor), periodically pausing the recording and asking learners to say what they had been thinking at that particular point in time. Stimulated recall has been argued to provide a window into learners' interpretations of the events that were observed as they were observed. They have been widely adopted as a data source by researchers interested in viewing some aspects of what might be going on in learners' minds. We provide a very detailed account of stimulated recall methodology, as well as considerations in applying it in classroom and laboratory studies, in Gass and Mackey (2015).

The study in the following Read It! box deals with stimulated recall in the classroom.

Read It!

Sato, R. (2016). Examining high-intermediate Japanese EFL learners' perception of recasts: Revisiting repair, acknowledgement, and noticing through stimulated recall. *The Asian EFL Journal Quarterly, 18*, 109–129.

"This study examined three high-intermediate Japanese university students' perceptions of recasts. The learners were engaged in an interview test in which recasts were given. Stimulated recall interviews were conducted after the interview test. The analysis of the stimulated recall found that in most cases of repair, which is correct reformulation of an error occurring immediately after recasts, learners noticed the recasts and that when they responded to recasts via verbal or non-verbal acknowledgement, such as "yes," "mm", or nodding, noticing rarely occurred. In addition, it was found that the learners were less likely to have noticed recasts when they failed to respond to them. The results suggested that a frequency count of learner repair after recasts is a valid measurement of their effectiveness. The analysis of comments obtained through the stimulated recall partially implied that learners mainly used their explicit knowledge in noticing recasts to repair their initial problematic utterances" (p. 109).

7.7 Using Journals in Studies of Interaction, Feedback, and Tasks in L2 Learning

Journals of learners enrolled in classes can produce useful data on a range of aspects of the second language learning process, as well as learners' and instructors' insights into their own learning and teaching processes. Learners can be given specific instructions about what to write about: in general, guided journals are more helpful at eliciting learners' thoughts than unstructured ones, which can prove intimidating. Journals can sometimes be oral (it's easy these days to ask learners to hit record and send their researchers or instructors a voice file). In interaction, feedback, and task research, journals can provide information on learners' views about interaction (e.g. whether they have interacted with anyone outside their instruction that week and what they recall about the interaction), about feedback (e.g. whether they noticed any feedback and what they noticed about it), and about tasks (e.g. task difficulty, sequencing, and so on). Journals can be used as a source of how perceptions change (or not) over time. However, as I alluded to in Chapter 4, we also need to think about some of the issues involved in the use of journals, including memory decay, and of course, how subjective the data are.

Some instructors integrate journals into their teaching practice, asking students to keep diaries as a part of coursework (and even sometimes the assessment). Focusing on specific aspects of the instruction, for example, whether they find it easier to notice a recast if it comes from a peer or a teacher, for example, can be an interesting way to use them.

Diaries kept by instructors have also provided interesting data in the second language research field more generally. For example, Bailey, Nunan and Swan (1996) used instructor diaries to investigate the role of language learning and teaching beliefs in decisions made by student instructors.

Keeping journals requires time from those who write or record them and for the researchers who code the data and look for patterns. Guidelines for the range and amount of writing or time of speech expected per entry can be given, and sample entries can be provided to help learners get started. Journal writers can be encouraged to keep a notebook or a smartphone to record insights as they occur and transfer them later to the diary (or leave them in an audio file in the case of oral diaries). Learners can also be reminded to include examples to illustrate their insights in the diary entries.

The study in the next Read It! box deals with diary research in the classroom.

Read It!

Lee, V. & Gyogi, E. (2015). *The reflective learning journal in the classroom.* [Paper presentation]. The Annual International Conference on Language Teaching and Learning and Educational Materials Exhibition, Shizuoka City, Japan.

[Paper abstract] "In this paper, we highlight the role of the reflective learning journal in 2 different classrooms: a translation classroom in Seoul and a Japanese-language classroom in London. In both classrooms, the learning journal was assigned to students for the duration of 5 classes. Excerpts from 5 students' journals from both classrooms are presented and discussed with reference to Moon's (1999, 2004) map of the reflection process to offer student perspectives and identify how the learning journal helped in the areas of interests identified, doubts encountered, and strategies explored for obstacles. The results from both classrooms show that reflective learning journals enabled a greater focus on the learner by both the teacher and the learner. By reflecting on their own work, learners can discover more about their selves during the process of learning. For the teacher, this reflection can provide insight to the learners' process of learning."

7.8 Group Assignments in Quasi-experimental Classroom Research on Interaction, Feedback, and Tasks

In classroom research, students in intact classes are often assigned to different groups. For example, one class may be assigned to be a treatment group, in which case they may receive a certain form of corrective feedback from the instructor and another comparable class may be assigned to serve as a second treatment group that receives a different form of corrective feedback, like prompts, while a third class serves as the control group and takes the same amount of time on activities and tasks as the experimental groups, but receives no feedback. The aim of this group assignment would be to isolate the effects of the variable under investigation (in this case, the type of feedback) on, for example, the students' morphosyntactic development. It is important to watch out for the fact that studies that require control groups can be ethically questionable in classroom-based research, as withholding something from learners where we have every expectation that they might benefit from it should lead us to ask questions about how fair that is to those learners, and to figure out how we might help them by adding in what they missed at a later point. This is certainly the case in corrective feedback studies; for example, in a longitudinal study of the course of an entire semester, it would be unethical for a control group to receive no corrective feedback, since we know that corrective feedback (in some form or another) is beneficial to SLA. In the case where a control group is required for the study design, it would be best to design the treatment to last only over the course of several tasks or activities or in controlled situations, to avoid withholding feedback from an entire class.

The studies in the next Read It! boxes deal with experimental classroom research.

Read It!

McKinnon, S. (2017). TBLT instructional effects on tonal alignment and pitch range in L2 Spanish imperatives versus declaratives. *Studies in Second Language Acquisition, 39*(2), 287–317.

"The present study investigates the prosody/pragmatics interface in TBLT by extending the traditional morphological focus-on-form to a focus on intonational forms, with Spanish declaratives and imperatives. Twenty-eight intermediate L2 Spanish learners were assigned to one of two conditions that differed in the type of focus-on-form present during the pre- and post-task phases of a focused, task-based intervention: focus on grammar (FOG) or focus on grammar + intonation (FOG + I). All participants were administered an oral discourse completion task in a pre- and a posttest that elicited Spanish imperatives and declaratives to measure gains. Results show that participants, regardless of condition, did not distinguish imperatives from declaratives using intonation in the pretest. However, participants in the FOG + I condition modified their pitch range and pitch accents in the posttest to signal a difference between imperatives and declaratives, though their use was different from the input provided by a native speaker instructor" (p. 287).

Read It!

Sippel, L. & Jackson, C. N. (2015). Teacher versus peer oral corrective feedback in the German language classroom. *Foreign Language Annals, 48*(4), 688–705.

"This classroom study investigated the effects of oral teacher and peer corrective feedback on the acquisition of the German present perfect tense, including auxiliary verb selection (a rule-based structure) and past participle formation (an item-based structure). Intermediate learners of German were assigned to a teacher feedback condition, a peer feedback condition, or a control group. Learners in the teacher feedback group were corrected by their course instructor, while learners in the peer feedback group were trained to provide guidance to each other at the beginning of a two-day instructional treatment. Results from both an immediate and delayed posttest showed that while both experimental groups significantly improved in grammatical accuracy with both auxiliary selection and the past participle, the largest improvement was seen among the learners in the peer feedback group. These findings suggest that peer corrective feedback heightens learners' awareness of linguistic forms and that learners who provide such feedback may benefit not only from receiving but also from providing it. The results further demonstrate that peer feedback can be effective with less-proficient learners and with different types of grammatical structures" (p. 688).

Try It!

Think about the following broad research question: "How are idioms acquired by ESL learners?" How would you set up a classroom research study using authentic tasks? What would you need to think about (e.g. recordings, materials, consent, etc.)? Now consider a similar study conducted in an elementary school EFL classroom in Japan. How would you change the study? What different issues might arise in this context?

7.9 Interaction, Tasks, and Feedback in Action Research

Action research is usually defined following Crookes (1993) as "teachers doing research on their own teaching and the learning of their own students" (p. 131). It is also generally referred to as *collaborative research, practitioner research,* or *teacher research.*

Action research tends to be more oriented to instructor and learner development than it is to theory building, although it can be used for the latter. Chaudron (2000) points out that action research does not "imply any particular theory or consistent methodology of research" (p. 4) and that the goals include wanting a better understanding of how second languages are learned and taught, together with a commitment to improving the conditions, efficiency, and ease of learning (Nunan, 1993). Putman and Rock's helpful book (2017) *Action Research Using Strategic Inquiry to Improve Teaching and Learning* provides a useful overview of the various methodologies that are associated with action research.

Read It!

Park, K. (2016). Employing TBLT at a military-service academy in Korea: Learners' reactions to and necessary adaptation of TBLT. *English Teaching, 71*(4), 105–139.

"The necessity to adapt theoretical second language pedagogies to a context of instruction has been argued in the literature for a long time. This case study introduces an attempt to realize a context approach (Bax, 2003) to Task-Based Language Teaching (TBLT) implemented at a Korean military-service academy. Considering the alleged need for studies that investigate learners' reaction to TBLT in actual English classrooms, an Action Research project was conducted at this institution. Based on the data collected through two surveys of 80 students, interviews with 25 students, video recordings of 10 lessons and the teacher's observation of the course throughout one semester, this study identifies several challenges for employing TBLT in this EFL context such as the learners' lack of L2 interactions and attention to feedback. This paper discusses ways to adapt TBLT to the English courses offered at Korean military service academies while cautioning against excessive optimism for the effects of TBLT in some EFL contexts. The findings would contribute to understanding the reality of English classrooms at a Korean college and drawing implications for designing English programs suitable for EFL college students" (p. 105).

Try It!

Teachers often decide to do action research in their own classrooms because they are interested in improving their own outcomes or teaching. If you are or have been an instructor, write some general questions about your own teaching that you might be interested in researching in relation to interaction, feedback, or tasks. Try to write at least three questions, the answers to which could lead to benefits in your classroom. If you haven't taught, think about a language learning class you've taken and come up with three questions that you would be interested in knowing the answer to. Think about how you would carry out this research while you read the rest of this section.

Doing action research entails busy teachers identifying problems or concerns in their own classrooms, and various researchers have written about how these should be problems that the teacher feels they can better understand and even solve if they do the research. In other words, action research is driven by the idea that teachers can improve things in their own classroom by doing the research. For example, an EFL instructor may be concerned that students seem to have particular problems with producing question forms in English orally, while not showing similar problems with written work. Next, the practitioner might do an observation in order to gather information about what is happening in the classroom; for instance, the instructor may carefully take note of what happens when the students are engaging in interactive tasks that require the oral formation of questions, figure out where problems seem to arise, with specific forms, with the oral genre, or with something else (or all three). At this stage it is common to create a dataset using information gathered from sources independent of the observations, for example other written work, relevant test scores, or something like questionnaires or interviews. This is known as triangulation – the process of obtaining data from more than one source – and it is important in many types of research, including qualitative, mixed methods, and action research.

What happens after the data are gathered in an action study like this is that the instructor might be able to come up with an intervention or treatment and see if that helps with the problem. This could be a special class on question formation, a workshop on listening for errors and providing feedback to peers, or other methods for drawing students' attention to their own issues with questions and suggesting resources to solve them. Finally, the instructor might work on a way to assess the effects of their interventions. This might involve another round of data gathering or even asking a colleague to observe the class to see if they draw the same conclusions. If the outcome is positive, the practitioner may share the results with other colleagues informally, or perhaps through newsletters, papers, blogs, or conferences. In disseminating results, it is worthwhile noting that action research is usually not intended for generalization and is not designed with that in mind. Rather, it is usually situated, or context dependent.

Read It!

Calvert, M. & Sheen, Y. (2015). Task-based language learning and teaching: An action-research study. *Language Teaching Research, 19*(2), 226–244.

"The creation, implementation, and evaluation of language learning tasks remain a challenge for many teachers, especially those with limited experience with using tasks in their teaching. This action-research study reports on one teacher's experience of developing, implementing, critically reflecting on, and modifying a language learning task to better address the needs of her students in an adult refugee English program. Task evaluation involved a response-based comparison of student success in task completion and qualitative student-based results. The results noticeably improved after the task modification and the successful implementation of the modified task led to changes in how the teacher viewed task-based teaching. The study serves as an example of how teachers can create their own tasks and of the importance of evaluating them empirically. The article concludes with the importance of action research as a means by which language teachers can address problems that arise in task-based instruction" (p. 226).

7.10 Practical and Logistical Considerations in Classroom Research on Interaction, Feedback, and Tasks

Classroom research comes in all sorts of shapes and sizes, ranging from highly ethnographic work in authentic classroom settings to quasi-experimental studies of the effects of specific instructional practices such as tasks and explicit feedback. There are, though, considerations, logistical and conceptual, that interaction, feedback, and task researchers might want to consider when designing and collecting data in instructional contexts. I also direct readers to the long discussion in Mackey and Gass (2015) on the logistics of collecting data in classrooms, and the helpful checklist reproduced in the Keep It in Mind! box below.

7.10.1 Recording

Choosing how to record the class is important. A large- or whole-class activity will need wide-angled video recording and a very sensitive microphone. Recording separate, simultaneous dyadic or small-group activities will mean trying not to pick up sound from adjacent groups, so pilot testing is important, as is seating groups in circles, as far away from each other as possible.

When recording younger learners in classrooms, as we note in Mackey and Gass (2015), we need to remember that, to children, our recorders or iPhones or indeed anything out of their usual classroom routine will be novel and a target for attention, including tampering with and playing. Following the same process I mentioned earlier in relation to observations, if the researcher starts coming to class before the data are collected, showing the equipment to the class a few days or weeks before the data collection begins, children can get used to the researcher and the equipment and, equally importantly, you the researcher will have a chance to meet the children which will give you a sense of which ones are prone to wandering attention (and therefore, perhaps, who should have recorders placed under their chairs rather than on the table in front of them). Avoiding temptation is always a good idea.

Keep It in Mind!

The following checklist (from Mackey & Gass, 2015, pp. 208–209) is helpful to consider when working out the logistics of classroom research.

- Select a recording format that will facilitate the ultimate uses of the data (e.g., transcription, analysis, presentation).
- Consider whose voices and actions need to be recorded, as well as how sensitively and distinguishably this needs to be done and in which situations.
- Determine what kinds of microphones and other equipment should be used for these purposes and where they should be placed to collect as much relevant data as possible.
- Supplement your primary recording method with a backup, but try to gauge what is necessary and sufficient for the job in order to avoid equipment malfunction or undue complexity. Pilot testing can help.
- Consider the amount of intrusion in the classroom caused by equipment and equipment operators.
- Take anonymity concerns seriously and act accordingly.
- Plan the physical arrangement beforehand, taking into account the suitability and adaptability of the environment.
- Consider human factors such as the age of the participants and how the equipment may affect them; acclimate learners if necessary.
- In all of these areas, pilot testing can be immensely useful.

7.10.2 Informed Consent

As with all research, obtaining the consent of participants is critical. In the case of research in instructional settings, this usually means from several parties. Obviously, consent must be obtained from learners (and also from their guardians or parents if the learners are children); consent also needs to come from the instructor, and often also from the program or school administrators. If the research is in a school setting, then usually an IRB (or equivalent regulator) at the researcher's institution and a school district IRB must be approved. In classroom research it is particularly important that students do not feel pressured, so it's best, if possible, to have someone other than their instructor ask them about participating. It is also important that they are assured that there will be no penalties if they do not participate. Finally, if they don't participate but others in the class do, it is important to reassure them that even if their voice or image is inadvertently captured (although they will be seated behind cameras and away from recorders), it will not be transcribed, coded, used, or shown in any way to anyone other than the researcher, who will ignore it.

CHAPTER EIGHT

Choosing and Using Eye-Tracking, Imaging, and Prompted Production Measures to Investigate Interaction, Feedback, and Tasks in L2 Learning

The tools discussed so far in this book have been fairly simple, mostly requiring only paper, pictures, a computer, smartphone, apps, and software. However, recent technological advancements are enabling researchers to examine L2 learning from innovative different angles. Newer studies have investigated corrective feedback and task-based interaction utilizing tools such as eye-trackers, brain-imaging, and ultrasound imaging, offering fresh perspectives on second language learners' L2 processing, development, and learning. While these technologies are unlikely to replace the traditional tools of investigation covered elsewhere in this book, it seems likely they will be increasingly used, possibly in conjunction with commonly used techniques in psycholinguistic approaches to research topics such as prompted production, reaction time, and priming, adding to our understanding of how interaction, feedback, and tasks impact L2 learning.

In 2006, I wrote: "In the future, the question of how interaction impacts learning might be investigated in collaboration with neuroscientists. Recent methodological advances in cognitive neuroscience permit investigation of cognitive processes in real time. Electroencephalography (EEG) and functional magnetic resonance imaging (fMRI) are noninvasive techniques that might prove particularly useful for interaction research... It is important to note that most research in cognitive neuroscience is in its infancy" (Mackey, 2006 pp. 369–379). Now, technology typically used in psychology and neuroscience has become increasingly commonly used in linguistics, and more specifically, second language research in contexts that can include interaction, feedback, and tasks, amongst other activities (e.g. Faretta-Stutenberg & Morgan-Short, 2018b; Morgan-Short, Faretta-Stutenberg et al., 2015).

Before getting too far into this topic, though, I would like to echo the same words of caution I sounded in reference to some of the more recent neurolinguistics techniques in the experimental and observational science areas. As I have written previously (e.g. King & Mackey, 2016; Mackey, 2016; Gass & Mackey, 2017), it is important to keep in mind that that even though some of these newer methods can provide a window for us to look through to gain insights into cognitive processes, what we think is going on may not be exactly what is actually going on. We may believe because we are using technologically advanced measures, like imaging, that our observations are cut and dried; however, we have to realize that much of this sort of work is in its early days. As applied linguists and L2 researchers, most of us were not trained as neuroscientists, and even neuroscientists express skepticism about the applicability of their own work to actual knowledge of understanding how learning occurs. More than ten years ago, researchers were warning that "educators' current fascination with synapses and brain images causes them to overlook a substantial body of psychological and behavioral research that could have immediate impact in the classroom" (Bruer, 2006, p. 105).

A recent paper concurs, admitting that "there is currently very little neurobiology research that might explain how concepts as important to learning as metacognition and knowledge organization might be expressed in the brain" and

> "a significant portion of our knowledge linking learning to cellular and molecular changes in the brain is indirect, deriving from animal studies or studies conducted in the confinement of a magnetic resonance imaging scanner. In the future, we may be able to look into the human brain in real time and get more direct information about how synapses and circuits change in students as they learn" (Owens & Tanner, 2017, p. 7).

So, it is important at the outset to recognize that as we try to learn more about what's going on in interaction, feedback, and task-based learning, while imaging is important and interesting, we are still in the early stages. As we also know, triangulating information is always helpful, as is often the case in studies involving working memory (see for example helpful research by Indrarathne & Kormos, 2018 and Révész & Gurzynski-Weiss, 2016).

8.1 Eye-Tracking in Interaction, Feedback, and Task Research

Eye-movement studies have played an important role in interaction, feedback, and task research, where many researchers have asked questions about what is actually going on in learners' heads as they interact, and receive and respond to feedback while carrying out tasks. With appropriate equipment and training, researchers can gain a wealth of data regarding the processes involved in interacting. As Frenck-Mestre (2005) notes, eye-tracking enables the recording of the "jumps, stops, and re-takes [and] provides a to-the-letter, millisecond-precise report of the readers' immediate syntactic processing as well as revisions thereof" (p. 175).

There are a number of research areas that can be investigated with eye-movement tracking. For example, researchers can determine sources of ambiguity (i.e. when and where negotiation for meaning during interaction becomes necessary) and what individuals do to resolve them. Eye-tracking can also be used to determine differences between contextual and lexical constraints on processing (Altarriba et al., 1996) or how working memory and eye movements are associated (Indrarathne & Kormos, 2018). Eye-tracking can also support task-based research from the teacher's perspective, as demonstrated by Révész and Gurzynski-Weiss (2016). They tracked teachers' eye movements while they evaluated the difficulty levels of a series of tasks, and how they might modify the tasks to make them easier or more difficult. Révész and Gurzynski-Weiss found that teachers' gazes rested proportionately more on the instructions than on the pictorial input when they were evaluating the difficulty of the tasks, and their eye movements were generally consistent with the think-aloud data collected at the same time.

Read It!

For a more thorough primer on eye-movement recording research, see Winke, Godfroid, and Gass's (2013) introduction to the special eye-tracking issue of *Studies in Second Language Acquisition* and Godfroid (2019) which provides an extremely comprehensive guide.

Read It!

Winke, P., Godfroid, A., & Gass, S. M. (2013). Introduction to the special issue: Eye-movement recordings in second language research. *Studies in Second Language Acquisition, 35*(2), 205–212.

"An important part of understanding how languages are learned is understanding the cognitive processes that underly acquisition. Many methodologies have been used over the years to understand these processes, but one method of recent prominence is eye-movement recording, colloquially referred to as eye-tracking. Because more and more attention is being paid to this methodology by SLA researchers, we believe the time is ripe for this special issue focusing on eye-movement recording and SLA. Eye-movement recording is a versatile research technique with implications that reach into diverse areas. Thus, within the field, eye-movement registration has already been used to investigate lexical access and representation in bilinguals (e.g., Blumenfeld & Marian, 2011; Duyck, Van Assche, Drieghe, & Hartsuiker, 2007; Felser, Sato, & Bertenshaw, 2009; Flecken, 2011; Van Assche, Drieghe, Duyck, Welvaert, & Hartsuiker, 2011; Van Assche, Duyck, Hartsuiker, & Diependaele, 2009), syntactic ambiguity resolution (e.g., Dussias & Sagarra, 2007; Frenck-Mestre & Pynte, 1997; Roberts, Gullberg, & Indefrey, 2008; see also reviews by Dussias, 2010 , and Frenck-Mestre, 2005), attention (Godfroid, Boers, & Housen, in press), and cognitive processes during specific tasks, such as second language (L2) testing (Bax & Weir, 2012) and video-based L2 listening (Winke, Gass, & Sydorenko, 2013). This special issue presents the reader with an up-to-date understanding of some of the current research questions being investigated through eye-movement registration. In so doing, this special issue affords an opportunity to pause and evaluate how some applied linguists are utilizing this novel data-collection method in our field" (p. 205).

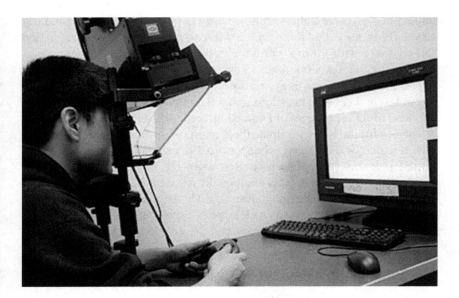

Figure 8.1 An eye-tracking machine (https://bit.ly/37Xudap)

> **Try It!**
>
> Even if you don't have access to an eye-tracking machine, take a few minutes to observe someone's eyes as they converse and then as they read a short paragraph. What do you think you might discern from their eye movements with advanced equipment?

8.2 Pupillometry Measures

Nascent second language research has begun to discuss the use of *pupillometry* (or measuring pupil size), which is an index of cognitive effort. Mathôt (2018) outlines pupillometry in cognition, explaining that pupils constrict in response to brightness (the pupil light response), in response to near fixation (the pupil near response), and dilate in response to increases in arousal and mental effort, either triggered by an external stimulus or spontaneously. He outlines how pupils provide information about high-level cognition. In the second language field, Schmidtke (2018) also provides a review for second language researchers, explaining pupillometry as "a welcome addition to other online methods such as eye-tracking and event-related potentials (ERPs)" (p. 529).

Pandža, Karuzis, Phillips, et al. (2020) used pupillometry to assess the impact of neurostimulation on how learners process and learn Mandarin tones. They used pupillometry growth-curve analysis, and triangulated this measure with a range of more traditional language outcome measures, including reaction times. For such studies, special pupillometry devices aren't required, as eye trackers can typically perform this function.

For researchers with questions about the impact on cognition and cognitive load of different types of interaction, feedback, and tasks, pupillometry might be a fruitful way to examine these questions in the future. For example, new research by Toivo and Scheepers (2019), using pupillometry, has supported previous survey-based studies about the emotional resonance of words in the L1 versus the less emotionally resonant L2, a good example of how pupillometry is being adopted and used in the bilingualism and linguistic fields. It might also be used as a measure of cognitive effort in comparisons between younger and older learners, and their performance on tasks.

8.3 Electroencephalogram (EEG) Tests

Event-related potentials (ERPs) are electrical responses generated by the brain in response to external stimuli (Luck, 2012) and are extracted from an electroencephalogram (EEG) test. EEGs use electrodes placed near the scalp to record the electrical potentials produced by the brain. Commonly employed in psychology research, this method of measuring online language processing can complement behavioral data by providing millisecond-by-millisecond information about how the brain responds to linguistic input. EEG is frequently employed to examine the similarities and differences between L1 and L2 processing (Dussias et al., 2019). EEG accomplishes this by examining the degree to which neural signals approximate those in native speakers. Studies of L2 to date have produced mixed results: some studies have found that L2 speakers are less sensitive to syntactic violations than NSs, whereas others have documented L2 speakers performing at the level of NSs and even exhibiting the same brain signatures (Dussias et al., 2019). Given these results, authors in this domain warn that there is a large amount of individual variation (for both NSs and NNSs) in terms of their responses to linguistic input and it might not be possible to generalize EEG data across all speakers.

EEGs have also been previously employed in second language research to investigate implicit versus explicit learning processes (e.g. Faretta-Stutenberg & Morgan-Short, 2018a, 2018b; Luque et al., 2018; Morgan-Short, Faretta-Stutenberg, et al., 2015). An advantage of this technique is that ERPs are recorded whether a participant responds outwardly to stimuli or not. ERPs also index whether and when a participant registers linguistic incongruities. This temporal information can distinguish automatic and controlled processes. In this way, ERPs can help answer questions related to implicit L2 learning. For example, a study by Faretta-Stutenberg and Morgan-Short (2018a) investigated the development of L2 Spanish grammatical gender agreement during study abroad. The authors used judgment and production tasks to assess the role of pre-departure proficiency and L2 use while abroad in behavioral development. They additionally used ERPs derived from EEG tests to examine the role of the same factors in the development of the learners' L2 processing signatures. Behaviorally, learners improved in terms of their scores on proficiency and grammatical judgment tests. However, on neurocognitive tests of language processing, the researchers did not find significant changes from pre- to post-testing. An examination of individual differences between learners identified a potential link between pre-departure proficiency and L2 contact and behavioral gains with the higher proficiency learners and learners who reported more L2 contact, experiencing greater gains. Processing results uncovered a link between time speaking the L2 and a positive shift in processing development.

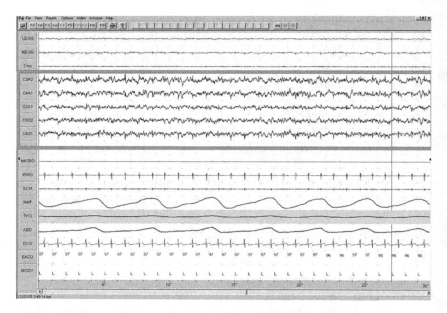

Figure 8.2 Example of an EEG scan of a sleeping person (https://bit.ly/35DJ0W8)

The researchers call for more research into individual differences in L2 performance and neurocognitive processing in longitudinal studies.

In the context of research on interaction, feedback, and tasks, we might be interested in the point at which a speaker decides repair is necessary or not, when and how a repair is formulated, or the extent to which mistakes are implicitly or explicitly noticed. ERPs might, for example, be used to investigate learners' reactions when they receive feedback. This is currently studied using a range of methods, for example using verbal protocols. However, ERPs would not give rise to the same sorts of concerns about memory, interference, reactivity, or veridicality although, of course, there would be a different set of concerns. A promising early ERP study showed lower-proficiency learners had altered activation patterns for grammatical violations they were unable to identify on paper-and-pencil tests (e.g. Tokowicz & MacWhinney, 2005). Studies that combine behavioral measures with neurocognitive processing observations in interaction- and task-based research could provide critical missing components to the puzzle of how, when, and why interaction and feedback work to promote L2 development. A useful method of collecting new kinds of data, fMRI might be used

for investigating a wider range of factors that might impact task, interaction, and feedback research than has currently been the case.

8.4 Functional Magnetic Resonance Imaging (fMRI) Tests

Although not as sensitive to temporal aspects of language as ERPs, fMRI
provides high-resolution information about the neural regions involved in
the processing of a language. Most fMRI studies measure blood flow;
when a certain brain region is active it will demonstrate increased blood
flow that is correlated with neural activity (Andrews, 2019), allowing
researches to localize brain activations. For example, in research on
sentence processing in a first language, when participants encounter different types of linguistic input, there is variance in the activation of specific
regions. When working memory is implicated in morphosyntactic processing certain frontal and subcortical regions are associated, whereas posterior regions are linked with lexicosemantic processes. In other words,
different parts of the brain are used for storing words and formulating
sentences. Looking at how these regions are activated during interaction
or task completion can help us understand how to design tasks to target
learners' strengths and weaknesses. Working with neuroscientists, questions about how language is processed and learned in the brain are in the
process of beginning to be answered more directly than has been the case
in second language research to date.

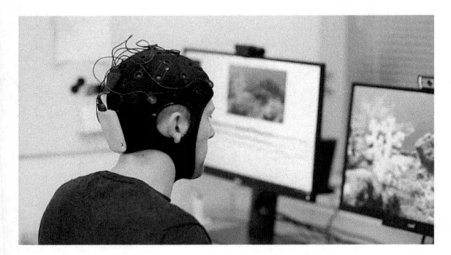

Figure 8.3 An EEG machine (https://bit.ly/30atwru)

It is fascinating to note also that beginner and near-native second language knowledge might also result in different regional activation differences or patterns. Early studies utilizing fMRIs claimed that "early" bilinguals (those who became bilingual at a young age) had different representations in the brain than L2 or "late" bilinguals; however, newer research has emerged that has indicated proficiency level is a more reliable factor for neural organization of language than age (Andrews, 2019).

Studies using fMRI routinely investigate brain activation while learning an artificial or previously unknown language (e.g. Morgan-Short, Deng, et al., 2015). For example, in a study of adult second language learners, Tagarelli (2014) found that when native speakers of English were trained from exposure to learn a subset of Basque to high proficiency, fMRIs captured activations that were associated with L1 processing. This suggests that late-L2 learners have access to L1 brain regions; however, other areas were also activated suggesting the L1 regions are not sufficient for L2 processing. Furthermore, Tagarelli (2014) found that at early stages of learning, participants relied on declarative memory and explicit processes for vocabulary and grammar learning; however, at later stages they relied on procedural memory and implicit processes for grammar learning. All of these results were thanks to fMRI, which highlighted the regions of the brain that were activated at various learning stages.

Read It!

Tagarelli, K. (2014). *The neurocognition of adult second language learning: An fMRI study* [Doctoral dissertation, Georgetown University]. At this permanent link: http://hdl.handle.net/10822/712460.

"Learners achieved very high proficiency in vocabulary and reasonably high proficiency in grammar, though morphosyntactic agreement was difficult to master. FMRI activation was found in areas associated with first language (L1) processing (e.g., BA45/47, and parietal cortex for lexical/semantics, and BA44 and 6 for grammar), suggesting that late-L2 learners have access to L1 regions. Additional areas were engaged, suggesting that L1 mechanisms are not sufficient for L2 learning and processing. At early stages of learning, hippocampal activation was found for both vocabulary and grammar. At later stages, basal ganglia activation was observed for grammar, particularly in the caudate nucleus. The findings suggest that early word and grammar learning relies on declarative memory (and more explicit processes), but that grammar later relies on procedural memory (and more implicit processes). These results highlight the utility of a mini-language model, have implications for neuro-cognitive theories of L2, and demonstrate the importance of integrating neural and behavioral methods in L2 research" (p. iii–iv).

In another example of a study like this, Jeong, Sugiura, Sassa, et al. (2010) used fMRI to determine differences between text-based and situation-based vocabulary learning. The fMRI allowed the researchers to see which areas of the brain were involved in various learning and retrieval functions in different modes. They found that the type of learning and use of lexical items affects how they are accessed and remembered. A later study, Jeong, Sugiura, Suzuki, et al. (2016) utilized fMRI to investigate a commonly researched individual difference – language anxiety. Language anxiety is one of the individual variables that researchers hypothesize might interact with willingness to communicate and/or the ability to benefit from corrective feedback obtained in communicative tasks. In Jeong et al.'s (2016) study, Japanese speakers who had learned English as an L2 participated in communicative and descriptive tasks in their L1 and L2 while in an fMRI scanner. The researchers found that the L2 communication tasks, where the participant was asked to interact with an actor in a video, rather than simply describe actions they saw, were the only tasks that recruited the region of the brain associated with goal-directed actions. The L2 communication, but not the description tasks, were also found to be sensitive to oral proficiency and anxiety levels as evidenced by brain activation in associated areas.

Read It!

Jeong, H., Sugiura, M., Suzuki, W., Sassa, Y., Hashizume, H., & Kawashima, R. (2016). Neural correlates of second-language communication and the effect of language anxiety. *Neuropsychologia, 84*, e2–e12.

"Communicative speech is a type of language use that involves goal-directed action targeted at another person based on social interactive knowledge. Previous studies regarding one's first language (L1) have treated the theory of mind system, which is associated with understanding others, and the sensorimotor system, which is associated with action simulation, as important contributors to communication. However, little is known about the neural basis of communication in a second language (L2), which is limited in terms of its use as a communication tool. In this fMRI study, we manipulated the type of speech (i.e., communication vs. description) and the type of language (L1 vs. L2) to identify the specific brain areas involved in L2 communication. We also attempted to examine how the cortical mechanisms underlying L2 speech production are influenced by oral proficiency and anxiety regarding L2. Thirty native Japanese speakers who had learned English as an L2, performed communicative and descriptive speech-production tasks in both L1 and L2 while undergoing fMRI scanning. We found that the only the L2 communication task recruited the left posterior supramarginal gyrus (pSMG), which may be associated with the action simulation or prediction involved in generating goal-directed actions. Further- more, the neural mechanisms underlying L2 communication, but not L2 description, were sensitive to both oral proficiency and anxiety levels;a) activation in the left middle temporal gyrus (MTG) increased as oral proficiency levels increased, and b) activation in the orbitofrontal cortex (OFC), including the left insula, decreased as L2 anxiety levels increased. These results reflect the successful retrieval of lexical information in a pragmatic context and an inability to monitor social behaviors due to anxiety. Taken together, the present results suggest that L2 communication relies on social skills and is mediated by anxiety and oral proficiency" (p. e2).

8.5 Research Using fMRI Techniques

Other research utilizing fMRI techniques has investigated questions related to bilingualism (Coderre et al., 2016; Mouthon et al., 2019). Research using fMRI can provide useful and interesting information about cognitive functioning and much has been used by researchers to weigh in on the debate of the "bilingual advantage," (i.e., whether or not bilingualism offers cognitive advantages such as increased executive control) (e.g., Bialystok, 2015; Pliatsikas & Luk, 2016; Mohades et al., 2014).

There are important limitations to brain-based research. As I noted at the beginning of this chapter, some have argued against making connections and assumptions in interpretation in this line of research, and of course, many point out that that imaging studies are extremely expensive in terms of equipment and time (time spent on training as well as running experiments). Some authors have pointed out the importance of experimental design (Andrews, 2019), noting that even simple changes between experimental and control groups in fMRI research can greatly impact the results in unexpected ways. Also, going back as far as a decade and half ago, there has been debate over what fMRI can and cannot tell us about second language learning (Paradis, 2004), with the most recent papers still noting that care should be taken when comparing fMRI-based results across studies (Andrews, 2019).

In summary then, fMRI technology is obviously much more costly in terms of equipment and training than second language researchers are used to. We have to learn how to develop stimuli, and work with neuroscientists to avoid the potential for misinterpretations and over-generalizations. Early research for the most part has been posing constrained questions and making cautious claims. It seems likely though that, with the huge potential to shed new light on the brain bases for SLA and interaction, these methodologies will increasingly be used in collaborations with neuroscientists to learn more about interaction, tasks, and feedback in the future.

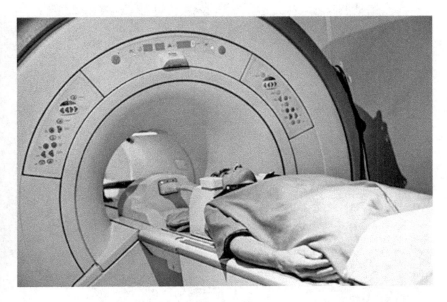

Figure 8.4 An fMRI machine (https://bit.ly/2sdeeFS)

8.6 Ultrasounds

While EEG and fMRI measure internal neural processing, ultrasound imaging, like eye-tracking, records or displays vocal tract movements that would otherwise be unobservable to researchers. Ultrasound, commonly utilized in the medical field, has recently been adapted by linguists to observe and record, for example, tongue articulations. Ultrasound imaging provides two-dimensional, real-time sagittal views of the moving tongue (Gick et al., 2008) and has been profitably applied to the teaching of segmental features in previous work (Gick et al., 2008, Tsui, 2012; Tateishi & Winters, 2013).

A recent study by Oakley (2019) utilized ultrasound tongue imaging and acoustic data including video recordings of the lips to investigate the articulatory strategies used by English speakers learning to produce French high vowels. Participants in this study performed two production tasks in both French and English while an ultrasound probe recorded their tongue movements and a camera and audio equipment recorded their lips and vocalizations. Oakley found that while NNSs of French are

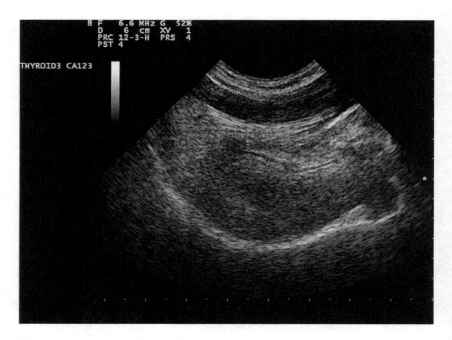

Figure 8.5 An ultrasound image of a tongue (© Nevit Dilmen [CC BY-SA 3.0 https://creativecommons.org/licenses/by-sa/3.0])

able to learn to use lip rounding like NSs, it was their tongue motions that caused their productions of French vowels to be nontarget-like.

Ultrasound, then, may be used not only for research but as feedback for instruction, as a tool to help learners understand where they should place their tongues to produce more native-like pronunciations. This is a common practice for speech-language pathologists who have used ultrasound tools when working with children and adults with speech delays and deficits (Barberena et al., 2014; Fabre et al., 2017). While to date, no empirical investigations in the field of SLA have investigated and compared interaction and corrective feedback utilizing ultrasound technology, Bryfonski (2019a) has argued for research that includes ultrasound as an additional form of corrective feedback. While oral corrective feedback is the type most commonly and easily employed in L2 classrooms, teachers and learners have recently become interested in how technology can be utilized to improve L2 outcomes, especially in pronunciation instruction, a notoriously difficult aspect of a second language to acquire. The impact of phonological feedback on L2 development has been studied previously (e.g. Bryfonski & Ma, 2019; Saito, 2019); however, biofeedback as provided by ultrasound imaging has yet to be investigated as an additional or alternative form of feedback for task-based interactions. As Bryfonski (2019a) suggests, one possibility would be to compare developmental and acoustic gains for learners who hear traditional oral corrective feedback for phonological errors during task-based interactions, with learners who see biofeedback from an ultrasound image, and also with those who receive both oral feedback and biofeedback. In this way, researchers could untangle the potential benefits and drawbacks of integrating ultrasound technology into L2 learning and teaching.

Keep It in Mind!

- Eye-tracking equipment can help researchers understand L2 users' thought processes, reactions to ambiguity, and even specific points of difficulty in tasks.
- EEG tracks brain activity in order to understand what parts of the brain learners are using at precise intervals, which helps understand how they deal with different types of interaction, feedback, or task challenges.
- fMRI provides actual images of the brain that reveal which areas are activated under certain conditions and how learners process language.
- Ultrasound imaging provides two-dimensional, real time sagittal views of the moving tongue.

8.7 Psycholinguistic Techniques: Reaction Time, Word Association, and Priming

In contrast to measures of eye, brain, or articulatory mechanism activity, prompted-response techniques present participants with stimuli which they must then respond to in some way. Interaction, feedback, and task researchers are often interested in these sorts of data collection measures because linguistic production is directly observable and obtaining it doesn't usually mean acquiring access to the expensive equipment and training required for the neurological and physical techniques described previously. I will focus on three that are commonly used: reaction times, word association, and priming.

8.7.1 Reaction Time

Reaction times are typically used in L2 research to shed light on how people process (certain aspects of) language. In other words, they are used as a measure that (indirectly) reflects processing. In reaction time experiments, times are generally measured in milliseconds, on the basis that the longer it takes to respond to something, the more processing load or "energy" is assumed to be required. For example, if we asked a learner to repeat an utterance containing a recast, where the original utterance was as follows "I see two big Siamese cat yesterday" we might predict that an utterance with several recasts, *I saw two big beautiful Siamese cats yesterday,* would take more time to repeat than an utterance with fewer recasts because the utterance with more recasts contains more changes to complex grammatical form than an utterance with fewer recast forms (and, hence, a greater processing load). Although this kind of study is traditionally conducted in a laboratory setting, researchers have recently measured reaction times in classroom and home settings, too. Cornillie, Van Den Noortgate, Van den Branden, et al. (2017) used reaction times as part of their study on corrective feedback. Tracking reaction times in a grammaticality judgment test embedded in an entertaining mini-game helped show that automaticity was improved with practice of the forms under study, and metalinguistic feedback did influence the outcomes. Another example of reaction times being used in a study of tasks is Lee's (2018) look at task complexity using a response time task.

Read It!

Lee, J. (2018). Task complexity, cognitive load, and L1 speech. *Applied Linguistics, 39*(3), 1–35.

"Relationships among task characteristics, L2 performance, and interlanguage development are of interest both for SLA research and the design of syllabuses and language teaching materials. Complexity has been identified as a promising, but methodologically problematic, task design feature. A study was conducted of the effects of progressive increases in the complexity (operationalized as number of elements) of three versions of each of three tasks on the syntactic complexity and lexical diversity of the speech of 42 English native speakers. Data on native speaker performance are important because they reveal task complexity effects unfiltered by non-native competence. Independent evidence that greater task complexity increased cognitive load was shown by participant self-ratings of perceived difficulty, mental effort, and stress, shorter prospective duration estimates and, using dual-task methodology, slower reaction times. Mid-complex versions of the three tasks elicited the most complex syntactic structures, and the most complex versions elicited the greatest lexical diversity. Implications are noted for the design of parallel studies with non-native speakers, along with suggested methodological improvements for future research with native and non-native populations" (p.1).

Reaction time measures are often used as a supplement to other kinds of elicitation techniques, for example, grammaticality or acceptability judgments used as means of determining linguistic knowledge. Underlying the use of reaction times in conjunction with these measures is the assumption that it takes longer to judge an ungrammatical sentence because a learner has to attempt to match the sentence with some structural description in the learner's grammar. In the case of an ungrammatical sentence, there is no structural description, hence the delay.

Try It!

Affordable or even free software such as PsychoPy and E-Prime are readily available to help researchers easily design and administer measures such as reaction time. Visit Psychology Software Tools at https://pstnet.com/products/e-prime/ to download a demonstration version of E-Prime software that will allow you to make your own tests. This type of software can often interface with other technology such as eye-tracking and fMRI (see above).

8.7.2 Word Association

Word association tasks have often been used in psychoanalysis as a way of gaining access to a patient's or client's mind. In interaction, feedback, and task research, a similar assumption can be made, the idea being that learning something about the word associations that learners make may provide a window into how their lexicon is organized. In other words, task and interaction researchers may be interested in understanding the semantic networks that learners have and how those networks are arranged.

In a typical word association task, respondents are presented with a word and asked to provide the first word that comes to mind. There are a number of linguistic bases for these associations. One type of response, in which the learner completes a phrase, suggests a syntagmatic relationship, akin to collocational knowledge. Thus, a word such as *comb* would evoke a response such as *hair*. Another type of response is a paradigmatic response, in which the response is part of the same word class as the stimulus. This category of responses includes synonyms and antonyms; thus, *hot* might elicit *cold*. Other responses, relying on word form, are known as clang associations, and are phonological or orthographic in nature. A response in this category might be seen in the case of the stimulus *nap* eliciting the response *nab*. The important point to remember about word association tasks is that they are able to provide information about the organization of the L2 lexicon as well as its relationship to the L1 lexicon and are thus of interest to task and interaction researchers who want to, for example, use tasks to raise awareness of lexical items that are unknown, or known but not automatic, and compare that knowledge before and after engaging in task-based interactions or receiving and responding to corrective feedback.

Read It!

Mann, W., Sheng, L., & Morgan, G. (2016). Lexical-semantic organization in bilingually developing deaf children with ASL-dominant language exposure: Evidence from a repeated meaning association task. *Language Learning*, 66(4), 872–899.

"This study compared the lexical-semantic organization skills of bilingually developing deaf children in American Sign Language (ASL) and English with those of a monolingual hearing group. A repeated meaning-association paradigm was used to assess retrieval of semantic relations in deaf 6-10-year-olds exposed to ASL from birth by their deaf parents, with responses coded as syntagmatic or paradigmatic. Deaf children's responses in ASL and English were compared at the within-group level, and their ASL was compared to the English responses of age-matched monolingual hearing children. Finally, the two groups were compared on their semantic performance in English. Results showed similar patterns for deaf children's responses in ASL and English to those of hearing monolinguals, but subtle language differences were also revealed. These findings suggest that sign bilinguals' language development in ASL and English is driven by similar underlying learning mechanisms rooted in the development of semantic frameworks" (p. 872).

8.7.3 **Priming**

In most priming experiments, two stimuli are typically presented successively, with the first one being the *prime* and the second the *target*. The participant must respond to the target in some way, and priming is said to occur when there is an influence of the prime on the target. A variant is *masked priming*, whereby the prime is presented immediately prior to the target with little intervening time and no intervening items. In masked priming experiments, participants are not aware of the prime, given the rapidity of the presentation. In fact, the prime is often presented for a short enough period of time that respondents are not even aware of its presence (Kinoshita & Lupker, 2003).

As explained by McDonough and Trofimovich (2008) in their comprehensive guide to priming research and methods in L2 studies, syntactic priming "refers to the phenomena in which prior exposure to specific language forms or meanings either facilitates or interferes with a speaker's subsequent language processing" (p. xvi). In other words, speakers have a tendency to repeatedly produce the structure, form, or meaning of a previously spoken or heard structure (Bock, 1990, 1995; Bock & Griffin, 2000; Pickering & Ferreira, 2008). Thus, when speakers have a choice between two structures, they are more likely to opt for the one that they have previously encountered, even when the newly produced utterance contains different lexical items. To take an example from the corrective feedback literature, in a study we carried out in 2006, Kim McDonough and I investigated the role of recasts and primed production in L2 development. In our research, Thai EFL learners carried out a series of communicative tasks and targeted question formation. We coded responses to recasts in two ways: either as a repetition of the recast or as primed production. In primed productions the learners showed a clear tendency to use the question form provided in the recast to ask a new question.

Example from McDonough and Mackey (2006):

> Learner: why he hit the deer? (stage 3 question)
> NS: why did he hit the deer?
>   He was driving home and the deer ran out in front of his car (recast, stage 5).
> Learner: What did he do after that? (primed production stage 5).

We found that recasts were a significant predictor of ESL question development and that learners' responses in the form of primed productions, but not direct repetitions, also predicted development. Priming has also been used in a variety of previous work (e.g. Trofimovich et al., 2013, see the next Read It! box).

Read It!

Trofimovich, P., McDonough, K., & Neumann, H. (2013). Using collaborative tasks to elicit auditory and structural priming. *TESOL Quarterly, 47*(1), 177–186.

"Interaction between second language (L2) learners in which the primary goal is the communication of meaning rather than the manipulation of language forms is widely regarded as beneficial for L2 learning from a variety of theoretical and pedagogical perspectives. Besides learning opportunities created through interactional feedback, modified output, and attention to language form, collaborative tasks may also promote L2 learning by generating the occurrence of priming. Priming refers to effects of speakers' previous experience with specific aspects of language. Collaborative priming activities provide models of target structures and elicit production of those structures with a variety of lexical items, without requiring that learners provide each other with feedback, produce modified output, or discuss language form. Consequently, these types of activities may be an innovative method for modeling and eliciting target structures through peer interaction in L2 classrooms. This study examined whether collaborative tasks can elicit auditory and structural priming during peer interaction in L2 classrooms" (p. 177).

As McDonough and Mackey (2006) pointed out, priming tasks can be conducted in a number of ways in interaction, feedback, and task research. One way is through a two-part experiment in which a sentence repetition segment is followed by a picture description task. In the first part, participants hear and repeat an item and then have to decide if they have heard it before. In the second part, they describe a picture that provides a context for the structure in question and then make a decision about whether or not they have seen the picture before. The recognition part of these tasks aims to deflect the participants' attention from the real task of describing.

A second technique involves presenting participants with written or oral sentence fragments that they are then asked to complete. Some of the fragments are primes and have been manipulated in such a way that the participants will produce a particular structure as they complete the sentences. This is followed by presenting them with shorter fragments that can be completed using one of two structures. The claim is that syntactic priming is evident when participants complete the shorter fragments using the same structure they used when completing the prime fragments more often than they use that same structure when the shorter fragments followed something different.

A third technique in syntactic priming research is sentence recall, which involves three parts: First, the computer screen quickly presents a sentence one word at a time. Second, there is a distractor task, and finally, participants repeat the original sentence aloud. At issue is the structure of the repeated sentence: Does it have the same structure as the one that was read, or does it have the structure of a previous sentence? For a detailed explanation of the many types of interpretation tasks available, see Ionin and Zyzik's (2014) discussion in the *Annual Review of Applied Linguistics.*

Keep It in Mind!

- Reaction time tasks can reveal processing time, which is useful information in studying task types and responses to types of feedback.
- Word association tasks can help researchers understand the organization of the L2 lexicon as well as its relationship to the L1 lexicon.
- Priming activities can help peers elicit target forms during classroom interaction and are a way to help learners access previous linguistic knowledge.

CHAPTER NINE

Working with Data in Interaction, Feedback, and Task Research

In interaction, feedback, and task research, data are often sourced from oral production, and sometimes from written production. In computer-aided interaction there may also be synchronous or asynchronous digital transcripts, which fall somewhere between oral and written data. Some kinds of data are, as part of the data collection process, already in digital formats (e.g., gestures as feedback in the form of teachers' movements during videos of their teaching). Data might also be visual, too, in the form of eye movements that indicate what learners are looking at or focusing on when they receive feedback, for example. Data can also consist of images, like those obtained via fMRI or EEG while learners carry out communicative tasks. Some types of data might be ready for analysis immediately or very soon after collection, for example CALL data of learner–learner chats showing how they modify their output during peer interaction over tasks, or in larger scale studies, like research syntheses or meta-analyses.

Data can include learners talking to themselves (e.g., microphones or smartphones can be used capture their inner monologues when receiving feedback or carrying out tasks) but more often, the data involve learners interacting with each other in pairs or small groups, with native speakers, teachers, or others. Feedback can come from any of these interlocutors, and tasks are typical vehicles for promoting interaction and feedback. Interaction, feedback, and task data may have been collected in a very wide range of ways, including, for example, interactions between native speakers and learners, learners in dyads or small groups carrying out communicative tasks in a laboratory setting, or learners and their teacher in intact classroom settings, as well as from observations or structured or unstructured interviews.

9.1 Transcribing Interaction, Feedback, and Task Data

Most spoken data in interaction, feedback, and task research involves transcription of some kind. It's helpful to understand that not everything in a recording always needs to be transcribed – it depends on the goals of the study. In some cases, only aspects of language that fit into coding

Table 9.1 Sample transcription conventions

?	indicates rising intonation at the end of a unit
.	indicates falling intonation
..	two dots indicate a noticeable pause
...	three dots indicate a significant pause
→	an arrow indicates the intonation unit continues to the next line
=	equals sign shows latching (second voice begins without perceptible pause)
[	brackets show overlap (two voices heard at the same time)
(??)	indicates inaudible utterance
(h)	indicates laughter during a word
<manner words>	angle brackets enclose descriptions of the manner in which an utterance is spoken, e.g. *<high-pitched>*, *<laughing>*, etc.
word	italics indicate emphatic stress
bold	indicates speech spoken loudly
:	colon following a vowel indicates elongated vowel sound
–	indicates an abrupt stop in speech; a truncated word or syllable

categories are transcribed. If, for example, you are doing research on a teacher's feedback on plural "s" and that's all you are interested in, then you might be able to simply transcribe all incidents of such feedback (and possibly the immediately preceding and following interactions, for some context). Occasionally it might even be possible to simply listen to the data and code while listening. It is generally a good idea, though, if not transcribing everything systematically, to keep an ear out and take notes (often known as field notes) if you hear any interesting examples or patterns, or even exceptions to patterns because these can come in handy when writing discussion and interpretation sections.

If you plan on using transcription conventions, it is always helpful to consult previous studies in the area to see how they transcribed. Also, be sure to include a description of the conventions you used in the study as part of any write-up. For instance, in their study of corrective feedback in study abroad, Bryfonski and Sanz (2018, p. 28) used transcription conventions, and further noted that they used the notations shown in Table 9.1, adapted from Tannen, Kendall, and Gordon (2007) to convey different meanings in their transcripts.

In interaction, feedback, and task data, you often hear overlap as learners talk over each other, or there are shorter or longer pauses, which might be interesting in considerations of what learners are paying attention to.

9.2 Describing Interaction, Feedback, and Task Data

Most research methodology books, mine included (see, for example, Mackey & Gass, 2015), provide quite complicated explanations of a wide range of different sorts of coding, but the basic information is usually the same. When we code, we're looking for patterns in data. Data of all different types can be coded and then classified. A basic step in classification is often describing the data in terms of whether it's nominal, ordinal, or interval. Data are also often viewed along the quantitative–qualitative paradigm, which can also impact how we go about coding. Ways to go about coding each of these types of interaction, feedback, and task data are discussed below.

Studies of interaction, feedback, and tasks often involve a dichotomous variable (i.e. a variable with only two values) or a variable with several values. When dealing with dichotomous variables, we can employ codes such as *Yes* or *No* (*Present* or *Absent*). For example, in the database illustrated in Table 9.2 from Teimouri's (2018) study of how learners report responding to certain scenarios (a method that can be used to gauge perceptions of interaction), the data were coded *Yes* or *No* in terms of participants' experiences. As shown in the table, sixty-four students reported that they had experienced language-learning scenario 1, whereas forty-five stated that they had not encountered such a situation.

When data involve dealing with one variable and several values, such data are considered non-dichotomous and in these cases, numbers can

---

Table 9.2 Sample of nominal coding

Have you ever experienced any of the following language-learning scenarios?	Yes	No
Language-learning scenario 1	64	45
Language-learning scenario 2	45	64
Language-learning scenario 3	38	49

sometimes be used to represent membership in different categegories. For instance, in interaction, feedback, and task research we are often interested in biographical data, such as the educational levels of participants in our studies set in instructional contexts. We might be interested in whether our participants experience tasks as more or less complex based on their levels of education. A numerical value could be assigned to each educational level (e.g. up to two years of college = 1, four years of college = 2, master's = 3, and so on). All of these examples are instances of nominal data collection.

Ordinal data are often coded using a ranking order. For example, if you want to understand the relationship between learners' ability to modify their output following recasts before and after studying abroad and their overall oral proficiency scores, one of the things you need to do, after coding them as "yes" or "no" for a specified study-abroad experience, is to rank the students based on their proficiency scores. The student with the highest oral proficiency score would be ranked "1", the student with the second-highest score would be ranked "2", and so on. For students with the same oral proficiency score, the ranking would be split. For example, if two learners each had the fourth-highest score on a Spanish oral proficiency test, both would be ranked "3.5."

We can also rank-order the students in groups. For example, we might be interested in learners' working memory scores and how these might impact their performance in interaction in terms of willingness to communicate and production of modified output. To do this, we first divide students' scores into groups and then assign a number to each group. For example, number 1 would be assigned to represent the top 25 percent, who scored the highest in working memory tests, whereas number 4 would be assigned to indicate the bottom 25 percent who scored the lowest. A student who is previously ranked as 5th on a 100-item list would usually be ranked as in group 1 (among the top 25 percent). Dividing learners into ranked groups can be advantageous if we want to compare the top and bottom, as is sometimes the case with working memory scores where we are particularly interested in those with high and low working memory scores, as well as those who participate frequently, or infrequently, in oral interaction. By using this sort of ordinal scale, for instance, we can see that two students who scored 69 and 54 on a particular test have similar performances and outperformed other groups of students. In a study using an anxiety questionnaire, to answer questions about how anxiety contributes (or does not) to learners' tendency to modify their output, a researcher might be curious to know if L2 production might be different for students with low, medium, and high levels of anxiety. This is not the only way to set a cut-off score. Research-ers can also set other cut-off points for classifying their data scores, using, for example, points based on measures of central tendency.

Interval scales, like ordinal scales, also provide a rank ordering. They also show the interval, or distance, between points in the ranking. In addition to showing us which scores are higher or lower (as in the ordinal scale), they also indicate the amount or degree to which they differ. Data that are typically coded in this way and are often considered as variables of interest in interaction, feedback, and task research include things like age and number of years of language study. The impact this data has on learning may be different at different intervals. For example, the differ-ence between language study of one and two years may have the same interval as the one between four and ten on a language test, but the impact is likely to be quite different given maturational constraints. Similarly, the difference between zero and one years of instruction may be the same interval as the difference between five and six years in that it's one year of difference, but that year might be very different in terms of the impact on language production for a learner who is a zero beginner versus one who is at a highly advanced level. This is particularly the case in a study of interaction, feedback, and tasks because the zero beginner learner is likely to be benefiting from instruction in quite different ways to the advanced learner, attending to different things, responding in different ways and able to do quite different tasks involv-ing completely different types of language.

9.3 How to Code Interaction, Feedback, and Task Data

As you will read in many a research methods textbook, in coding, it is always best to code as narrowly as possible, meaning code everything you can. This is recommended because, while you can collapse categor-ies quite easily later if you need to, it is much more time-consuming to have to go back to re-code if you realize partway through that your categories are not fine-grained enough. Looking at an example in the context of interaction, feedback, and task research, if you code inter-actional feedback as including recasts, explicit correction, and negotiation for meaning all into one "interactional feedback category" but later decide that you want to separate out implicit and explicit feedback (placing recasts and negotiation into the implicit category and explicit correction into an explicit category), you would need to go back to the data and recode. In other words, it is much easier to combine categories after the fact than to recode. Also, coding finely can allow

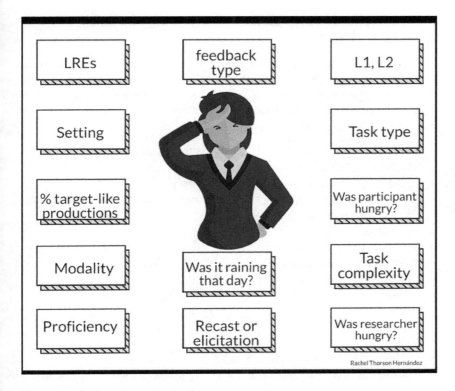

Figure 9.1 Coding category chaos

more patterns to be viewed, although it's important to keep in mind that separating out absolutely everything might lead to a "not seeing the wood for the trees" scenario.

Other things to bear in mind when coding data is whether there is a standard coding system available through reading other research in your area of interest, or whether you need to develop a tailor-made system for your study. If you follow someone else's coding system this will make comparison of findings easier, and strengthen the generalizability of your findings, because they have been used by at least one and possibly even a range of researchers. A review of all of the many rich and excellent coding schemes existing in the field of interaction, feedback, and tasks is beyond the scope of this one chapter, but a few examples appear below. In general, I recommend using existing coding schemes or modifying them slightly if they already exist and make sense for the research questions in your study.

9.4 Examples of Ways to Code Interaction, Feedback, and Task Data

Meta-analyses are good places to look for examples of the different sorts of coding units that have been used in these studies over the years. For example, depending on the research questions being asked and the nature of the study, interaction and feedback data have been coded using the following units, just to name a few:

- Recasts (more or less explicit, longer, shorter and so on)
- Responses (immediate, delayed and so on)
- Opportunities for responses (present, absent)
- Negotiations for meaning (clarification requests, comprehension checks, confirmation checks)
- Explicit metalinguistic feedback
- Implicit metalinguistic feedback
- Language related episodes
- Turns
- Utterances
- Clauses
- Type–token ratios
- Task type
- Setting (dyadic, triadic, and so on)
- Complexity, accuracy, and fluency (CAF) measures of production
- Target-like usage counts

9.4.1 Recasts

In her study on the use of recasts and gestures on the acquisition of English locative prepositions, Nakatsukasa (2016) used stimulated recall to code for whether or not a subset of the participants noticed the recasts/gestures, and an immediate post-test to code for another subset's use of the target structure.

Read It!

Nakatsukasa, K. (2016). Efficacy of recasts and gestures on the acquisition of locative prepositions. *Studies in Second Language Acquisition, 38*, 771–779.

"This study investigates whether gestures can be used during recasts to enhance the saliency of a target structure (locative prepositions) and to lead to better production of the target structure. Forty-eight low-intermediate

English as a second language (ESL) students partook in communicative activities during which they received either no feedback (control), verbal recasts only (R), or recasts plus gesture (RG), and a subset of participants completed a stimulated recall session. Then the pretest, immediate, and delayed posttest scores of grammar and oral production tests were used to analyze the linguistic development. The results showed that no one commented on recasts or locative prepositions during the stimulated recall session and that there were no significant changes in grammar test scores in all conditions; however, the R and RG conditions performed significantly better in the production test than the control in the immediate posttest. Furthermore, the RG condition maintained the development in the delayed posttest, whereas the R condition did not" (p. 771).

In their study on single and multiple recasts, Hassanzadeh, Marefat, and Ramezani (2019) used an elicited oral imitation task (EOIT), a timed grammaticality judgment task (TGJT) to test participants' implicit knowledge, and an untimed grammaticality judgment task (UGJT) to test their explicit knowledge. For their rating procedure, they coded correct responses as "1" and incorrect responses as "0."

Read It!

Hassanzadeh, M., Marefat, F., & Ramezani, A. (2019). The impact of single versus multiple recasts on L2 learners' implicit and explicit knowledge. *Heliyon, 5*(5), e01748.

"Recasts have been the object of extensive theoretical and empirical investigation in second language acquisition research since the mid-1990s. Despite being acknowledged to have a facilitative effect on second language (L2) learning, the extent of their acquisitional contribution is a matter of controversy. This study examined the effectiveness of single and multiple recasts (SR & MR) on the acquisition of a planned target structure, as represented on the learners' implicit and explicit knowledge. The participants were three intact groups of English as a foreign language (EFL) learners at a language institute in Iran. The two experimental conditions received respective recasting on errors of English unreal conditionals. All groups – including a third control condition – were then tested via three discrete tasks aimed at measuring their implicit and explicit knowledge: an elicited oral imitation task, a timed grammaticality judgment task, and an untimed grammaticality judgment task. The results revealed that both groups exhibited improvements on both measures along immediate and delayed occasions. However, their performance over

the two implicit knowledge measures yielded dissimilar outcomes. Pedagogic-
ally speaking, it must be realized that recasting would not necessarily lead to
acquisition unless L2 teachers become more conscious of where and how to
orchestrate them" (p. 1).

9.4.2 Interactional Features

A more qualitative, interpretive approach to coding interaction data can
be found in the next article, which is worth comparing with the one
above to see how different perspectives can provide interesting windows
on the data.

Read It!

Youn, S. (2020). Interactional features of L2 pragmatic interaction in role-play
speaking assessment. *TESOL Quarterly*, *54*(1), 201–233.

"This study explicates the nature of second language (L2) pragmatic interaction focusing on the quantitative function of interactional features.
A relationship between the fine-grained interactional features elicited
from learners' role-play performances at varying levels and trained raters'
scores was investigated. The corpus of 102 learners' role-play performances
was transcribed turn by turn and analyzed qualitatively to identify
recurrent interactional phenomena, which formed the basis of data-driven
coding schemes that are grounded in conversation analysis. Three levels
of interactional features – *length of interaction, engaging with interaction*,
and *sequential organizations* – were coded. The coded data were
extracted using the CLAN program and analyzed quantitatively to examine
what interactional features distinguished among varying performance levels.
The linear regression analysis indicated that the combination of nine
significant interactional features accounted for 74.7% of the variance in the
raters' scores. The discriminant function analysis revealed that the interactional
features elicited from the role-plays that involve formal pragmatic functions
were important variables in distinguishing among the performance levels. This
study confirms that the interactional features deserve a prominent place in
defining L2 pragmatic interaction. The author discusses practical implications
for teaching and assessing interactive pragmatic performance, as well as
methodological issues underlying quantifying spoken interaction" (p. 201).

9.4.3 Metalinguistic Feedback

Metalinguistic feedback is a type of feedback sometimes considered in interaction, feedback, and task research which involves "either comments, information, or questions related to the well-formedness of the student utterance, without explicitly providing the correct answer" (Long, 1996, p. 46). In his study on the role of feedback explicitness, Nassaji (2009) first coded written transcriptions of interaction data to identify nontarget-like forms and the feedback given to those forms. The feedback was then coded as either (1) recast or (2) elicitation and then coded again as being an example of either implicit or explicit feedback.

Read It!

Nassaji, H. (2009). Effects of recasts and elicitations in dyadic interaction and the role of feedback explicitness. *Language Learning, 59*(2), 411–452.

"The present study investigated the effects of two categories of interactional feedback – recasts and elicitations – on learning linguistic forms that arose incidentally in dyadic interaction. The study also identified implicit and explicit forms of each feedback type and examined their subsequent effects immediately after interaction and after 2 weeks. Data came from 42 adult English as a second language learners who participated in task-based interaction with two native-speaker English language teachers and received various forms of recasts and elicitations on their nontargetlike output. The effects of feedback were measured by means of learner-specific preinteraction scenario descriptions and immediate and delayed postinteraction error identification/correction tasks. The results showed a higher degree of immediate postinteraction correction for recasts than for elicitations. The results also showed that in both cases the more explicit forms of each feedback type led to higher rates of immediate and delayed postinteraction correction than the implicit forms. However, the effects of explicitness were more pronounced for recasts than for elicitations. These latter findings suggest that although both recasts and elicitations may be beneficial for second language learning, their effectiveness might be closely, but differentially, related to their degree of explicitness" (p. 411).

9.4.4 Task Complexity

Task complexity involves cognitive factors affecting the intrinsic cognitive difficulty of a task (e.g., doing simple addition versus calculus).

There are two subcategories of task complexity: resource directing and resource dispersing (Robinson, 2001, 2007). In their synthesis/meta-analysis, Jackson and Suethanapornkul (2013) found that studies in this area used a wide variety of measures when coding L2 production, including clauses per C-unit, clauses per T-unit, percent of error-free clauses, percent of target-like production, and disfluency episodes.

Read It!

Jackson, D. O. & Suethanapornkul, S. (2013). The cognition hypothesis: A synthesis and meta-analysis of research on second language task complexity. *Language Learning, 63*(2), 330–367.

"This study employed synthetic and meta-analytic techniques to review the literature on the Cognition Hypothesis, which predicts that increasing task complexity influences the quality of second language production. Based on 8 inclusion criteria, 17 published studies were synthesized according to key features. A subset of these studies (k = 9) was also meta-analyzed to investigate the overall effects of raising resource-directing task demands on learner output during monologic tasks. The synthesis of 17 primary studies revealed an assortment of treatments and measures. Among the 9 comparable studies, the meta-analysis uncovered small positive effects for accuracy and small negative effects for fluency. This lends support to the Cognition Hypothesis; however, the present study also disconfirms predictions regarding syntactic complexity. Implications for research and pedagogy are discussed" (pg. 330).

Keep It in Mind!

Coding used in typical recast and meta-linguistic feedback studies includes, but is not limited to:

- L1, L2
- Proficiency (beginner, intermediate, advanced)
- Setting (classroom, laboratory)
- Context (FL versus SL)
- Task type (drill, communicative, miscellaneous)
- Outcome measures (free constructed, constrained constructed, GJT, selected response)
- Target feature (grammar, vocabulary, etc.)

Coding used in task complexity studies includes, but is not limited to:

- Modality (spoken or written)
- Conditions (narrative or interactive)
- Resource-directing dimension (+/– here-and-now, +/– few elements, +/– reasoning
- Task complexity level (simple, mid, complex)
- Reliability score

9.5 Coding Qualitative and/or Interpretive Data in Interaction, Feedback, and Task Research

Just as with primarily quantitative studies, researchers doing qualitative, or interpretive, analyses are usually interested in patterns. However, in these paradigms, coding is usually grounded in the data, with researchers asking themselves questions like these: Why does a phenomenon occur? How does the research context affect participants and vice versa? How does the positionality of the researcher affect the research context and the interpretation of the data? As such, qualitative coding, or patterns, are typically seen as emergent, that is, they arise out of data as opposed to being worked out and imposed before data are collected or coded. When initial categories come out of a first pass through the data, the process is sometimes called *open coding*. An example might be a researcher noticing that learners respond to providers of feedback in different ways depending on who is present at that time, and then they investigate potential connections among and between categories. As the process of coding continues, how much variation there is can also be observed. Identifying themes of interest so that the data can be reflected and represented appropriately in the analysis is the goal.

9.6 Mixed-Methods Data in Interaction, Feedback, and Task Research

A mixed-methods study usually means that researchers use more than one approach. For example, in their study of corrective feedback in a study-abroad context, Bryfonski and Sanz (2018) took an interpretive perspective on coding. Their data consisted of semi-structured interviews conducted with their participants. After transcribing their interviews, they used grounded theory to thematically code and categorize reflections or perceptions that emerged from the interviews.

In engaging with interview data as they did, an interaction, feedback, and task study can involve (re)assigning paraphrases, questions, headings, labels, or overviews in a second or subsequent pass through the data. Some researchers approach coding the data by reminding themselves of the need to justify the labels and coding system they used, and so maintaining field notes about where insights came from is important. This is so that data from those insights themselves can, if later deemed important, also often be coded. After a first round of coding, themes and trends in the data often yield further insights into the data. After this usually comes a consideration of what segments of data might be combined, and which, if any, are independent categories. The final stages often involve overall organizational orders becoming clearer. At this point, researchers often ask themselves if their data are telling an interesting story. If they are, coding can lead into writing. There is no one way to approach coding in the interpretive paradigm, so, with that in mind, this section should be read purely as an example.

9.7 Coding Mechanics in Interaction, Feedback, and Task Data

How data are coded is something that differs among researchers because of factors like how they were trained, the research questions being answered, and coding systems already found in the literature, among others. For example, in their study on task modality and L1 use in EFL oral interaction, Azakarai and García Mayo (2015) categorized the L1 functions in their study based on two previous studies with similar EFL settings, allowing them to more easily compare their findings to these previous studies.

Read It!

Azkarai, A. & García Mayo, M. D. P. (2015). Task-modality and L1 use in EFL oral interaction. *Language Teaching Research, 19*(5), 550–571.

"This study examines whether task-modality (speaking vs. speaking+writing) influences first language (L1) use in task-based English as a foreign language (EFL) learner–learner interaction. Research on the topic has shown that different task-modality triggers different learning opportunities with collaborative speaking tasks drawing learners' attention to meaning and tasks that also incorporate a written component drawing attention more to formal linguistic aspects. Research has also shown that a balanced L1 use might be positive in learner–learner interaction, as it helps learners maintain their interest in the task and acts as a strategy to make difficult tasks more manageable. This

---

article analyses L1 use and the functions it served during the oral interaction of 44 EFL Spanish learners while they completed four collaborative tasks: two speaking tasks (picture placement and picture differences) and two speaking +writing tasks (dictogloss and text editing). Findings point to a clear impact of task-modality on L1 use, as speaking+writing tasks made learners fall back on their L1 more frequently. L1 functions were also task dependent with grammar deliberations more frequent in speaking+writing tasks and vocabulary searches in speaking tasks" (p. 550).

When coding, some researchers may work directly on transcripts and mark, for example, recasts in one color pen and uptake in another. Others, as I noted earlier in this chapter, may decide to listen to or watch recordings without transcribing and instead only code the phenomena in which they are interested. Working out how much of the data to code is also important. This process is sometimes known as data sampling or data segmentation. When deciding how much/what data to code we need to keep in mind that the data to be analyzed should be representative of the dataset as a whole. For example, taking the middle section of the data (e.g., the central ten minutes) ensures you don't get warming up or cooling down issues.

9.8 Ensuring Reliability in Interaction, Feedback, and Task Data

When individual researchers code data, they need to make decisions about how to classify and categorize data. If a study involves only one coder, or rater, without any inter-rater measures of the agreement between them being reported, wondering about the conclusions of the study is warranted on the basis that we don't know if we or others would code the data the same way. To increase confidence, it is important to carefully train an additional rater or raters who do not know what part of the data (e.g., pre-test or post-test) or for which group (experimental or control) they are coding, and have them code the data to see how far they agree (and don't) with yours. If, for example, a study involves coding data from three communicative tasks to identify and rate various types of corrective feedback provided by teachers, researchers may decide to carefully train other raters in a way that involves explaining the goals of the study with an overview of how to use the coding scheme to code different types of corrective feedback, providing sample coding schemes and some pre-coded data, as well as some sample data for raters to practice coding on before they judge the study data.

9.9 Simple Percentages and Cohen's Kappa for Reliability in Interaction, Feedback, and Task Research

I am often asked questions about the minimum amount of data that should be coded by second or third coders. Quite a few reference books, including mine, and many research methods books supply answers like "as much as is feasible given the time and resources available for the study." If all the data can be coded by two or more people, the confidence of readers in the reliability of the coding categories will be enhanced, assuming the reliability scores turn out to be high. However, if resources aren't sufficient to get all the data coded twice, and scores turn out to be very high (95 percent plus), then it's often considered acceptable to only cross-code something like 20 percent of the data. At the end of this section, I provide some examples of reliability reports from studies in interaction and task research.

Inter-rater reliability can be measured by methods like simple percentages, as in the Azkarai and García Mayo (2016) study discussed previously, where they reported that an independent rater coded twelve task-based reactions from their dataset and that the inter-rater reliability percentage was 95 percent, meaning that there was disagreement over only 5 percent of the data. Using a percentage like this, that is easy to calculate, is particularly useful with continuous data where codes that can theoretically involve any value in a possible range are used. Discrete data, on the other hand, involve using codes that are limited, for example, to integer values. A limitation of simple percentage agreement is the tendency to discount the notion that some of the agreement may have occurred by chance. To correct for this concern about chance, another calculation is often employed, known as Cohen's kappa (Cohen, 1960). This involves calculating the average rate of agreement for a complete set of scores taking into account the frequency of agreements and disagreements by category. In a dichotomous coding scheme (e.g., coding feedback as explicit or implicit), calculating Cohen's kappa means researchers will know how much of the feedback two or more raters coded as explicit, how much was coded as explicit by the first rater and as implicit by the second, and so on. Cohen's kappa involves more detail on agreement and disagreement than simple percentage modes of calculating agreement, while also taking chance into account.

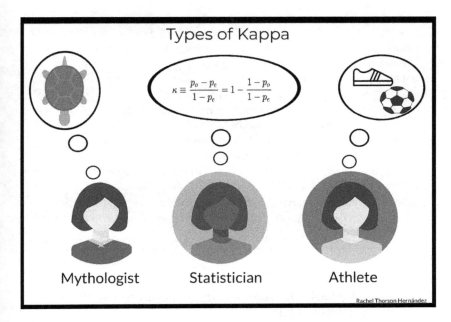

Figure 9.2 Types of kappa

Other measures of calculating reliability include Spearman Rank Correlation Coefficients and Pearson's Product Moment. Both are based on measures of correlation and both reflect the degree of association between the ratings provided by more than one rater.

Try It!

Look at the following excerpts and notice how each study reported on reliability and how much of the data were subject to inter-rater reliability scoring. Do you notice anything else?

[Study A] "The inter-rater reliability of scoring was calculated for the three tests based on the pretest scores. A second rater independently reviewed about 20% of the randomly selected portions of the oral description and the written story-telling tasks. The inter-rater reliability based on percentage agreement and Cohen's kappa was 97.8% (k=.946) for the oral picture description task and 98.1% (k=.962) for the written story-telling task. For the grammaticality judgment task, a second scorer scored the entire pretest and the correlation coefficient was .99" (Nassaji, 2017, p. 359).

[Study B] "A trained rater coded a subsample (20%) of the identified feedback moves for both coding features (whether the feedback provider was an NS or NNS and whether the feedback was implicit or explicit), and any differences were discussed for an initial reliability estimate of 85%. The remaining 15% were considered again by the two coders, and a final agreement of 100% was reached" (Bryfonski & Sanz, 2018, p. 13).
[Study C] "An independent researcher also analysed all the oral interactions transcribed. Different rounds of coding resulted in an agreement of 96%. The remaining 4% of the utterances were considered again by the two researchers and a final agreement of 100% was reached" (Azkarai & García Mayo, 2016, p. 6).
[Study D] "Another researcher independently scored 15% of the data set: The inter-rater reliability using Cronbach's alpha yielded α = .89" (Sato & Lyster, 2012, p. 604).

9.10 Using Reliable Instruments in Interaction, Feedback, and Task Research

We need to ensure that the instruments we are using to collect interaction, feedback, and task data are reliable. One example of how the assessment of instruments can be found in Teimouri's (2018) work, where he assessed the reliability of a newly-developed L2-TOSGA questionnaire (Second Language Test of Shame and Guilt Affect) – a scenario-based questionnaire in which shame-proneness and guilt-proneness of learners were assessed in a set of L2 interactional situations – by re-administering the questionnaire one month later. He computed test–retest reliability of the sub-scales by determining correlation coefficients between the two administrations.

Other ways of looking at reliability can involve two parallel forms of a task being developed and administered to the same sample. Then, correlational coefficients between the two tasks can be calculated and reported as a measure of reliability. This method of reliability estimation is common in pre-post design studies, where researchers administer two parallel tasks or even tests (before and after the treatment) to assess learners' linguistics gains (e.g., to measure the effects of recasts on the acquisition of a targeted grammatical form). Finally, tests can be administered to a sample with their reliability being calculated based on how well each item measures the target construct and yields similar results. There are various measures of internal consistency, such as Average Item-Total correlation, Split-Half reliability, and Cronbach's Alpha (α).

9.11 Different Types of Validity in Interaction, Feedback, and Task Research

Interaction, feedback, and task researchers want to ensure (along with questions of reliability) that the results of their study are actually what they believe they are, as well as meaningful in that they apply not only to the participants in the study itself, but also, at least for most experimental research, to a wider population. The wide range of different types of validity include content, face, construct, criterion-related, and predictive validity.

- **Content validity** refers to the representativeness of our measurement regarding the phenomenon about which we want information. For example, if we are interested in the effect of recasts on the acquisition of English modals, we need to make sure that all English modals are represented in the study.
- **Face validity** means how familiar an instrument is, and how easy it is to convince others that there is content validity to it. If, for example, learners are presented with more and less complex tasks in dyads as part of an experiment and are already familiar with these sorts of tasks in dyadic settings, because they have used them in their classrooms, we can assume that the task has face validity for those learners.
- **Construct validity**, often considered one of the most complex types, means how far the study captures the construct of interest, for example, time on task.
- **Criterion-related validity** refers to the extent to which tests used in a research study are comparable to other well-established tests of the construct in question. For example, if you want to assess the complexity of students' output by using a set of interactional tasks, you should make sure your tasks have criterion-related validity in eliciting similar output. Should there be good correlations between students' output across different tasks, one can then say that those tasks have criterion-related validity.
- **Predictive validity** is the use that a researcher might eventually want to make of a particular measure. For example, returning to the previous example, if output complexity in a task predicts performance on some other dimension, such as scores on language proficiency test), the task can be said to have predictive validity.

Try It!

In the following excerpt from Awwad and Tavakoli (2019, p. 10), the authors discuss connections between task complexity (TC) and language proficiency

(LP). Which type(s) of validity do the authors discuss? How does their study seek to remedy the issues they describe?

"[T]he limited approach to assessing proficiency in previous studies that examined TC across different levels of LP is a source of ambiguity in understanding and interpreting the results of the studies summarized above. To make up for such limitations and to develop a more in-depth insight into the effects of LP on TC, two tests were used to investigate explicit and implicit knowledge. The Oxford Placement Test (OPT) (Alan, 2004) is assumed to measure learners' L2 explicit knowledge, and elicited imitation tasks (EIT) (Wu & Ortega, 2013) are supposed to assess their implicit knowledge (Ellis, 2009; Erlam, 2006)" (p. 10).

9.11.1 Internal Validity in Interaction, Feedback, and Task Research

Questions of internal validity ask: To what extent are the differences that have been found for a dependent variable directly related to the independent variable? In other words, we want to exclude possible factors that could potentially account for the results, or at least control any such factors we find. For example, in a CALL-feedback study, if we wanted to observe learners' reaction times to feedback on different types of form, we might develop a program that captures keystrokes, so that we can measure how long it took the participants to respond. After we have completed the study, though, we might realize we did not ask if participants were touch typists, or frequent computer users. Some might be very used to their smartphones and have spent little time on the sort of keyboards we asked them to use, whereas others might use computers daily. Our results would be compromised. We would have to conclude that there was little internal validity.

Some of the most common and typical ways that validity can be impacted include not adequately considering learners' individual characteristics or their (in)attention and attitudes, as well as not adequately thinking through our data collection methods and tools.

9.11.2 External Validity in Interaction, Feedback, and Task Research

Quite a bit of existing interaction, feedback, and task research would like to extend its reach further than the individual study's research setting and participants. Questions about external validity relate to the generalizability of our findings. By this we mean how relevant the findings of a specific study are to a broader population of learners than the ones included in the study.

If the findings of a feedback study, for instance, suggested that high school students' acquisition of English plurals at a public school can be improved through recasts, we would not want to automatically claim we could generalize such a finding to elementary school students. Neither could we generalize the findings of the study to students learning English at private high schools. We need to balance the IRB-approved anonymity of participants with enough information so that other researchers could estimate the generalizability of our research findings. For example, you often see sentences in published research like the following: "We collected the data from 150 college-aged students enrolled in a second-year Japanese program at a large Midwestern U.S. university."

9.12 WEIRD Participants and Representation in Interaction, Feedback, and Task Research

To date, much of the research in applied linguistics and other social sciences has relied heavily on the participation of North American and European college students (often referred to by the acronym "WEIRD" – Western, Educated, Industrialized, Rich, Democratic). The heavy reliance on this type of research participant is due mainly to convenience – most college students are required to take a language and can be asked to participate in language studies as part of class and a great deal of researchers work in these settings. This is problematic, however, for issues of external validity and generalizability, as so many of the world's language learners are not WEIRD. In recent years, as attention has been brought to this issue, members of the SLA research community are turning their attention to asking questions about the WEIRD issue and encouraging more research using non-academic participants (see McDonough & Mackey, 2013 and Plonsky, 2016), while some scholars have been sounding the warning bell for even longer (see Tarone & Bigelow, 2005). In 2019, Sible Andringa and Aline Godfroid, with the support of the Open Science initiative, put out a call in for replication studies using non-WEIRD participants in a direct effort to engage the SLA community in addressing the issue of sample bias associated with the longstanding and continued use of WEIRD participants. Hopefully, this signals a raising of awareness in the interaction, feedback, and task

Name: _____   Research Code: _____

Gender: ___Male ___Female ___Other   First language(s): _____

Age _____ Prefer not to say age _____

How many years have you been learning Spanish? _____

How old were you when you started learning Spanish?

_____

What Spanish classes are you taking now?

_____

What Spanish classes will you take next semester?

_____

How many hours per week do you spend using Spanish outside class to...

Do homework	0	1-2	3-4	5-6	7 or more
Prepare for quizzes/tests	0	1-2	3-4	5-6	7 or more
Listen to music, podcasts, etc.	0	1-2	3-4	5-6	7 or more
Watch movies, series, YouTube, etc.	0	1-2	3-4	5-6	7 or more
Read for fun	0	1-2	3-4	5-6	7 or more
Talk to friends	0	1-2	3-4	5-6	7 or more
Talk to family	0	1-2	3-4	5-6	7 or more
Talk to tourists	0	1-2	3-4	5-6	7 or more

Have you ever been to a Spanish-speaking country (Spain, Mexico, Colombia, etc.)?

Yes__No__

If yes, how long were you there? _____

What were you doing there? _____

Besides your first language(s) and Spanish, do you know any other languages? Yes___ No___

If yes, what language(s)? _____

How well do you know the language(s) you listed in the previous question?

_____

Figure 9.3 Sample biodata form

community that, where possible, it would be preferable to think about recruiting more non-WEIRD populations and participants.

9.13 Collecting Biodata in Interaction, Feedback, and Task Research

While we are talking about participant characteristics, it seems helpful to think about how we collect and report biodata (i.e., biographical data). In terms of how much and which biodata should be reported, we should think about including enough information to enable our work to be replicated, in enough detail that readers can make up their own minds about how generalizable our findings are. As I mentioned above, it is also important to consider the privacy and anonymity of our participants when writing papers and reports including biodata. A sample biodata form appears in Figure 9.3.

Learners sometimes need clarification of items on biodata forms. For instance, learners might have difficulty understanding what "first language(s)" means. Does it mean chronologically first? Does it mean best language? Learners often find it easier to answer more specific questions, such as which language they speak at home, or what their "mother tongue" is. Researchers can also use biographical information to better understand and interpret their findings. For example, a researcher might find the high performance of some learners is not what they had expected based on the treatment, and then by examining their biodata information, realize that these students had visited Spanish-speaking countries on several occasions prior to data collection or that certain students were in fact heritage speakers of Spanish who listed their first languages as Spanish and English.

Try It!

For each of the excerpts provided below, describe the sample used for the study, including the number of participants and any other information that would be necessary to judge if the sample is representative and/or to replicate the study. In addition, note down how many of the studies used WEIRD participants.

[Study A] "The participants were 48 students at a private secondary school in Jordan. Since the school was a single-sex school, all the participants were males. They were aged 16, with Arabic as their first language. The demographic data showed they had very similar schooling and language instruction experiences, i.e. they had studied English for about ten years at school and had never lived in an English-speaking country" (Awwad & Tavakoli, 2019, p. 9).

[Study B] "Forty-five third-year L2 Spanish learners enrolled in introductory Spanish content courses (i.e. institutionally defined as intermediate learners) at a large American university volunteered to participate in the present study in exchange for extra credit. Sixteen participants were excluded because they were heritage speakers of Spanish or because all of their productions contained disfluencies and/or a creaky voice.1 The final sample of 28 L2 Spanish learners were L1 English speakers and began acquiring Spanish in a foreign language classroom beginning at ages 12–13" (McKinnon, 2017, p. 295).

[Study C] "The participants were 81 English language learners (41 females and 40 males) enrolled in an intensive English program (IEP), also known as an English-for-academic-purposes program at a large public university in the United States... The participants came from 15 different countries, ranged in age from 17 to 52 (M = 26.20), and had spent, on average, 6.8 years studying English (including instruction in their home countries). At the time of the study, all participants were enrolled at the intermediate level (i.e. Levels 3–4)" (Kim, Payant, & Pearson, 2015, pp 558–559).

[Study D] "The participants of this study were 42 Spanish EFL learners attending the same school in a major Spanish city. They were in 4th primary grade (9–10 years old) and had started learning English at the age of 4 (mean age: 4.18), with 5 hours of instruction in English per week. In order to assess their English level, participants completed the Cambridge Young Learners of English Starters Test. The average score was 17.32 out of 25 total Points" (Azakaria & García Mayo, 2016, p. 5).

9.14 Outliers in Interaction, Feedback, and Task Data

Outliers are usually seen as data that seem to be atypical of the rest of the dataset and can significantly impact findings. In the L2 field in general, the definition of what exactly outliers are and how they should be handled is unclear (Nicklin & Plonsky, 2020). Having outliers in a dataset sends alarm signals to researchers, who typically respond with a careful review to work out whether data collected from the outlying participants, and their characteristics, seem consistent with patterns in data from the whole group. Occasionally, researchers find principled reasons not to include outlier data in the final analysis, discovering for example, on a closer look that the top scorer had five times more experience with the language than others. If researchers find principled reasons for eliminating outlying data, a detailed explanation should always be given in the report. An example follows, which shows the difficulty of making these decisions.

Study target structure: Adjective/noun gender agreement for a discrete list of 20 animal terms in Spanish.

Data elicitation: Participants are divided into two groups: one that received oral corrective in the form of recasts, and one that received corrective feedback in the form of metalinguistic feedback. Acquisition of the target forms was measured with an error correction test (ECT), a writing task (WT), and an oral production task (OPT).

Problem: Pre-test and post-test scores reveal that one student has done wildly better than the other students.

Reason: In a stimulated recall session, the participant in question mentions that they have a private Spanish tutor and that they spent the last two weeks learning the gender of common animals in Spanish and how to describe them.

Decision: Delete this individual's data.

Justification: The student in question's performance was influenced by their private classes and their acquisition of the forms cannot be clearly linked to the corrective feedback they received in class.

This example shows the process and product of excluding outlying data. The data are not typically removed immediately. Rather, because there were outliers, the researchers decided to examine more data, including the transcript from the stimulated-recall participants. After a detailed second look, they were able to determine that the outlier's data was not based on a valid operationalization of the construct of interest, so in this case, the researchers decided that it was appropriate not to include the data in the final construction of the set for analysis. It is always important to include a full explanation for decisions like this in the report of the study.

9.15 The Importance of Triangulation in Interaction, Feedback, and Task Data

A common definition of triangulation is that it entails the use of multiple, independent methods of obtaining data in a single investigation in order to arrive at one set of research findings. In interaction, feedback, and task research, stimulated recall is often used to triangulate data and test the validity of research findings. For example, in their study on inter-action, task complexity, and working memory, Kim, Payant, and Pearson (2015) used stimulated recall "to test the validity of task complexity manipulation through learners' cognitive processes" (p. 559). Collecting data through multiple means and even modes allows us to alleviate some of the concerns that researchers point to when listing issues with data collection in general. While one particular technique or elicitation or source of data may lead to questions, multiple methods, like the legs on a stool, help to support each other.

CHAPTER TEN

Common Problems, Pitfalls, and How to Address Them in Research on Interaction, Corrective Feedback, and Tasks in L2 Learning

As we have seen in the preceding chapters, there are quite a few issues that need to be addressed when doing interaction, feedback, and task research. In this final chapter, I discuss several of the most common problems and pitfalls faced by novice and experienced researchers alike. I have included stories of my own, from my colleagues, and from my students. The stories are roughly based on the notes I made after they were recounted or sent to me. They recount "research fails" that people were kind enough to share with me. I present them anonymously and I thank everyone who talked and laughed with me over our could-do-better stories which are shared in the hope that they can help others not to fall into the same traps we did. To protect identities, I have randomized my use of pronouns, merged and changed some details. I am, of course, fully responsible for any misinterpretations. These stories are presented not only to illustrate how things can and do go wrong, but to focus on how there is nearly always a way to resolve difficulties you might encounter along the way.

10.1 What Can Go Wrong When We Are Designing Studies?

10.1.1 Pitfall 1: Skipping the Pilot Testing

Even though we design our studies with as much care as possible, we cannot assume that how we plan the data collection tools and methods automatically guarantees how, or indeed whether, they will work. In other words, we should never underestimate how important it is to do a pilot study. A pilot study is a small-scale trial of the design, including the procedures, materials, coding, and analysis techniques for our research. Testing out all of these aspects of a study beforehand, with a population similar to the one we will study, is important to help us understand what sorts of issues may arise (and they will) and come up with different ways to address them before we carry out the high-stakes study and invest all the resources of our time and attention (and that of our participants). Pilot research is essential to see how feasible our data sampling and collection methods (among other things) will be and to make any necessary changes before they are used with our research participants. Sometimes piloting, making revisions, and then repiloting is necessary. However time-consuming this process may be, it is not by any means as time-consuming as having to redo an entire study (after finding different participants), or developing revised data collection tools or different analytic or coding methods. It is of critical importance to allocate time for pilot tests. Below I explain about a pitfall a colleague and I faced in a study where we aimed to see if and how far the positive outcomes we had seen of certain types of interaction with adults could also hold true for children who were acquiring their second language in home and classroom contexts. We were less interested in the "age effects" question, and more interested in practical aspects, such as whether children would respond in the same ways as adults to picture-based description tasks, carried out with peers and with researchers, in both classroom and experimental contexts. Here is what happened in our pilot testing phase.

The Importance of Extensive Pilot Testing: Teddy Bears and Imaginative Children

A colleague and I had decided that she would be in charge of collecting the data for our study with children using research assistants to help her, and, on my end, I would take the lead in transcribing and coding the data. We decided to pilot-test the tasks, mostly to ensure the language we hoped to elicit was not too complicated for the children's levels, and to check that the ten minutes we'd assigned to the task was realistic. At first, I thought all was going well, but when I started listening to one of the children's picture descriptions, it sounded like she had given the child the wrong picture. I was expecting a description of a basic house, a walkway, and flowers. Instead, the child was describing a crazy scene with flying teddy bears, airplanes, and parrots. I followed up with my co-author to see what happened and she confirmed she didn't have anything like the picture the child was describing in her experimental materials folder. She investigated further by returning to the classroom, even though she already suspected she knew what had happened, and she was right. As it turned out, the child had an active imagination. On being gently questioned about how he liked the activity and the task, he said he thought the picture he was asked to describe was boring – so he just made up what he wanted to see. Interestingly, he used some of the morpho-syntactic structures we were trying to elicit (locative constructions), but we realized we should have more specifically explained to the children that they needed to describe the actual picture in front of them, not an imaginary picture, and to remind the research assistant to check that the picture was to be described literally, rather than as a stimulus to talk (which is what she had assumed). More extensive pilot testing resulted in us using a more interesting picture and giving better instructions.

It's sometimes the case that while doing a pilot, researchers obtain data that is extremely pertinent and relevant to the main study. In other words, researchers can end up with pilot data that they would really like to use for the main study. What is important in these cases is to pay attention to any constraints imposed by human subjects committees, institutional review boards (IRBs), or other regulatory bodies in the field of research. Some researchers choose to seek permission from their IRBs ahead of piloting, so that as they carry out their pilots, if they do not encounter problems with their pilot-testing, they may include those data in their main study as long as exactly the same procedures are used. If problems arise during the pilot phase, and they make revisions, then they ask the IRB, who approved the main study, to also approve those revisions. Others ask for IRB approval specifically to include the pilot data where possible. Some IRBs may ask for pilot data in order to approve the study. Therefore, knowing what your IRB requires and planning ahead of time is important in case you decide that pilot data (which doesn't have serious issues) would be best included in your study. Not all institutions will give blanket permission for the use of pilot data. Some IRBs are hesitant to approve the use of data retroactively. As a final word, it is a rare pilot study that does not result in some sort of revision of materials or methods, however minor. Below is a description of how, in a study investigating learners' perspectives on differing types of classroom interaction, excellent data were obtained, and were eventually not usable.

IRB Rules Are Important: Technicolor Versus Shades of Grey
A colleague told a story about how, many years before, she had done a study involving interview and focus-group data. She was asking participants for their opinions about specific types of feedback, and she had randomly chosen three participants for her pilot study, all from the same intact classroom she was studying. She explained how "utterly frustrating" it was that these three pilot participants who'd been selected using the names-out-of-a-hat technique had turned out to provide the richest, and most comprehensible data. She described how listening to their interviews was exciting and stimulating; they reported insights she had expected and been looking for, as well as insights that had not occurred to her. She was unable to get her IRB to give permission to retroactively include the data in her analysis, and she described it like this: "I felt as though the pilot participants were

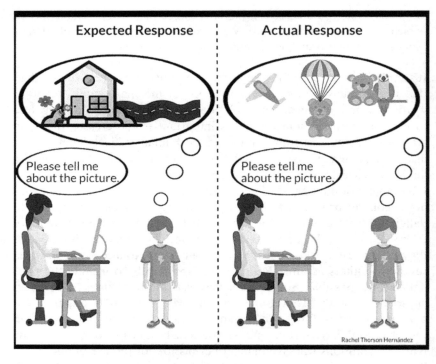

Figure 10.1 The importance of extensive pilot testing

giving me full, technicolor answers, and the IRB-approved participants, their data seemed more like shades of grey. I got my answers, but it could have been so much more eye-poppingly interesting if I'd been able to include their data. Lesson learned."

10.1.2 Pitfall 2: Access and Research Responsibilities

One of a teacher's most valuable and rightly-guarded resources is time. As such, convincing language teachers that your research is worth giving up their class time and/or access to their students can be a challenge. Many teachers also are nervous about being watched while teaching, even when researchers assure them that it's the students they are interested in, not the teachers. Methods books remind us that we bear a responsibility to all participants – especially parents, instructors, and administrators – to continue contact after the conclusion of the study to not only properly thank them, but also to let them know about the outcomes of the research. It's helpful, for example, to send a letter to parents summarizing the outcomes of a study. Administrators also often appreciate a letter, phone call, or meeting to discuss the results of the research. This can reassure them that their efforts in facilitating research have been a productive use of their program, and of their instructors' limited time and resources. Sometimes, L2 research is more theoretical and less practical in terms of its aim at informing teaching, but even so, a carefully explained and motivated research project should be able to contribute to what we know about second language learning, and so result in some insights into second language instruction. It's often the case, too, that instructors like hearing about how research conducted in their school context fits into what they know about how second languages are learned and taught. In other words, going beyond a small token of thanks immediately after the data are collected by letting all stakeholders know about the actual outcomes of the research is always a good idea. It also helps us, as researchers, to put the practical applications of our research, assuming there are outcomes, into words. In interaction, feedback, and task research in particular, this is often easier than in other areas. However, see below for a potential pitfall in this process in relation to task, interaction, and feedback research.

The Research-Weary Classroom

A former director of an English language program was responsible for approving all research conducted in classrooms that fell under the umbrella of the English language program. This director explained in an email to applied linguistics professors at the university that all newly proposed studies that students and faculty wanted to conduct in the English language program would be rejected for a semester, and possibly a year, since the classrooms had been "over-studied" and, through student surveys and instructor meetings, it had become clear that ESL students and their instructors were "weary" of experiments in their classrooms. The applied linguistics faculty initially panicked. While projects conducted by master's students could be re-situated or redesigned, there were PhD students with approved proposals who had been counting on the availability of students and classes at the English language program. A few faculty members had obtained grants to do research with the English language program's population. In the end, the colleagues pooled resources, and helped their students find alternative research sites. However, they also asked what led to this situation and launched an informal internal review to try to answer that question. It turned out that neither graduate students nor their mentors had been very consistent about communicating the findings of their studies, big or small, to the teachers and students who had opened up their classrooms and given up their time, and had not communicated at all with the director of the program, who had approved all the studies. Consequently, the university faculty launched a training and education initiative which required all researchers to explain how their findings could be used to benefit specific classrooms where applicable and encouraged researchers to debrief instructors and administrators in 'findings for the field' sessions. They required that the English language program be explicitly acknowledged and thanked in every available forum from grant proposals to conference papers to publications, and each acknowledgment was collected and sent to the director, for potential use in the wider university context. They also ran sessions for the teachers, explaining how they could use results from studies that had been done in their own classrooms. Perhaps the most successful outcome of this was a new project involving teachers and researchers as partners, where task-based materials were designed in collaboration, based on the curriculum, and then trialed in classrooms. The director commented that perhaps this was the first project at the English language program that actually lessened the teacher's day-to-day workload. The lesson to be learned, then, is that we are all partners to varying degrees in research we carry out in instructional contexts, and that situations can be turned around with careful planning. In interaction, feedback, and task research, our studies in classrooms quite often relate closely to the context of the classroom and findings often have utility for teachers.

10.1.3 Pitfall 3: Language Barriers

One interesting issue related to interaction, feedback, and task-based research is that this kind of research involves a high degree of variability of a myriad of factors; activities and interactive treatments, input and output of linguistic form, interactional modification, and others will vary based on what is going to be measured and how it is measured. It is imperative to keep this variability in mind when planning research, as it can make studies complicated and even have unintended consequences for the data.

Before beginning a study, we need to make sure that the learners who will participate in our research fully understand the instructions and expectations. To do this and obtain informed consent, we need to make sure that not only do they understand what we intend to do in the study, but also that they are able to ask any necessary clarifying questions about the study. Sometimes, this will mean soliciting the help of interpreters so that participants can have their questions answered in their L1s. Enlisting the help of research assistants who speak the participants' L1 can be particularly valuable. When the use of L1s is not practical (e.g., when the researcher is studying a large population with multiple L1s), we need to think about the complexity of the language in the all of the participants' documents, ensuring that all text is widely comprehensible and not a block of intimidating "legalese" (i.e., dense, formal language in agreements that is often hard to understand).

"Legalese" and Obtaining Participant Consent
A colleague brought me an interesting story related to language barriers. In this colleague's study, they realized that participants, who were doing activities in small groups, often negotiated with each other to try to make sense of the instructions. This was puzzling, because the instructions for completing the activities were played on audio and then supplied in writing, and then participants were asked if they had any questions. But the researcher noticed that the first few minutes of every activity seemed to involve the more proficient members of the group explaining what to do to the less proficient members, sometimes with appeals to the researcher to check they understood. During transcription and coding, they began to ask themself: If participants could not understand the instructions for the task, had they fully understood the consent forms? They said they did, and they signed, but the researcher still felt uneasy. Before using the data, the researcher asked the participants again, after the study, to review the consent forms and make sure they agreed to allow use of the data.

If participants seem not to be able to understand language employed in the tasks of the study, and that language is less complex than that used in the consent forms, it is a good idea for researchers to check with their own institutional review board for guidelines on how to make consent forms more comprehensible and possibly re-present consent forms to their participants, to make sure participants understand what they agree to for the study.

10.2 What Can Go Wrong While We Are Collecting Data?

10.2.1 Pitfall 4: Logistical Surprises

Interaction, feedback, and task research often requires researchers to be flexible and ready to handle the unexpected. Even very well piloted and designed studies often don't follow the exact path originally designed for the second language classroom, laboratory, or other context to be studied. These kinds of unexpected surprises necessitate creative and adaptive thinking on the part of the researcher. For example, what happens when an experiment calls for three students to do a task and provide feedback to each other but only two show up? Thinking on our feet, and having anticipated these things ahead of time, is a valuable skill. Sometimes the researcher might decide that dyads are still appropriate methods, other times a researcher might fill in for the missing participant, and not say much. Either way, any modifications need to be fully disclosed in data analysis. Working with a population you don't usually study can also bring its own challenges.

A Case of the Wiggles
Another colleague told me:
> "As I was readying a set of computers for a classroom activity with young children, I was delighted to see from their chatter and energy that they were eager to start. One child in particular was raising his hand and wiggling with excitement. I asked him if he could be patient and said I would be very quick getting his machine ready. However, when I turned around a minute or two later, expecting to find him begging to be the first with his hand on the mouse, instead I found a little puddle under his chair. We visited the health room where a lovely nurse who knew him well helped him to clean up and gave him spare clothes and a lollipop, and while I waited, I remembered (again) not to underestimate the importance of paying close attention to everything when working with children. My data collection was slightly delayed, as it should have been given my lack of preparedness for the unexpected."

A Flowerbed for Your Thoughts?
In a pilot for one of the studies I did with older adults (who told me they preferred that description rather than "elderly adults"), I tried many times to get one lady in her eighties (who I knew from a British-American club) to agree to a time when I could collect some follow-up data. She drove a hard bargain, eventually saying if I could give her some help digging her garden first, this would then free up her time to sit around doing nothing but chatting to me, as she put it. I did give that help, and I reflected on how it made a nice change from the usual participant compensation. I did also report it to the IRB as a change.

A researcher more used to dealing with children or older people would probably have been less surprised than I was to hear about and then to participate in these two occurences. However, the main point is that being patient, flexible, and compassionate, as well as ready to consider alternatives, is the best way forward.

10.2.2 Pitfall 5: Wrong Method/Wrong Use of Method

As we have discussed, there are multiple ways to collect appropriate data to answer our questions. Research questions can guide researchers into selecting one particular technique over another. However, in addition to inadvertently choosing techniques that turn out to be inappropriate for the data we are trying to collect, it is also possible that we might inadvertently misuse techniques that are otherwise considered generally suitable. When we use a data collection technique inappropriately, this can result in data that may be unusable or difficult to interpret. Below is an example of the use of a technique that went wrong, leading to data that could not be used, but also some valuable lessons.

Read between the Lines
In one of my early studies using stimulated recall with two colleagues, I had zeroed in on an interesting bit of interaction with a student. I played the clip two or three times, but the student kept saying, "I don't know, I don't know what I was thinking about," when I asked him to talk about it. I was interpreting that as "it's difficult in a second language, so I'm not going to try." I asked nicely, then again, then suddenly he unpinned his microphone and said, "I'm sorry, this makes me uncomfortable," and left. Looking back on it, I could see his "I don't know" was likely a signal that "I don't want to talk about it," and he was uncomfortable with the experience. I realized we were being quite demanding of all our participants, because we wanted them to tell us precisely what they were thinking every time they modified output or received feedback. In retrospect, we realized it was too much digging for data. As we explained in our book on stimulated recall (Gass and Mackey, 2005), when learners say they don't know, you should leave them alone and stop asking. We realized we could prepare participants better, and encourage them to self-select out, if we showed them a video of stimulated recall taking place, including clips where the participants clearly have nothing to say. In the end, we viewed this episode positively because we realized our participants can withdraw from a study at any time, and this one had exercised his right to do just that.

10.2.3 Pitfall 6: Technology Failure

Almost all interaction, corrective feedback, and task-based research is dependent to some degree on technology. Even at the most basic level, unless we are using uptake sheets or real time field notes, some sort of recording device is often necessary.

Whose Recording Is It Anyway?
A colleague reported on a study that involved a lot of research assistants collecting data at the same time (in a lab, with the tables well spaced). Learners were working together in pairs to carry out picture-sequencing

tasks. One of the RAs asked my colleague if they should start a new audio file for each dyad's oral activity, or just pause between dyads so that they would all be on one file. The colleague told her RAs it didn't matter, that they could do whatever was easiest for them. Most put all of the oral interactions on one file, but one RA started a new file for each dyad. When it was time to transcribe and code the data, however, a problem arose. One of the RAs who had used the continuous recording approach had been so careful to protect participants' anonymity (a laudable goal), that the participants in the dyads weren't even identified by participant number. However, the one RA who had started new files for each dyad recorded each participant's number at the beginning of individual files, which made the analysis simple. Sorting out the others required listening to hours of narratives and working through stacks of sign-up sheets to figure out which participants were on which recording. Because they had not been asked to say their numbers or pseudonyms early on the recordings, distinguishing who was speaking and when was an additional problem. Eventually, some of the data had to be discarded and new participants found.

This story illustrates a valuable lesson: Identifying participants on audio recordings is very important. Usually, with technology, we think about things like when the batteries will be exhausted, if the stop button will be pressed by mistake, the likelihood of participants not showing up, the right cords not being there, the lab password being changed, etc., so we make a series of backup plans to account for those possible problems. For example, most methods books recommend using two recording devices for every data collection session, bringing extra chargers, and having alternate meeting times and places in mind. However, specifying who is who, transcribing, and coding very soon after the data are collected are also essential.

10.3 What Can Go Wrong When We Are Analyzing Data?

10.3.1 Pitfall 7: Data Segmentation and Coding

Once we have collected the data, we need to analyze them and present them in a manner that is accessible to interested parties. The aims of the research as well as context should always determine units of analysis for task, feedback, and interaction data. So when researchers want to investigate linguistic forms used by learners in classrooms, small groups, or pairs, one unit of analysis might be the turn (how many forms per turn). If, on the other hand, if the researcher wants to analyze feedback, they might compare more and less explicit feedback that occurs in each turn.

Missing the Trees for the Code
When I worked out the coding scheme for one of my large feedback studies, it seemed like distinguishing between confirmation checks and clarification checks was a relatively outdated approach, and I was interested in other forms of feedback, so I coded them both as questions. After coding was complete, I realized that clumping them all together as questions made the category too broad. I had coded straight from the recordings instead of transcribing, so I had to listen to every minute of data again and recode into those smaller categories. It's okay to code from recordings if you're absolutely sure about your system, but if you're not, then you really run the risk of having to listen to everything again or re-read everything, and code again. Another way to put this is to code as narrowly as possible the first time and then collapse categories afterwards if you need to do that.

10.4 Summary

In pointing out these concerns and telling these stories, my intent is to encourage (and perhaps even amuse) novice as well as experienced researchers as they carry out studies of interaction, feedback, and tasks, and to emphasize that there are always difficulties or unexpected things that arise, and that they can almost always be overcome, in one way or another, with an open mind and a bit of flexibility. What can't be overcome becomes a lesson to be learned and not repeated.

Glossary

Abstract   A brief summary of research that typically includes the research questions, the methods used (including participants), and a brief indication of the results.

Action research   Studies carried out by practitioners (often teachers) to gain a better understanding of the practical aspects of how second languages are learned and taught, typically focusing on improving the conditions and efficiency of learning and teaching.

Aptitude   A measure of an individual's potential to succeed (at learning a second or foreign language).

Availability bias   A bias in which the publication process may favor studies that report statistically significant results, see also *Publication bias*.

Biodata   Basic information about a participant. Information gathered/reported depends on the goal of a study. Age, amount, and type of prior L2 study, gender, first language(s), and proficiency in L2s are typical examples.

Blog   A journal kept online, typically visible to the public or a select group of others, see also *Journal*.

Case study   A detailed description of a single participant or group, for example an individual learner or a class within a specific population and setting.

Classroom observation   Researcher viewing what is going on, often in a classroom setting. Can use a structured scheme or tally sheet for recording data.

Closed-ended question   Survey item that provides finite choices for respondents, i.e. multiple choice or scales.

Coding   The process by which data (of any kind) are organized (in various ways) to make them manageable, analyzable, and to allow researchers to search for and mark patterns in the data.

Cohen's kappa   A statistic typically used to measure rater reliability on categorical data. Cohen's kappa represents the average rate of (dis)agreement by coders and takes chance agreement into account.

Computer-mediated communication (CMC)   Communicative exchanges between participants using a computer. Can be synchronous (real-time) or not. Exchanges can be recorded and information on performance such as keystrokes, or erasures, and times can be documented.

Confidentiality   An ethical standard in research to keep any identifiable information from research participants private.

Construct validity The degree to which research adequately captures the construct of interest.

Content validity The extent to which a test or measurement device adequately measures the knowledge, skill, or ability that it was designed to measure.

Counting span A numerical test of working memory that involves counting shapes and remembering the total number of shapes for later recall.

Credibility A term used by qualitative researchers to ensure that the picture provided by the research is as full and complete as possible.

Criterion-related validity The extent to which tests used in a study are comparable to other well-established tests of the construct in question.

Data In interaction, the source material used to investigate and answer research questions. Data may be oral, and audio or video recorded, written, in the form of essays, test scores, diaries, or check marks on observation schemes and so on, electronic, such as responses to a computer-assisted accent modification program; or visual, for example, eye movements made while reading text at a computer or gestures made by a teacher in a classroom. Other types also exist.

Data collection The general process of gathering data pertaining to a particular research question, problem, or area.

Data elicitation A subset of data collection, data elicitation refers to the process of directly obtaining information from individuals, for example, through an interview or a task.

Data sampling Selecting and segmenting data into relevant units (e.g. recasts, language-related episodes), sometimes using only a portion of data in a procedure known as reduction or segmentation.

DCT Discourse completion task. A data collection tool that typically presents a learner with a scenario, followed by a blank space that elicits a targeted speech act utterance. DCTs may be written, spoken, or technology-enhanced.

Debriefing Providing information to participants after a study or data collection period. For example, participants may be informed about research findings, questions, or the content of observations.

Descriptive statistics Numerical values that summarize, describe, and categorize data. Common measures include means (i.e., the average of a dataset) and standard deviations (i.e., the variability of a dataset).

EEG Electroencephalography. A means of capturing brain activity by time and region of the brain that is used to research speech production.

Effect size A measure that can be used to determine the magnitude of an observed relationship or effect.

Elicited imitation A procedure for collecting data where a participant is presented with a sentence, clause, or word and is asked to repeat (imitate) it.

ERP   Event-related potential. EEG-based data that provide millisecond-by-millisecond information about linguistic processing.

Ethics review board   See *Institutional Review Board.*

Exclusion criteria   Characteristics that researchers use to disqualify prospective subjects (or studies, in the case of meta-analysis) from inclusion in a study. Examples of exclusion criteria in meta-analysis include the language in which the study was published, and the publication date.

External validity   The extent to which the results of a study are relevant to a wider population.

Face validity   The familiarity of an instrument and the ease with which the validity of the content is recognized.

fMRI   Functional magnetic resonance imaging. See also *Magnetic resonance imaging.*

Forest plot   A visual technique used to display meta-analytic effects for the included studies.

Funnel plot   A visual technique used to plot meta-analysis results and check them for publication bias.

Generalizability   The extent to which the results of a study can be extended to a greater population.

Hi-LAB   High-Level Language Aptitude Battery. A second language learning aptitude test designed to test the capacity of adult language learners to learn languages to advanced levels.

Human subjects committee   See *Institutional Review Board.*

Hypothesis   A prediction made regarding the outcome of a research study.

Inclusion criteria   Characteristics that researchers use to qualify prospective subjects (or studies, in the case of meta-analysis) for inclusion in a study.

Information-gap task   A task in which one individual usually has a gap in his/her information. For example, a picture drawing activity, where one person describes and another person draws, is a type of information-gap task.

Informed consent   Voluntary agreement to participate in a study about which the potential subject has enough information and understands enough to make an informed decision.

Institutional Review Board   A committee established to review research involving human subjects to ensure it is in compliance with ethical guidelines laid down by government and funding agencies. (This term is often used interchangeably with *Human subjects committee* and *Ethics review board.*)

Instrument reliability   The consistency of a particular instrument over time.

Internal validity   The extent to which the results of a study are a function of the factor that is intended by the researcher.

Inter-rater reliability The degree of agreement there is in the ratings given by different coders.

Interval data Data that can be ordered and where the exact difference between variables can be calculated. For example, age, years of schooling, and years of language study.

Interval scale A scale in which there is an ordering of variables and in which there is an equal interval between variables.

Interview A data collection tool that aims to elicit information by asking participants open-ended questions.

Intra-rater reliability The degree of consistency within a single rater's coding across episodes or the range of data.

Introspective methods A set of data elicitation techniques that encourage learners to communicate about their internal processing and/or perspectives about language learning experiences.

IRIS Instruments for Research into Second Languages. A collection of instruments, materials, and stimuli used to elicit data for research into second and foreign languages. www.iris-database.org/

Journal Written, recorded, or internet-based diary entries typically recording participants' impressions and language learning experiences.

Likert scale A form of response to a question that provides participants with choices from a range of numerical values that represent progressive options. For example, 1 = completely disagree and 5 = completely agree.

Map task A type of jigsaw task in which participants are given two different parts or versions of a map and asked to solve tasks like giving instructions to a certain location or communicating which streets in a city are closed.

Mean A measure of central tendency, the mean is a value obtained by summing all the scores in a score distribution and dividing the sum by the number of scores in the distribution.

Measures of central tendency A way of providing quantitative information about the typical behavior of individuals with respect to a particular phenomenon, usually given through means, modes, and medians.

Median A measure of central tendency, the median is a value that represents the midpoint of all the scores. Half of the scores are above the median and half below it.

Meta-analysis A statistical tool used in research synthesis to convert the methods and/or findings of individual studies to comparable values in order to estimate an overall observed finding about a given treatment or condition across studies.

Meta-meta-analysis A statistical tool used in research synthesis to convert the methods and/or findings of individual meta-analyses to comparable values in order to estimate an overall observed finding about a given treatment or condition across meta-analyses.

Mixed methods   Research in which authors present and discuss quantitative and qualitative/interpretive data, or use methods associated with both types of research in collecting data or conducting studies.

MLAT   Modern Language Aptitude Test. A five-part test that is used to determine an individual's capacity to learn a foreign language.

MRI   Magnetic resonance imaging. A means of capturing high-resolution information about the neural regions involved in language processing.

Needs analysis   A process used to determine the real-world language needs of a learner or group of learners, often used with task-based learning.

Nominal data   Data with no inherent quantitative value. For example, part of speech, native language, and gender.

Nominal scale   A scale used to place nominal attributes into two or more categories (e.g., age).

Null hypothesis significance testing   Commonly known by the acronym NHST, this statistical method involves testing an experimental factor against the assumption that there is no relationship between two or more variables.

Objectivity   The idea that researchers should distance themselves from what they're studying so that their findings are based on facts and not beliefs, opinions, or feelings.

Observation   Researchers systematically observe different aspects of a setting in which they are immersed, for example, the interactions, relationships, language, and events in which learners engage. The aim is to provide careful descriptions of learners' activities without unduly influencing the events in which the learners are engaged.

Obtrusive observer   A researcher that affects the research environment and the participants therein via their presence and/or actions. See also *Unobtrusive observer.*

Open-ended question   A question that allows respondents to answer freely, as opposed to a closed-ended question, which gives respondents a set of responses from which they must choose.

Operation span   A measure of working memory that requires participants to solve mathematical operations and recall words presented in a sequence.

Ordinal data   Data that can be ranked. For example, test scores.

Ordinal scale   A scale in which there is an ordering of variables. There is no implication that there is an equal interval between variables.

Outlier   A score that is different from the other scores in a set. It may be considerably larger or smaller than all the other scores.

Participant   An individual whose behavior is being measured or investigated.

Pedagogic task   A task that resembles a real-world task in some way, but which is designed for use in the classroom.

Picture-description task A task in which one person describes a picture to another person who, in turn, tries to draw what the first person described.

Picture-sequencing task A task in which one person describes a series of actions to another person with mixed-up pictures of the actions. The second person orders the pictures based on the sequence described by the first person.

Pilot study A small-scale trial of the proposed procedures, materials, and methods. It may also include a trial of the coding sheets and analytic categories.

Priming A prompted response activity in which two stimuli are presented successively, with the first one being the prime and the second the target. The participant must respond to the target in some way, and priming is said to occur when there is an influence of the prime on the target.

PSTM Phonological short-term memory. A measure of sound-related storage and processing capacity.

Publication bias The likelihood that a study is more likely to be published if it presents statistically significant findings.

Questionnaire An instrument for collecting data from participants through a series of questions that is the same for each participant.

Random-effects model In meta-analysis, a model that directly estimates the meta-analytic variance in effect sizes instead of assuming it is zero.

Random sampling Sampling in which each member of a population has an equal chance of being selected.

Reaction time The time between a stimulus and a learner's response. Reaction time experiments are usually computer-based and can also be used to investigate processing.

Reliability The degree to which there is consistency in results.

Replication Conducting a research study again, in a way that is either identical to the original procedure or with small changes (e.g. different participants), to test the original findings. Many different types of replication exist, for example, conceptual replication (the main concept or idea is the same) and partial replication (where one aspect of the original study might be changed).

Representativeness The extent to which an individual who could be selected for a study has the same chance of being selected as any other individual in the population.

Research synthesis The process of combining existing research and findings on an issue or hypothesis with the aim of increasing the generalizability and applicability of the findings.

Scoping review A type of research synthesis that surveys the literature on a certain topic in order to present an overview of the literature on the topic, key concepts, gaps in the research, etc.

Sequence span   A working-memory test in which participants must recall a list of stimuli based on the particular order in which the stimuli were presented to them.

Standard deviation   A measure of dispersion, it is a numerical value that indicates how scores are spread around the mean.

Stimulated recall   A technique in which a researcher plays a recording or video or shows other illustrative data of an individual's language learning or use and asks the individual to reflect on and describe what their thought processes were during the experience.

Stimulated recall – delayed   An introspective technique for gathering data in which learners are asked to reflect on language learning or use while viewing or hearing a stimulus to prompt their recollections of the learning or use.

Stimulated recall – immediate   An introspective technique for gathering data that can yield insights a learner's thought processes during language learning experiences.

Subjectivity   In research, the idea that the interpretation of the data in a study, and thus the results, are influenced by beliefs, opinions, or feelings.

Survey   A method of data collection that uses the same instruments on a number of participants determined to be an appropriate sample of a larger population.

Target language (TL)   The language being learned.

Task-based language teaching (TBLT)   An educational framework for the theory and practice of teaching second or foreign based in syllabi grounded in the real-world daily tasks a specific group of learners needs to accomplish in their second language.

Think-aloud   A type of research method in which participants speak about their thoughts while completing a task.

Triangulation   Using multiple research techniques and multiple sources of data in order to explore an issue from all feasible perspectives.

Unobtrusive observers   A researcher who takes care not to affect the research environment and the participants therein via their presence and/or actions. See also *Obtrusive observer*.

Uptake sheets   Learners' reports about their learning, illustrating what they take up from the language learning opportunities they have through instruction.

Validity   The extent we can make correct generalizations based on the results from a particular measure.

Verbal reporting   A type of introspection that consists of gathering information by asking individuals to say what is going through their minds as they are solving or after they have solved a problem or doing a task.

Verbal reporting – concurrent   A type of introspection that consists of gathering information by asking individuals to say what is going through their minds as they are solving a problem or doing a task.

Verbal reporting – retrospective   A type of introspection that consists of gathering information by asking individuals to say what was going through their minds after they finish solving a task.

Verbal reporting – self-report   A type of introspection where a learner comments on their general approaches to language learning and/or use.

Working memory   Memory that involves both processing capacity and storage capacity.

References

Abbuhl, R. (2018). Research replication. In A. Phakiti, P. I. De Costa, L. Plonsky, & S. Starfield (Eds.), *The Palgrave Handbook of Applied Linguistics Research Methodology* (pp. 145–162). Palgrave Macmillan.

Abbuhl, R., Mackey, A., Ziegler, N., & Amoroso, L. (2018). Interaction and learning grammar. In J. I. Liontas (Ed.), *The TESOL Encyclopedia of English Language Teaching* (pp. 1–7). Wiley-Blackwell.

Abrahamsson, N. & Hyltenstam, K. (2008). The robustness of aptitude effects in near-native second language acquisition. *Studies in Second Language Acquisition*, *30*(4), 481–509.

Albert, Á. & Kormos, J. (2004). Creativity and narrative task performance: An exploratory study. *Language Learning*, *54*(2), 277–310.

(2011). Creativity and narrative task performance: An exploratory study. *Language Learning*, *61*(Suppl. 1), 73–99.

Alcón-Soler, E. (2017). Pragmatic development during study abroad: An analysis of Spanish teenagers' request strategies in English emails. *Annual Review of Applied Linguistics*, *37*, 77–92.

Allwright, R. L. (1984). Why don't learners learn what teachers teach? The interaction hypothesis. In D. M. Singleton and D. G. Little (Eds.), *Language Learning in Formal and Informal Contexts* (pp. 3–18). IRAAL.

(1987). Classroom observation: Problems and possibilities. In B. K. Das (Ed.), *Patterns of Classroom Interaction in Southeast Asia* (pp. 88–102). SEAMEO Regional Language Centre.

Altarriba, J., Kroll, J. F., Sholl, A., & Rayner, K. (1996). The influence of lexical and conceptual constraints on reading mixed-language sentences: Evidence from eye fixations and naming times. *Memory and Cognition*, *24*(4), 477–492.

Ammar, A. & Spada, N. (2006). One size fits all? Recasts, prompts, and L2 learning. *Studies in Second Language Acquisition*, *28*(4), 543–574.

Andrews, E. (2019). Cognitive neuroscience and multilingualism. In J. W. Schwieter (Ed.), *The Handbook of the Neuroscience of Multilingualism* (pp. 19–47). John Wiley and Sons.

Awwad, A. & Tavakoli, P. (2019). Task complexity, language proficiency and working memory: Interaction effects on second language speech performance. *International Review of Applied Linguistics in Language Teaching*.

Azkarai, A. & García Mayo, M. D. P. (2015). Task-modality and L1 use in EFL oral interaction. *Language Teaching Research*, 19(5), 550–571.

(2016). Task repetition effects on L1 use in EFL child task-based interaction. *Language Teaching Research*, 21, 480–495.

Baddeley, A. D. (1986). *Working Memory*. Oxford University Press.

Bailey, K. M., Nunan, D., & Swan, M. (Eds.) (1996). *Voices From the Language Classroom: Qualitative Research in Second Language Education*. Cambridge University Press.

Baralt, M. (2015). Working memory capacity, cognitive complexity and L2 recasts in online language teaching. In Z. Wen, M. B. Mota, & A. McNeill (Eds.), *Working Memory in Second Language Acquisition and Processing* (pp. 248–269). Multilingual Matters.

Barberena, L. S., Brasil, B. C., Melo, R. M., Mezzomo, C. L., Mota, H. B., & Keske-Soares, M. (2014). Ultrasound applicability in speech language pathology and audiology. *CoDAS*, 26(6), 520–530.

Barkhuizen, G. P., Benson, P., & Chik, A. (2014). *Narrative Inquiry in Language Teaching and Learning Research*. Routledge.

Bax, S. (2003). The end of CLT: A context approach to language teaching. *ELT Journal*, 57, 278–287.

Benson, P. (2015). Commenting to learn: Evidence of language and intercultural learning in comments on YouTube videos. *Language Learning and Technology*, 19(3), 88–99.

Beretta, A. & Davies, A. (1985). Evaluation of the Bangalore Project. *ELT Journal*, 39(2), 121–127.

Bialystok, E. (2015). Bilingualism and the development of executive function: The role of attention. *Child Development Perspectives*, 9(2), 117–121.

Bialystok, E., Kroll, J. F., Green, D. W., MacWhinney, B., & Craik, F. I. (2015). Publication bias and the validity of evidence: What's the connection? *Psychological Science*, 26(6), 944–946.

Block, D. (2000). Problematizing interview data: Voices in the mind's machine? *TESOL Quarterly*, 34(4), 757–763.

(2010). Researching language and identity. In B. Paltridge & A. Phakiti (Eds.), *Continuum Companion to Research Methods in Applied Linguistics* (pp. 337–349). Continuum International Publishing Group.

Blum-Kulka, S. (1982). Learning to say what you mean in a second language: A study of the speech act performance of learners of Hebrew as a second language. *Applied Linguistics*, 3, 29.

Bock, K. (1990). Structure in language: Creating form in talk. *American Psychologist*, 45(11), 1221–1236.

(1995). Sentence production: From mind to mouth. In J. L. Miller & P. D. Eimas (Eds.), *Handbook of Perception and Cognition: Speech, Language, and Communication* (2nd ed., pp. 181–216). Academic Press.

Bock, K. & Griffin, Z. M. (2000). The persistence of structural priming: Transient activation or implicit learning? *Journal of Experimental Psychology: General, 129*(2), 177–192.

Borenstein, M., Hedges, L., Higgins, J., & Rothstein, H. (2005). *Comprehensive Meta-Analysis* [computer software]. Biostat.

Bowles, M. (2010). Features that make a task amenable to think-aloud: A meta-analysis of studies investigating the validity of think-alouds on verbal tasks. In *The Think-Aloud Controversy in Second Language Research* (pp. 67–112). Routledge.

Brown, D. (2016). The type and linguistic foci of oral corrective feedback in the L2 classroom: A meta-analysis. *Language Teaching Research, 20*(4), 436–458. 10.1177/1362168814563200

Bruer J. T. (2006). Points of view: On the implications of neuroscience research for science teaching and learning: Are there any? A skeptical theme and variations: The primacy of psychology in the science of learning. *CBE–Life Sciences Education, 5*(2), 104–110. DOI:10.1187/cbe.06-03-0153

Brunfaut, T. & Révész, A. (2015). The role of task and listener characteristics in second language listening. *TESOL Quarterly, 49*(1), 141–168.

Bryfonski, L. (2019a). "Is seeing believing? The role of ultrasound tongue imaging and oral corrective feedback in L2 pronunciation development," unpublished manuscript, Department of Linguistics, Georgetown University, Washington, DC.

(2019b). *Task-based teacher training: Implementation and evaluation in Central American bilingual schools*(Publication No. 13811093), [Doctoral dissertation, Georgetown University]. ProQuest Dissertations Publishing.

Bryfonski, L. & Ma, X. (2019). Effects of implicit versus explicit feedback on Mandarin tone acquisition in a SCMC learning environment. *Studies in Second Language Acquisition*, 1–28.

Bryfonski, L. & McKay, T. (2017). TBLT implementation and evaluation: A meta-analysis. *Language Teaching Research*, 1–30.

Bryfonski, L. & Sanz, C. (2018). Opportunities for corrective feedback during study abroad: A mixed methods approach. *Annual Review of Applied Linguistics, 38*, 1–32.

Bygate, M. (2001). Effects of task repetition on the structure and control of oral language. In M. Bygate, P. Skehan, & M. Swain (Eds.), *Researching Pedagogic Tasks: Second Language Learning, Teaching, and Testing* (pp. 23–48). Longman.

Bygate, M. (Ed.) (2015). *Domains and Directions in the Development of TBLT: A Decade of Plenaries from the International Conference.* John Benjamins.

Bygate, M., Norris, J., & Van den Branden, K. (2015). Task-based language teaching. In C. Chapelle (Ed.), *The Encyclopedia of Applied Linguistics.* Wiley-Blackwell.

Calvert, M. & Sheen, Y. (2015). Task-based language learning and teaching: An action-research study. *Language Teaching Research, 19*(2), 226–244.

Carroll, J. B. & Sapon, S. M. (1959). *Modern Language Aptitude Test.* Psychological Corporation.

Carroll, S. & Swain, M. (1993). Explicit and implicit negative feedback: An empirical study of the learning of linguistic generalizations. *Studies in Second Language Acquisition, 15*(3), 357–386.

Chaudron, C. (2000). Contrasting approaches to classroom research: Qualitative and quantitative analysis of language use and learning. *Second Language Studies, 19*, 1–56.

Cleophas, T. & Zwinderman, A. (2017). *Modern Meta-Analysis Review and Update of Methodologies.* Springer International Publishing.

Cobb, M. (2010). *Meta-analysis of the effectiveness of task-based interaction in form-focused instruction of adult learners in foreign and second language teaching* [Unpublished doctoral dissertation]. University of San Francisco.

Coderre, E. L., Smith, J. F., Van Heuven, W. J., and Horwitz, B. (2016). The functional overlap of executive control and language processing in bilinguals. *Bilingualism: Language and Cognition, 19*(3), 471–488.

Cohen, J. (1960). A coefficient of agreement for nominal scales. *Educational and Psychological Measurement, 20*, 37–46.

Coombe, C. and Davidson, P. (2015). Constructing questionnaires. In J. D. Brown and C. A. Coombe (Eds.), *The Cambridge Guide to Research in Language Teaching and Learning* (pp. 217–223). Cambridge University Press.

Cooper, H. (2017). *Research Synthesis and Meta-Analysis: A Step-By-Step Approach* (5th ed.). SAGE.

Cornillie, F., Van Den Noortgate, W., Van den Branden, K., & Desmet, P. (2017). Examining focused L2 practice: From in vitro to in vivo. *Language Learning and Technology, 21*(1), 121–145.

Cowan, N., Towse, J. N., Hamilton, Z., Saults, J. S., Elliott, E. M., Lacey, J. F., Moreno, M. V., & Hitch, G. J. (2003). Children's working-memory processes: A response-timing analysis. *Journal of Experimental Psychology: General, 132*(1), 113–132.

Creswell, J. W. (2015). *A Concise Introduction to Mixed Methods Research.* Sage.

Creswell, J. W. & Creswell, J. D. (2018). *Research Design: Qualitative, Quantitative, and Mixed Methods Approaches* (5th ed.). Sage.

Creswell, J. W. & Plano Clark, V. L. (2007). *Designing and Conducting Mixed Methods Research*. Sage.

Creswell, J. W., Plano Clark, V. L., & Garrett, A. L. (2008). Methodological issues in conducting mixed methods research designs. In M. Bergman (Ed.), *Advances in Mixed Methods Research* (pp. 66–84). Sage Publishing.

Crookes, G. (1993). Action research for second language teaching: Going beyond teacher research. *Applied Linguistics, 14*, 130–142.

Culpeper, J., Mackey, A., & Taguchi, N. (2018). *Second Language Pragmatics: From Theory to Research*. Routledge.

Daneman, M. and Case, R. (1981). Syntactic form, semantic complexity, and short-term memory: Influences on children's acquisition of new linguistic structures. *Developmental Psychology, 17*(4), 367–78.

de Bruin, A., Treccani, B., & Della Sala, S. (2015). Cognitive advantage in bilingualism: An example of publication bias? *Psychological Science, 26*(1), 99–107.

Dewey, D., Belnap, R., & Steffen, P. (2018). Anxiety: Stress, foreign language classroom anxiety, and enjoyment during study abroad in Amman, Jordan. *Annual Review of Applied Linguistics, 38*, 140–161.

Dörnyei, Z. (2003). *Questionnaires in Second Language Research Construction, Administration, and Processing*. Lawrence Erlbaum Associates.

(2010). *Questionnaires in Second Language Research: Construction, Administration, and Processing* (2nd ed.). Routledge.

Dörnyei, Z. & Csizér, K. (2012). How to design and analyze surveys in second language acquisition research. In A. Mackey & S. M. Gass. (Eds.), *Research Methods in Second Language Acquisition: A Practical Guide* (pp. 74–94). Wiley-Blackwell.

Dörnyei, Z. & Skehan, P. (2005). Individual differences in L2 learning. In C. Doughty & M. H. Long (Eds.), *The Handbook of Second Language Acquisition* (pp. 589–630). Wiley-Blackwell.

Doughty, C. (2018). Cognitive language aptitude. *Language Learning, 69*, 101–126.

Doughty, C. J., Bunting, M. F., Campbell, S. G., Bowles, A. R., & Haarmann, H. (2007). The development of the High-Level Language Aptitude Battery. *Center for Advanced Study of Language Technical Report (TTO 2105 M. 4)*. University of Maryland.

Doughty, C. & Varela, E. (1998). Communicative focus-on-form. In C. Doughty & J. Williams (Eds.), *Focus on Form in Classroom Second Language Acquisition* (pp. 114–138). Cambridge University Press.

Duff, P. (2012). Identity, agency, and second language acquisition. In S. Gass & A. Mackey (Eds.), *The Routledge Handbook of Second Language Acquisition* (pp. 410–426). Routledge.

Dussias, P. E., Valdés Kroff, J. R., Beatty-Martínez, A. L., & Johns, M. A. (2019). What language experience tells us about cognition: Variable input and interactional contexts affect bilingual sentence processing. In J. W. Schwieter (Ed.), *The Handbook of the Neuroscience of Multilingualism* (pp. 467–484). John Wiley and Sons.

Edwards, A. W. F. (1972). *Likelihood: An Account of the Statistical Concept of Likelihood and Its Application to Scientific Inference.* Cambridge University Press.

Egi, T. (2010). Uptake, modified output, and learner perceptions of recasts: Learner responses as language awareness. *The Modern Language Journal, 94*, 1–21.

Ellis, R. (2000). Task-based research and language pedagogy. *Language Teaching Research, 4*(3), 193–220.

(2003). *Task-Based Language Learning and Teaching.* Oxford University Press.

(2008). A typology of written corrective feedback types. *ELT journal, 63* (2), 97–107.

(2018). Taking the critics to task: The case for task-based teaching. In I. Walker, D. Chan, M. Nagami, & C. Bourguignon (Eds.), *New Perspectives on the Development of Communicative and Related Competence in Foreign Language Education* (pp. 103–117). De Gruyter Mouton.

Ellis, R., Basturkmen, H., & Loewen, S. (2001). Learner uptake in communicative ESL lessons. *Language Learning, 51*(2), 281–318.

Ellis, R., Skehan, P., Li, S., Shintani, N., & Lambert, C. (2019). *Task-Based Language Teaching: Theory and Practice.* Cambridge University Press.

Erard, M. (2014). Secret military test, coming soon to your Spanish class: A powerful, precise language aptitude test is entering civilian life. *Nautilus, 12.* Retrieved from https://bit.ly/2QHYCDD

Fabre, D., Hueber, T., Girin, L., Alameda-Pineda, X., & Badin, P. (2017). Automatic animation of an articulatory tongue model from ultrasound images of the vocal tract. *Speech Communication, 93*, 63–75.

Faretta-Stutenberg, M. & Morgan-Short, K. (2018a). Contributions of initial proficiency and language use to second-language development during study abroad: Behavioral and event-related potential evidence. In C. Sanz & A. Morales-Front (Eds.), *The Routledge Handbook of Study Abroad Research and Practice* (pp. 421–435). Routledge.

(2018b). The interplay of individual differences and context of learning in behavioral and neurocognitive second language development. *Second Language Research, 34*(1), 67–101.

Fetters, M. D. & Molina-Azorin, J. F. (2019). A checklist of mixed methods elements in a submission for advancing the methodology of mixed methods research. *Journal of Mixed Methods Research, 13*(4), 414–423.

Fortune, T. & Ju, Z. (2017). Assessing and exploring the oral proficiency of young Mandarin immersion learners. *Annual Review of Applied Linguistics, 37,* 264–287. 10.1017/S0267190517000150

Foster, P. & Skehan, P. (1996). The influence of planning and task type on second language performance. *Studies in Second Language Acquisition, 18*(3), 299–323.

Frenck-Mestre, C. (2005). Eye-movement recording as a tool for studying syntactic processing in a second language: A review of methodologies and experimental findings. *Second Language Research, 21*(2), 175–198.

Fukuya, Y. J. & Zhang, Y. (2002). Effects of recasts of EFL learners' acquisition of pragmalinguistic conventions of request. *Second Language Studies, 21*(1), 1–47.

García Mayo, M. D. P. & Alcón Soler, E. (2013). Negotiated input and output / interaction. In J. Herschensohn & M. Young-Scholten (Eds.), *The Cambridge Handbook of Second Language Acquisition* (pp. 209–229). Cambridge University Press.

García Mayo, M. D. P. & Labandibar, U. (2017). The use of models as written corrective feedback in English as a foreign language (EFL) writing. *Annual Review of Applied Linguistics, 37,* 110–127.

Gass, S. M. (1997). *Input, Interaction, and the Second Language Learner.* Lawrence Erlbaum.

(2010). Interactionist perspectives on second language acquisition. In R. B. Kaplan (Ed.), *The Oxford Handbook of Applied Linguistics* (2nd ed., pp. 217–231). Oxford University Press.

(2017). *Input, Interaction, and the Second Language Learner* (2nd ed.). Routledge.

Gass, S. M., Behney, J. N., & Uzum, B. (2013). Inhibitory control, working memory, and L2 interaction. In K. Droździał-Szelest & M. Pawlak (Eds.), *Psycholinguistic and Sociolinguistic Perspectives on Second Language Learning* (pp. 91–114). Springer.

Gass, S. M. & Mackey, A. (2005). *Stimulated Recall Methodology in Second Language Research* (2nd ed.). Lawrence Erlbaum Associates.

(2006). Input, interaction, and output: An overview. *AILA Review, 19*(1), 3–17.

(2015). Input, interaction and output in second language acquisition. In B. VanPatten & J. Williams (Eds.), *Theories in Second Language Acquisition* (2nd ed., pp. 180–206). Routledge.

(2017). *Stimulated Recall Methodology in Applied Linguistics and L2 Research*. Routledge.

Gass, S. M. & Varonis, E. M. (1989). Incorporated repairs in nonnative discourse. In M. Eisenstein (Ed.), *Variation and Second Language Acquisition* (pp. 71–86). Springer.

Gick, B., Bernhardt, B., Bacsfalvi, P., & Wilson, I. (2008). Ultrasound imaging applications in second language acquisition. In J. G. Hansen Edwards & M. L. Zampini (Eds.), *Phonology and Second Language Acquisition* (pp. 315–328). John Benjamins.

Godfroid, A. (2019). *Eye Tracking in Second Language Acquisition: A Research Synthesis and Methodological Guide*. Routledge.

Goetze, J. (2018). *Linking cognition and emotion: An appraisal study of foreign language teacher anxiety* [Unpublished doctoral dissertation]. Georgetown University.

Goo, J. (2012). Corrective feedback and working memory capacity in interaction-driven L2 learning. *Studies in Second Language Acquisition, 34*(3), 445–474.

Goo, J. & Mackey, A. (2013a). The case against the case against recasts. *Studies in Second Language Acquisition, 35*(1), 127–165.

(2013b). The case for methodological rigor: A Response to Lyster and Ranta. *Studies in Second Language Acquisition, 35*(1), E1. 10.1017/S0272263113000028

Gordon, C. (2012). Beyond the observer's paradox: The audio-recorder as a resource for the display of identity. *Qualitative Research, 13*(4), 299–317

Grigorenko, E. L., Sternberg, R. J., & Ehrman, M. E. (2000). A theory-based approach to the measurement of foreign language learning ability: The Canal-F theory and test. *The Modern Language Journal, 84*(3), 390–405.

Guilford, J. P. (1967). *The Nature of Human Intelligence*. McGraw Hill.

Gurevitch, J., Koricheva, J., Nakagawa, S., & Stewart, G. (2018). Meta-analysis and the science of research synthesis. *Nature, 555*(7695), 175–182.

Gurzynski-Weiss, L. (2016a). Factors influencing Spanish instructors' in-class feedback decisions. *The Modern Language Journal, 100*(1) 255–275.

(2016b). Spanish instructors' operationalization and interpretation of task complexity and sequencing in non-experimental foreign language lessons. *The Language Learning Journal, 44*(4), 467–486.

Gurzynski-Weiss, L. & Plonsky, L. (2017). Look who's interacting: A scoping review of research involving non-teacher/non-peer interlocutors. In L. Gurzynski-Weiss (Ed.), *Expanding Individual Difference Research in the Interaction Approach: Investigating Learners, Instructors, and Other Interlocutors* (pp. 305–324). John Benjamins.

Harrington, M. & Sawyer, M. (1992). L2 working memory capacity and L2 reading skill. *Studies in Second Language Acquisition, 14*(1), 25–38.

Hashemi, M. & Babii, E. (2013). Mixed methods research: Toward new research designs in applied linguistics. *The Modern Language Journal, 97*(4), 828–852.

Hassanzadeh, M., Marefat, F., & Ramezani, A. (2019). The impact of single versus multiple recasts on L2 learners' implicit and explicit knowledge. *Heliyon, 5*(5), e01748.

Hoff, E. (Ed.) (2011). *Research Methods in Child Language: A Practical Guide*. Wiley-Blackwell.

Hyltenstam, K. & Abrahamsson, N. (2003). Maturational constraints in SLA. In C. J. Doughty & M. H. Long (Eds.), *The Handbook of Second Language Acquisition* (pp. 539–588). Blackwell.

Indrarathne, B. & Kormos, J. (2018). The role of working memory in processing L2 input: Insights from eye-tracking. *Bilingualism: Language and Cognition, 21*(2), 355–374.

Ionin, T. & Zyzik, E. (2014). Judgment and interpretation tasks in second language research. *Annual Review of Applied Linguistics, 34*, 37–64.

Jackson, D. O. & Suethanapornkul, S. (2013). The cognition hypothesis: A synthesis and meta-analysis of research on second language task complexity. *Language Learning, 63*(2), 330–367.

Jang, E., Wagner, M., & Park, G. (2014). Mixed methods research in language testing and assessment. *Annual Review of Applied Linguistics, 34*, 123–153.

Jegerski, J. & VanPatten, B. (2013). *Research Methods in Second Language Psycholinguistics*. Routledge.

Jeong, H., Sugiura, M., Sassa, Y., Wakusawa, K., Horie, K., Sato, S., & Kawashima, R. (2010). Learning second language vocabulary: Neural dissociation of situation-based learning and text-based learning. *Neuroimage, 50*(2), 802–809.

Jeong, H., Sugiura, M., Suzuki, W., Sassa, Y., Hashizume, H., & Kawashima, R. (2016). Neural correlates of second-language communication and the effect of language anxiety. *Neuropsychologia, 84*, e2–e12.

Juffs, A. (2004). Representation, processing, and working memory in a second language. *Transactions of the Philological Society, 102*(2), 199–225.

Juffs, A. & Harrington, M. (2011). Aspects of working memory in L2 learning. *Language Teaching, 44*(2), 137–166.

Kartchava, E. (2016). Learners' beliefs about corrective feedback in the language classroom: Perspectives from two international contexts. *TESL Canada Journal, 33*(2), 19–45. 1018806/tesl.v33i2.1233

Katz, A. N. & Hussey, K. A. (2011). Psycholinguistics. In M. Runco & S. Pritzker (Eds.), *Encyclopedia of Creativity* (2nd ed., pp. 271–278). Elsevier.

Keck, C. M., Iberri-Shea, G., Tracy-Ventura, N., & Wa-Mbaleka, S. (2006). Investigating the empirical link between task-based interaction and acquisition: A meta-analysis. In J. M. Norris & L. Ortega (Eds.), *Synthesizing Research on Language Learning and Teaching* (pp. 91–131). John Benjamins.

Kim, Y., Payant, C., & Pearson, P. (2015). The intersection of task-based interaction, task complexity, and working memory: L2 question development through recasts in a laboratory setting. *Studies in Second Language Acquisition, 37*, 549–581.

Kim, Y. & Taguchi, N. (2015). Promoting task-based pragmatics instruction in EFL classroom contexts: The role of task complexity. *The Modern Language Journal, 99*(4), 656–677.

King, K. & Bigelow, M. (2018). East African transnational adolescents and cross-border education: An argument for local international learning. *Annual Review of Applied Linguistics, 38*, 187–193. 10.1017/S0267190518000041

King, K. & Mackey, A. (2016). Research methodology in second language studies: Trends, concerns, and new directions. *The Modern Language Journal, 100*(Supp. 1), 209–227.

Kinginger, C. & Wu, Q. (2018). Learning Chinese through contextualized language practices in study abroad residence halls: Two case studies. *Annual Review of Applied Linguistics, 38*, 102–121.

Kinoshita, S. & Lupker, S. J. (2003). Priming and attentional control of lexical and sublexical pathways in naming: A reevaluation. *Journal of Experimental Psychology: Learning, Memory, and Cognition, 29*(3), 405–415.

Kirkham, S. & Mackey, A. (2015). Research, relationships, and reflexivity: Two case studies of language and identity. *Ethics In Applied Linguistics Research* (pp. 103–120). Routledge.

Klein, R. A. (2018). Many Labs 2: Investigating variation in replicability across samples and settings. *Advances in Methods and Practices in Psychological Science, 1*(4), 443–490.

Krashen, S. (1977). Some issues relating to the monitor model. In H. Brown, C. Yorio, & R. Crymes (Eds.), *Teaching and Learning English As a Second Language: Trends in Research and Practice* (pp. 144–158). TESOL.

(1980). The input hypothesis. In J. Alatis (Ed.), *Current Issues in Bilingual Education* (pp. 168–180). Georgetown University Press.

Labov, W. (1972). Some principles of linguistic methodology. *Language in Society, 1*, 97–120.

Lantolf, J., Thorne, S. L., & Poehler, M. (2015). Sociocultural theory and second language development. In B. VanPatten and J. Williams (Eds.), *Theories in Second Language Acquisition* (pp. 207–226). Routledge.

Lardiere, D. (2007). *Ultimate Attainment in Second Language Acquisition: A Case Study*. Routledge.

Larsen-Freeman, D. & Tedick, D. J. (2016). World language teaching: Thinking differently. In D. Gitomer & C. Bell (Eds.), *Handbook of Research on Teaching* (5th ed., pp. 1335–1388). American Educational Research Association.

Laws, K. R. (2016). Psychology, replication, and beyond. *BMC Psychology, 4*(30), 1–8.

Lee, J. (2018). Task complexity, cognitive load, and L1 speech. *Applied Linguistics, 39*(3), 506–539.

Lee, V. & Gyogi, E. (2015). The reflective learning journal in the classroom, [Paper presentation]. Annual International Conference on Language Teaching and Learning and Educational Materials Exhibition, Shizuoka City, Japan.

Leeman, J. (2003). Recasts and second language development: Beyond negative evidence. *Studies in Second Language Acquisition, 25*(1), 37–63.

Leow, R. & Donatelli, L. (2017). The role of (un)awareness in SLA. *Language Teaching, 50*(2), 189–211.

Li, S. (2010). The effectiveness of corrective feedback in SLA: A meta-analysis. *Language Learning, 60*(2), 309–365.

(2013). The interactions between the effects of implicit and explicit feedback and individual differences in language analytic ability and working memory. *The Modern Language Journal, 97*(3), 634–654.

(2015). The associations between language aptitude and second language grammar acquisition: A meta-analytic review of five decades of research. *Applied Linguistics, 36*, 385–408.

Li, S., Zhu, Y., & Ellis, R. (2016). The effects of the timing of corrective feedback on the acquisition of a new linguistic structure. *The Modern Language Journal, 100*(1), 276–295.

Lightbown, P. M. & Spada, N. (1990). Focus-on-form and corrective feedback in communicative language teaching: Effects on second language learning. *Studies in Second Language Acquisition, 12*(4), 429–448.

Linck, J. A., Osthus, P., Koeth, J. T., & Bunting, M. F. (2014). Working memory and second language comprehension and production: A meta-analysis. *Psychonomic Bulletin and Review, 21*(4), 861–883.

Lipsey, M. W. & Wilson, D. B. (2001). *Practical Meta-Analysis.* Sage.

Llinares, A. & Lyster, R. (2014). The influence of context on patterns of corrective feedback and learner uptake: A comparison of CLIL and immersion classrooms. *The Language Learning Journal, 42*(2), 181–194.

Loewen, S. & Sato, M. (2018). Interaction and instructed second language acquisition. *Language Teaching, 51*(3), 285–329.

Long, M. H. (1980). *Input and interaction in second language acquisition* [Unpublished doctoral dissertation]. University of California at Los Angeles.

(1981). Input, interaction, and second language acquisition. *Annals of the New York Academy of Sciences, 379*(1), 259–278. 10.1111/j.1749-6632.1981.tb42014.x

(1985). Input and second-language acquisition theory. In S. M. Gass & C. Madden (Eds.), *Input in Second Language Acquisition* (pp. 377–393). Newbury House.

(1996). The role of the linguistic environment in second language acquisition. In W. C. Ritchie & T. K. Bhatia (Eds.), *Handbook of Second Language Acquisition* (pp. 413–468). Academic Press.

(2000). Focus on form in task-based language teaching. In R. Lambert & E. Shohamy (Eds.), *Language Policy and Pedagogy: Essays in Honor of A. Ronald Walton* (pp. 179–192). John Benjamins.

(2015). *Second Language Acquisition and Task-Based Language Teaching.* John Wiley and Sons.

(2016). In defense of tasks and TBLT: Non-issues and real issues. *Annual Review of Applied Linguistics, 36*, 5–33.

Long, M. H., & Crookes, G. (1992). Three approaches to task-based syllabus design. *TESOL Quarterly, 26*(1), 27–56.

Long, M. H., Lee, J., & Hillman, K. (2019). Task-based language learning. In P. Malovrh & A. Benati (Eds.), *Cambridge Handbook of Language Learning* (pp. 500–527). Cambridge University Press.

Long, M. H. & Robinson, P. (1998). Focus on form: Theory, research, and practice. In C. Doughty & J. Williams (Eds.), *Focus on Form in Classroom Second Language Acquisition* (pp. 15–41). Cambridge University Press.

Luck, S. J. (2012). Event-related potentials. In H. Cooper, P. M. Camic, D. L. Long, A. T. Panter, D. Rindskopf, & K. J. Sher (Eds.), *APA Handbook of Research Methods in Psychology: Foundations, Planning, Measures, and Psychometrics* (Vol. 1, pp. 523–546). American Psychological Association.

Luque, A., Mizyed, N., & Morgan-Short, K. (2018). Event-related potentials reveal evidence for syntactic co-activation in bilingual language processing: A replication of Sanoudaki and Thierry. In L. López (Ed.), *Code-Switching–Experimental Answers to Theoretical Questions: In Honor of Kay González-Vilbazo* (pp. 177–194). John Benjamins.

Lyster, R. (1998a). Negotiation of form, recasts, and explicit correction in relation to error type and learner repair in immersion classrooms. *Language Learning, 48*(Suppl. 1), 183–218.

(1998b). Recasts, repetition, and ambiguity in L2 classroom discourse. *Studies in Second Language Acquisition, 20*(1), 51–81.

(2004). Differential effects of prompts and recasts in form-focused instruction. *Studies in Second Language Acquisition, 26*(3), 399–432.

(2019). Roles for corrective feedback in second language instruction. In C. A. Chapelle (Ed.), *The Encyclopedia of Applied Linguistics*. Wiley-Blackwell.

Lyster, R. & Ranta, L. (1997). Corrective feedback and learner uptake: Negotiation of form in communicative classrooms. *Studies in Second Language Acquisition, 19*(1), 37–66.

(2013). Counterpoint piece: The case for variety in corrective feedback research. *Studies in Second Language Acquisition, 35*(1), 167–184. 10.1017/S027226311200071X

Lyster, R. & Saito, K. (2010). Oral feedback in classroom SLA: A meta-analysis. *Studies in Second Language Acquisition, 32*(2), 265–302.

Mackey, A. (1999). Input, interaction, and second language development: An empirical study of question formation in ESL. *Studies in Second Language Acquisition, 21*(4), 557–587.

(2006). Feedback, noticing, and instructed second language learning. *Applied Linguistics, 27*(3), 405–430.

(2012a). *Input, Interaction, and Corrective Feedback in L2 Learning*. Oxford University Press.

(2012b). Why (or why not), when, and how to replicate research. In G. Porte (Ed.), *Replication Research in Applied Linguistics*, 34–69. Cambridge University Press.

(2016). Practice and progression in second language research methods. *AILA Review*, *27*, 80–97.

Mackey, A., Abbuhl, R., & Gass, S. M. (2012). Interactionist approaches. In S. Gass & A. Mackey (Eds.), *The Routledge Handbook of Second Language Acquisition* (pp. 7–23). Routledge.

Mackey, A., Adams, R., Stafford, C., & Winke, P. (2010). Exploring the relationship between modified output and working memory capacity. *Language Learning*, *60*(3), 501–533.

Mackey, A. & Gass, S. M. (2005). *Second Language Research: Methodology and Design* (1st ed.). Lawrence Erlbaum.

(2015). Interaction approaches. In B. VanPatten & J. Williams (Eds.), *Theories in Second Language Acquisition* (pp. 180–207). Routledge.

(2016). *Second Language Research: Methodology and Design* (2nd ed.). Routledge.

Mackey, A. & Gass, S. M. (Eds.) (2012). *Research Methods in Second Language Acquisition: A Practical Guide*. Basil Blackwell.

Mackey, A., Gass, S. M., & McDonough, K. (2000). How do learners perceive implicit negative feedback? *Studies in Second Language Acquisition*, *22*(4), 471–497.

Mackey, A. & Goo, J. (2007). Interaction research in SLA: A meta-analysis and research synthesis. In A. Mackey (Ed.), *Conversational Interaction in Second Language Acquisition: A Collection of Empirical Studies* (pp. 407–452). Oxford University Press.

(2012). Interaction approach in second language acquisition. In C. Chapelle (Ed.), *The Encyclopedia of Applied Linguistics* (pp. 2748–2758). Wiley-Blackwell.

Mackey, A., McDonough, K., Fujii, A., & Tatasumi, T. (2001). Investigating learners' reports about the L2 classroom. *International Review of Applied Linguistics in Language Teaching*, *39*(4), 285–308.

Mackey, A., Park, H. I., Akiyama, Y., & Pipes, A. (2014, March). The role of cognitive creativity in L2 learning processes, [Paper presentation]. Georgetown University Round Table, Washington, DC.

Mackey, A. & Philp, J. (1998). Conversational interaction and second language development: Recasts, responses, and red herrings? *The Modern Language Journal*, *82*(3), 338–356.

Mackey, A., Philp, J., Egi, T., Fujii, A., & Tatsumi, T. (2002). Individual differences in working memory, noticing of interactional feedback, and

L2 development. In P. Robinson (Ed.), *Individual Differences and Instructed Language Learning* (pp. 181–209). John Benjamins.

Mackey, A., Philp, J. & Teimouri, Y. (2015, September). *The relationships amongst working memory, cognitive creativity and second language production during communicative tasks.* Task-Based Language Teaching Conference. Leuven, Belgium.

Mackey, A. & Sachs, R. (2012). Older learners in SLA research: A first look at working memory, feedback, and L2 development. *Language Learning, 62*(3), 704–740.

Mann, W., Sheng, L., & Morgan, G. (2016). Lexical-semantic organization in bilingually developing deaf children with ASL-dominant language exposure: Evidence from a repeated meaning association task. *Language Learning, 66*(4), 872–899. 10.1111/lang.12169

Markee, N. (2017). Are replication studies possible in qualitative second/foreign language classroom research? A call for comparative re-production research. *Language Teaching, 50*(3), 367–383.

Marsden, E. & Mackey, A. (2014). IRIS: A new resource for second language research. *Linguistic Approaches to Bilingualism, 4*(1), 125–130.

Marsden, E., Mackey A., & Plonsky, L. (2016). The IRIS repository: Advancing research practice and methodology. In A. Mackey & E. Marsden (Eds.), *Advancing Methodology and Practice: The IRIS Repository of Instruments for Research Into Second Languages* (pp. 1–21). Routledge.

Marsden, E., Morgan-Short, K., Thompson, S., & Abugaber, D. (2018). Replication in second language research: Narrative and systematic reviews and recommendations for the field. *Language Learning, 68*(2), 321–391.

Mathôt, S. (2018). Pupillometry: Psychology, physiology, and function. *Journal of Cognition, 1*(1), 1–23.

McDonough, K., Crawford, W. J., & Mackey, A. (2015). Creativity and EFL students' language use during a group problem-solving task. *TESOL Quarterly, 49*(1), 188–199.

McDonough, K. & Mackey, A. (2006). Responses to recasts: Repetitions, primed production, and linguistic development. *Language Learning, 56*(4), 693–720.

(2013). *Second Language Interaction in Diverse Educational Contexts.* John Benjamins.

McDonough, K. & Trofimovich, P. (2008). *Using Priming Methods in Second Language Research.* Routledge.

McKinnon, S. (2017). TBLT instructional effects on tonal alignment and pitch range in L2 Spanish imperatives versus declaratives. *Studies in Second Language Acquisition, 39*(2), 287–317.

Meara, P. (2005). *LLAMA Language Aptitude Tests: The Manual.* Lognostics.

Menon, V. & Muraleedharan, A. (2016). Salami slicing of data sets: What the young researcher needs to know. *Indian Journal of Psychological Medicine, 38*(6), 577–578.

Miller, P. C. (2003). *The effectiveness of corrective feedback: A meta-analysis* [Unpublished doctoral dissertation]. Purdue University.

Miller, P. C. & Pan, W. (2012). Recasts in the L2 classroom: A meta-analytic review. *International Journal of Educational Research, 56,* 48–59.

Miyake, A. & Friedman, N. P. (1998). Individual differences in second language proficiency: Working memory as language aptitude. In A. F. Healy & L. E. Bourne, Jr. (Eds.), *Foreign Language Learning: Psycholinguistic Studies on Training and Retention* (pp. 339–364). Lawrence Erlbaum Associates.

Mohades, S. G., Struys, E., Van Schuerbeek, P., Baeken, C., Van De Craen, P., & Luypaert, R. (2014). Age of second language acquisition affects nonverbal conflict processing in children: An fMRI study. *Brain and Behavior, 4*(5), 626–642.

Morgan-Short, K., Deng, Z., Brill-Schuetz, K. A., Faretta-Stutenberg, M., Wong, P. C., & Wong, F. C. (2015). A view of the neural representation of second language syntax through artificial language learning under implicit contexts of exposure. *Studies in Second Language Acquisition, 37*(2), 383–419.

Morgan-Short, K., Faretta-Stutenberg, M., & Bartlett-Hsu, L. (2015). Contributions of event-related potential research to issues in explicit and implicit second language acquisition. In P. Rebuschat (Ed.), *Implicit and Explicit Learning of Languages* (pp. 349–384). John Benjamins.

Mouthon, M., Khateb, A., Lazeyras, F., Pegna, A. J., Lee-Jahnke, H., Lehr, C., & Annoni, J. M. (2019). Second-language proficiency modulates the brain language control network in bilingual translators: An event-related fMRI study. *Bilingualism: Language and Cognition,* 1–14.

Nakatsukasa, K. (2016). Efficacy of recasts and gestures on the acquisition of locative prepositions. *Studies in Second Language Acquisition, 38,* 771–779.

Nassaji, H. (2009). Effects of recasts and elicitations in dyadic interaction and the role of feedback explicitness. *Language Learning*, *59*(2), 411–452.

(2016). Anniversary article: Interactional feedback in second language teaching and learning: A synthesis and analysis of current research. *Language Teaching Research*, *20*(4), 535–562.

(2017). The effectiveness of extensive versus intensive recasts for learning L2 grammar. *The Modern Language Journal*, *101*, 353–368.

(2019). The effects of recasts versus prompts on immediate uptake and learning of a complex target structure. In R. M. DeKeyser & G. P. Botana (Eds.), *Doing SLA Research with Implications for the Classroom: Reconciling Methodological Demands and Pedagogical Applicability* (pp. 107–126). John Benjamins.

Nassaji, H. & Kartchava, E. (Eds.) (2017). *Corrective Feedback in Second Language Teaching and Learning: Research, Theory, Applications, Implications*. Taylor and Francis.

(Eds.) (2019). *The Cambridge Handbook of Corrective Feedback in Language Learning and Teaching*. Cambridge University Press.

Nicklin, C. & Plonsky, L. (2020). Outliers in L2 research: A synthesis and data re-analysis from self-paced reading. *Annual Review of Applied Linguistics, 40*.

Norris, J. M. (2012). Meta-analysis. In C. Chapelle (Ed.), *The Encyclopedia of Applied Linguistics* (pp. 1–10). John Wiley.

Norris, J. M., Brown, J. D., Hudson, T. D., & Bonk, W. (2002). Examinee abilities and task difficulty in task-based second language performance assessment. *Language Testing*, *19*(4), 395–418.

Norris, J. M. & Ortega, L. (2000). Effectiveness of L2 instruction: A research synthesis and quantitative meta-analysis. *Language Learning*, *50*(3), 417–528.

(Eds.) (2006). *Synthesizing Research on Language Learning and Teaching*. John Benjamins.

Nosek, B. A. & Lakens, D. (2014). Registered reports: A method to increase the credibility of published results. *Social Psychology*, *45*(3), 137–141.

Nunan, D. (1993). Action research in language education. In J. Edge & K. Richards (Eds.), *Teachers Develop, Teachers Research: Papers on Classroom Research and Teacher Development* (pp. 39–50). Heinemann International.

Oakley, M. (2019, October). Ultrasound tongue imaging and the acquisition of the French /y/–/u/ contrast, [Paper presentation]. Second Language Research Forum, Montréal, Québec.

Oswald, F. L. & Plonsky, L. (2010). Meta-analysis in second language acquisition research: Choices and challenges. *Annual Review of Applied Linguistics*, *30*, 85–110.

Ottó, I. (1998). The relationship between individual differences in learner creativity and language learning success. *TESOL Quarterly*, *32*(4), 763–773.

Owens, M. T. & Tanner, K. D. (2017). Teaching as brain changing: Exploring connections between neuroscience and innovative teaching. *CBE–Life Sciences Education*, *16*(2). 10.1187/cbe.17-01-0005

Paradis, M. (2004). *A Neurolinguistic Theory of Bilingualism*. John Benjamins.

Park, K. (2016). Employing TBLT at a military-service academy in Korea: Learners' reactions to and necessary adaptation of TBLT. *English Teaching*, *71*(4).

Pandža, N., Karuzis,V., Phillips, I., O'Rourke, P., & Kuchinsky, S. (2020). Neurostimulation and pupillometry: New directions for learning and research in applied linguistics. *Annual Review of Applied Linguistics, 40*.

Parlak, Ö. & Ziegler, N. (2017). The impact of recasts on the development of primary stress in a synchronous computer-mediated environment. *Studies in Second Language Acquisition, 39*(2), 257–285.

Phakiti, A., De Costa, P. I., Plonsky, L., & Starfield, S. (Eds.) (2018). *The Palgrave Handbook of Applied Linguistics Research Methodology*. Palgrave.

Pham, M. T., Rajić, A., Greig, J. D., Sargeant, J. M., Papadopoulos, A., & McEwen, S. A. (2014). A scoping review of scoping reviews: Advancing the approach and enhancing the consistency. *Research Synthesis Methods*, *5*(4), 371–385.

Philp, J. (2003). Constraints on "noticing the gap": Nonnative speakers' noticing of recasts in NS-NNS interaction. *Studies in Second Language Acquisition*, *25*, 99–126. 10.1017/S0272263103000044

Philp, J., Adams, R., & Iwashita, N. (2013). *Peer Interaction and Second Language Learning*. Routledge.

Pica, T. (1994). Research on negotiation: What does it reveal about second language learning conditions, processes, and outcomes? *Language Learning*, *44*(3), 493–527.

Pica, T., Kanagy, R., & Falodun, J. (1993). Choosing and using communication tasks for second language instruction. In G. Crookes & S. M. Gass (Eds.), *Tasks and Language Learning: Integrating Theory and Practice* (pp. 9–34). Multilingual Matters.

Pickering, M. J. & Ferreira, V. S. (2008). Structural priming: a critical review. *Psychological Bulletin, 134*(3), 427–459. 10.1037/0033-2909.134.3.427

Pimsleur, P. (1966). *Pimsleur Language Aptitude Battery (PLAB)*. Harcourt Brace Jovanich.

Pipes, A. (2017, July). Examining cognitive creativity as an interlocutor individual difference [Paper presentation]. AILA Research Network on Interlocutor and Instructor Individual Differences in Cognition and SLA Symposium, Rio de Janeiro, Brazil.

(2019). *Examining creativity as an individual difference in second language production* [Unpublished doctoral dissertation]. Georgetown University.

Pliatsikas, C. & Luk, G. (2016). Executive control in bilinguals: A concise review on fMRI studies. *Bilingualism: Language and Cognition, 19*(4), 699–705.

Plonsky, L. (2011). The effectiveness of second language strategy instruction: A meta-analysis. *Language Learning, 61*(4), 993–1038.

(2015). Quantitative considerations for improving replicability in CALL and applied linguistics. *CALICO Journal, 32*(2), 232–244.

(2016, February). The N crowd: Sampling practices, internal validity, and generalizability in L2 research, [Conference presentation] University College London, United Kingdom.

(2017). Quantitative research methods in instructed SLA. In S. Loewen & M. Sato (Eds.), *The Routledge Handbook of Instructed Second Language Acquisition* (pp. 505–521). Routledge.

Plonsky, L. & Brown, D. (2015). Domain definition and search techniques in meta-analyses of L2 research (Or why 18 meta-analyses of feedback have different results). *Second Language Research, 31*(2), 267–278. 10.1177/0267658314536436

Plonsky, L. & Gass, S. (2011). Quantitative research methods, study quality, and outcomes: The case of interaction research. *Language Learning, 61*(2), 325–366.

Plonsky, L. & Han, S. (in preparation). Meta-analysis in language testing: A second order review and call for future research. Retrieved from https://lukeplonsky.wordpress.com/projects/

Plonsky, L. & Kim, Y. (2016). Task-based learner production: A substantive and methodological review. *Annual Review of Applied Linguistics, 36*, 73–97.

Plonsky, L. & Oswald, F. L. (2012). How to do a meta-analysis. In A. Mackey & S. M. Gass (Eds.), *Research Methods in Second Language Acquisition: A Practical Guide* (pp. 275–295). Wiley-Blackwell.

(2014). How big is "big"? Interpreting effect sizes in L2 research. *Language Learning, 64*(4), 878–912.

(2015). Meta-analyzing second language research. In L. Plonsky (Ed.), *Advancing Quantitative Methods in Second Language Research* (pp. 106–128). Routledge.

Porte, G. (2012). *Replication Research in Applied Linguistics*. Cambridge University Press.

Porte, G. & McManus, K. (2019). *Doing Replication Research in Applied Linguistics*. Routledge.

Préfontaine, Y. & Kormos, J. (2015). The relationship between task difficulty and second language fluency in French: A mixed methods approach. *The Modern Language Journal, 99*(1), 96–112.

Putman, M. S. & Rock, T. (2017). *Action Research: Using Strategic Inquiry to Improve Teaching and Learning*. Sage Publications.

Qureshi, M. (2016). A meta-analysis: Age and second language grammar acquisition. *System, 60*, 147–160.

Rebuschat, P. & Williams, J. N. (2012). Implicit and explicit knowledge in second language acquisition. *Applied Psycholinguistics, 33*(4), 829–856.

Reiterer, S. (Ed.) (2018). *Exploring Language Aptitude: Views from Psychology, The Language Sciences, and Cognitive Neuroscience*. Springer International Publishing.

Révész, A. (2012). Working memory and the observed effectiveness of recasts on different L2 outcome measures. *Language Learning, 62*, 93–132.

Révész, A. & Brunfaut, T. (2013). Text characteristics of task input and difficulty in second language listening comprehension. *Studies in Second Language Acquisition, 35*(1), 31–65.

Révész, A. & Gurzynski-Weiss, L. (2016). Teachers' perspectives on second language task difficulty: Insights from think-alouds and eye tracking. *Annual Review of Applied Linguistics, 36*, 182–204.

Riazi, A. M. (2016). Innovative mixed-methods research: Moving beyond design technicalities to epistemological and methodological realizations. *Applied Linguistics, 37*(1), 33–49.

(2017). *Mixed Methods Research in Language Teaching and Learning*. Equinox Publishing.

Riazi, A. M. & Candlin, C. N. (2014). Mixed-methods research in language teaching and learning: Opportunities, issues, and challenges. *Language Teaching, 47*(2), 135–173.

Robinson, P. (1995). Attention, memory, and the 'noticing' hypothesis. *Language Learning, 45*, 283–331.

(2001). Task complexity, cognitive resources, and syllabus design:
A triadic framework for examining task influences on SLA. In P.
Robinson (Ed.), *Cognition and Second Language Instruction*
(pp. 114–127). Cambridge University Press.

(2005). Aptitude and second language acquisition. *Annual Review of
Applied Linguistics, 25*, 46–73.

(2007). Task complexity, theory of mind, and intentional reasoning:
Effects on L2 speech production, interaction, uptake, and perceptions
of task difficulty. *International Review of Applied Linguistics in
Language Teaching, 45*(3), 193–213.

Robinson, P. & Gilabert, R. (2012). Task-based learning: Cognitive
underpinnings. In C. Chapelle (Ed.), *The Encyclopedia of Applied
Linguistics*. Wiley-Blackwell.

Robinson, P., Mackey, A., Gass, S. M., & Schmidt, R. (2012). Attention and
awareness in second language acquisition. In S. Gass & A. Mackey
(Eds.), *The Routledge Handbook of Second Language Acquisition*
(pp. 247–267). Routledge.

Roothooft, H. (2014). The relationship between adult EFL teachers'
oral feedback practices and their beliefs. *System, 46*(1), 65–79. 10.1016/
j.system.2014.07.012.

Rosenthal, R. (1979). File drawer problem and tolerance for null results.
Psychological Bulletin, 86(3), 638–41.

Ross, S. (1998). Self-assessment in second language testing: A meta-
analysis and analysis of experiential factors. *Language Testing, 15*(1),
1–20.

Rothstein, H. R., Sutton A. J., & Borenstein, M. (Eds.) (2005). *Publication
Bias in Meta-Analysis: Prevention, Assessment, and Adjustments*.
Wiley.

Russell, J. & Spada, N. (2006). The effectiveness of corrective feedback
for the acquisition of L2 grammar: A meta-analysis of the research.
In J. M. Norris & L. Ortega (Eds.), *Synthesizing Research on Language
Learning and Teaching* (pp. 133–164). John Benjamins.

Sachs, R. & Suh, B-R. (2007). Textually enhanced recasts, learner
awareness, and L2 outcomes in synchronous computer-mediated
interaction. In A. Mackey (Ed.), *Conversational Interaction in Second
Language Acquisition: A Collection of Empirical Studies* (pp. 199–227).
Oxford University Press.

Sagarra, N. (2007). From CALL to face-to-face interaction: The effect of
computer-driven recasts and working memory on L2 development. In
A. Mackey (Ed.), *Conversational Interaction in Second Language
Acquisition: A Series of Empirical Studies* (pp. 229–248). Oxford
University Press.

Saito, K. (2019). Corrective feedback and the development of L2 pronunciation. In H. Nassaji & E. Kartchava (Eds.), *The Cambridge Handbook of Corrective Feedback in Language Learning and Teaching*. Cambridge University Press.

Saito, K., Macmillan, K., Mai, T., Suzukida, Y., Sun, H., Magne, V., Ilkan, M. & Murakami, A. (2020). Open source: Developing, analyzing, and sharing multivariate datasets: Individual differences in L2 learning revisited. *Annual Review of Applied Linguistics, 40.*

Samuda, V. (2001). Guiding relationships between form and meaning during task performance: The role of the teacher. In M. Bygate, P. Skehan, & M. Swain (Eds.), *Researching Pedagogic Tasks: Second Language Learning, Teaching, and Testing* (pp. 119–140). Longman.

Sasayama, S., Malicka, A., & Norris, J. M. (2015). Primary challenges in cognitive task complexity research: Results of a comprehensive research synthesis, [Paper presentation]. International Conference on Task-Based Language Teaching (TBLT), Leuven, Belgium.

Sato, R. (2016). Examining high-intermediate Japanese EFL learners' perception of recasts: Revisiting repair, acknowledgement, and noticing through stimulated recall. *The Asian EFL Journal Quarterly, 18*, 109–129.

Sato, M. & Lyster, R. (2012). Peer interaction and corrective feedback for accuracy and fluency development: Monitoring, practice and proceduralization. *Studies in Second Language Acquisition, 34,* 591–626.

Schmidt, R. (1990). The role of consciousness in second language learning. *Applied Linguistics, 11*, 129–58.

Schmidtke, J. (2018). Pupillometry in linguistics research: An introduction and review for second language researchers. *Studies in Second Language Acquisition, 40*, 529–549.

Scovel, T. (2000). A critical review of the critical period research. *Annual Review of Applied Linguistics, 20*, 213–223.

Sheen, Y. (2004). Corrective feedback and learner uptake in communicative classrooms across instructional settings. *Language Teaching Research, 8*, 263–300.

(2010). Introduction: The role of oral and written corrective feedback in SLA. *Studies in Second Language Acquisition, 32*(2), 169–179.

Sippel, L. & Jackson, C. N. (2015). Teacher vs. peer oral corrective feedback in the German language classroom. *Foreign Language Annals, 48*(4), 688–705.

Skehan, P. (1996). A framework for the implementation of task-based instruction. *Applied Linguistics, 17*(1), 38–62.

(1998). *A Cognitive Approach to Language Learning*. Oxford University Press.

(2015). Language aptitude. In S. Gass & A. Mackey (Eds.), *Routledge Handbook of Second Language Acquisition* (pp. 381–395). Routledge.

Smith, B. (2012). Eye tracking as a measure of noticing: A study of explicit recasts in SCMC. *Language Learning and Technology*, *16*(3), 53–81.

Spada, N. & Tomita, Y. (2010). Interactions between type of instruction and type of language feature: A meta-analysis. *Language Learning*, *60*, 263–308.

Stanley, T. D., Carter, E. C., & Doucouliagos, H. (2018). What meta-analyses reveal about the replicability of psychological research. *Psychological Bulletin*, *144*, 1325–1346.

Süß, H. M., Oberauer, K., Wittmann, W. W., Wilhelm, O., & Schulze, R. (2002). Working-memory capacity explains reasoning ability – and a little bit more. *Intelligence*, *30*(3), 261–288.

Swain, M. (1985). Communicative competence: Some roles of comprehensible input and comprehensible output in its development. In S. Gass & C. Madden (Eds.), *Input in Second Language Acquisition*. Newbury House.

(2005). The output hypothesis: Theory and research. In E. Hinkel (Ed.), *Handbook on Research in Second Language Teaching and Learning* (pp. 471–484). Erlbaum.

Swain, M. & Lapkin, S. (2002). Talking it through: Two French immersion learners' response to reformulation. *International Journal of Educational Research*, *37*(3–4), 285–304.

Swain, M., Lapkin, S., Knouzi, I., Suzuki, W., & Brooks, L. (2009). Languaging: University students learn the grammatical concept of voice in French. *The Modern Language Journal*, *93*(1), 5–29.

Sydorenko, T. (2015). The use of computer-delivered structured tasks in pragmatic instruction: An exploratory study. *Intercultural Pragmatics*, *12*(3), 333–362.

Sykes, J. (2014). TBLT and synthetic immersive environments: What can in-game task restarts tell us about design and implementation? In M. González-Lloret & L. Ortega (Eds.), *Technology-Mediated TBLT: Researching Technology and Tasks* (pp. 149–182). John Benjamins.

Szucs, D. & Ioannidis, J. (2017). When null hypothesis significance testing is unsuitable for research: A reassessment. *Frontiers in Human Neuroscience*, *11*, 1–21.

Tagarelli, K. (2014). *The neurocognition of adult second language learning: An fMRI study* [Doctoral dissertation, Georgetown University]. At this permanent link: http://hdl.handle.net/10822/712460.

Tannen, D., Kendall, S., & Gordon, C. (Eds.) (2007). *Family Talk: Discourse and Identity in Four American Families.* Oxford University Press.

Tarone, E. (2010). Second language acquisition by low-literate learners: An under-studied population. *Language Teaching, 43*(1), 75–83.

Tarone, E. & Bigelow, M. (2005). Impact of literacy on oral language processing: Implications for second language acquisition research. *Annual Review of Applied Linguistics, 25,* 77–79.

Tashakkori, A. & Creswell, J. W. (2007). Editorial: The new era of mixed methods. *Journal of Mixed Methods Research, 1*(1), 3–7.

Tashakkori, A. & Teddlie C. (Eds.) (2010). *Handbook of Mixed Methods in Social and Behavioral Research* (2nd ed.). Sage.

Tateishi, M. & Winters, S. (2013, June). "Does ultrasound training lead to improved perception of a non-native sound contrast? Evidence from Japanese learners of English," in Proceedings of the 2013 Annual Conference of the Canadian Linguistic Association, 1–15.

Teimouri, Y. (2017). L2 selves, emotions, and motivated behaviors. *Studies in Second Language Acquisition, 39*(4), 681–709.

(2018). Differential roles of shame and guilt in L2 learning: How bad is bad? *The Modern Language Journal, 102*(4), 632–652.

Thompson, A. S. (2013). The interface of language aptitude and multilingualism: Reconsidering the bilingual/multilingual dichotomy. *The Modern Language Journal, 97*(3), 685–701.

Thorson Hernández, R. & Subtirelu, N. (2018, March). Everyday experiences of policy: Exploring the appropriation of educational language policy through teachers' narratives, [Unpublished paper presentation]. Georgetown University Round Table, Washington, DC.

Tokowicz, N. & MacWhinney, B. (2005). Implicit and explicit measures of sensitivity to violations in second language grammar: An event-related potential investigation. *Studies in Second Language Acquisition, 27*(2), 173–204.

Toivo W. & Scheepers, C. (2019). Pupillary responses to affective words in bilinguals' first versus second language. *PLoS ONE, 14*(4), e0210450. 10.1371/journal.pone.0210450

Torrance, E. (1970). *Encouraging Creativity in the Classroom.* William C. Brown.

Trofimovich, P., Ammar, A., & Gatbonton, E. (2007). How effective are recasts? The role of attention, memory, and analytical ability. In A. Mackey (Ed.), *Conversational Interaction in Second Language Acquisition: A Series of Empirical Studies* (pp. 171–195). Oxford University Press.

Trofimovich, P., McDonough, K., & Neumann, H. (2013). Using collaborative tasks to elicit auditory and structural priming. *TESOL Quarterly, 47*(1), 177–186. 10.1002/tesq.78

Truscott, J. (2007). The effect of error correction on learners' ability to write accurately. *Journal of Second Language Writing, 16*, 255–272.

Tsui, H. M. L. (2012). *Ultrasound speech training for Japanese adults learning English as a second language*, [Unpublished doctoral dissertation]. University of British Columbia.

Van Avermaet, P. & Gysen, S. (2006). From needs to tasks: Language learning needs in a task-based approach. In K. Van den Branden, M. Bygate, & J. M. Norris (Eds.), *Task-Based Language Education: From Theory to Practice* (pp. 46–61). John Benjamins.

Van den Branden, K. (Ed.) (2006). *Task-Based Language Education: From Theory to Practice*. Cambridge University Press.

Van den Branden, K., Bygate, M., & Norris, J. (Eds.). (2009). *Task-Based Language Teaching: A Reader*. John Benjamins.

Wang, W. & Loewen, S. (2016). Nonverbal behavior and corrective feedback in nine ESL university-level classrooms. *Language Teaching Research, 20*(4), 459–478.

Wen, Z. (2016). *Working Memory and Second Language Learning: Towards an Integrated Approach*. Multilingual Matters.

Wen, Z., Biedroń, A., & Skehan, P. (2017). Foreign language aptitude theory: Yesterday, today, and tomorrow, *Language Teaching, 50*(1), 1–31.

Williams, J. N. & Lovatt, P. (2003). Phonological memory and rule learning. *Language Learning, 53*(1), 67–121.

Williams, S. & Menard-Warwick, J. (2014). Qualitative research interviews in second language acquisition. In C. Chappelle (Ed.), *The Encyclopedia of Applied Linguistics* (pp. 1–5). Blackwell.

Willis, J. (1996). *A Framework for Task-Based Learning*. Pearson Education.

Winke, P. (2013). An investigation into second language aptitude for advanced Chinese language learning. *The Modern Language Journal, 97*(1), 109–130.

    (2018). Aptitude testing. *The TESOL Encyclopedia of English Language Teaching*, 1–7.

Winke, P., Godfroid, A., & Gass, S. M. (2013). Introduction to the special issue: Eye-movement recordings in second language research. *Studies in Second Language Acquisition, 35*(2), 205–212.

Winke, P. M. & Teng, C. (2010). Using task-based pragmatics tutorials while studying abroad in China. *Intercultural Pragmatics, 7*(2), 363–399.

Yilmaz, Y. (2013). Relative effects of explicit and implicit feedback: The role of working memory capacity and language analytic ability. *Applied Linguistics, 34,* 344–368.

Yilmaz, Y. & Granena, G. (2016). The role of cognitive aptitudes for explicit language learning in the relative effects of explicit and implicit feedback. *Bilingualism, 19*(1), 147–161.

Yilmaz, Y. & Sağdıç, A. (2019). The interaction between inhibitory control and corrective feedback timing. *International Journal of Applied Linguistics, 170*(2), 204–227.

Youn, S. (2020). Interactional features of L2 pragmatic interaction in role-play speaking assessment. *TESOL Quarterly, 54*(1), 201–233.

Zacharias, N. T. (2012). *Qualitative Research Methods for Second Language Education: A Coursebook.* Cambridge Scholars Publishing.

Zalbidea, J. (2017). "One task fits all"? The roles of task complexity, modality, and working memory capacity in L2 performance. *The Modern Language Journal, 101*(2), 335–352.

Ziegler, N. (2016). Synchronous computer-mediated communication and interaction: A meta-analysis. *Studies in Second Language Acquisition, 38*(3), 553–586. 10.1017/S027226311500025X

Ziegler, N., Seals, C., Ammons, S., Lake, J., Hamrick, P., & Rebuschat, P. (2013). Interaction in conversation groups: The development of L2 conversational styles. In K. McDonough & A. Mackey (Eds.), *Second Language Interaction in Diverse Educational Contexts* (pp. 269–292). John Benjamins.

Index

CPSIA information can be obtained
at www.ICGtesting.com
Printed in the USA
LVHW082002090820
662760LV00005B/69

9 781108 499637